Studies in Disorders of Communication

General Editors:

David Crystal
Honorary Professor of Linguistics, University College of North Wales, Bangor

Ruth Lesser
Head of Speech Department, University of Newcastle-upon-Tyne

Margaret Snowling
Principal, National Hospitals College of Speech S

BAMFORD AND SAUNDERS

HEARING IMPAIRMENT, AUDITORY PERCEPTION AND LANGUAGE DISABILITY

STUDIES IN DISORDERS OF COMMUNICATION

SECOND EDITION

WHURR PUBLISHERS
LONDON JERSEY CITY

First published 1985 by
Edward Arnold (Publishers) Ltd
Second edition 1991 published by
Whurr Publishers Ltd
19b Compton Terrace, London N1 2UN

British Library Cataloguing in Publication Data
Bamford, John
  Hearing impairment, auditory perception and language
  disability.–2nd ed.
  1. Hearing disordered persons. Language skills.
  I. Title II. Saunders, Elaine
  401:93

ISBN 1-870332-01-6

Typeset by Coleset Pte Ltd, Singapore
Corrections to second edition by Scribe Design, Gillingham, Kent
Printed and bound in Great Britain by Athenaeum Press Ltd, Newcastle-upon-Tyne

Contents

Acknowledgements

We wish to record our thanks to our various friends, relations and colleagues for their encouragement and forbearance during the time this book was conceived, thought through, written and corrected. Particular mention should be made of the general editors of the series, David Crystal and Jean Cooper; to our families; and to Christine Palmer for her clerical and administrative help and for her typing of the final manuscript.

JMB
ES

The publishers would like to thank the following for permission to reproduce copyright material:

Academic Press for Figs. 4.2 and 6.2; *Acta Oto-Laryngologica* and N.Y.S. Kiang for Fig. 1.6; Alpha Academic for Fig. 3.1; American Psychological Association and S. Trehub, B. Schneider and D. Bull for Fig. 2.2; American Speech-Language-Hearing Association and R.L. Cooper for Table 6.1, and D. Power and S.P. Quigley for Fig. 6.1; *Audiology* and E.F. Evans for Fig. 5.7; British Journal of Applied Physics and CBS College Publishing for Fig. 1.2; *British Journal of Audiology* for Figs. 1.3 and 4.3; College Hill Press for Figs. 10.1 and 10.2; Croom Helm Ltd Publishers for Fig. 6.3; D. Crystal, P. Fletcher and M. Garman for Figs. 3.2 and 3.3; Kay L. Gribben (1981) 'Psychoacoustical Tuning Curves in Normal and Impaired Hearing' M.Sc Dissertation, ISVR, University of Southampton for Figs. 1.5 and 5.6; *Journal of the Academy of Rehabilitative Audiology* for Fig. 9.1; *Journal of the Acoustical Society of America* and R.A.W. Bladon, B. Lindblom for Fig. 5.5 and J.P. Egan, H.W. Hake for Fig. 1.4; *Journal of Auditory Research* for Figs. 5.7 and 5.8; Kingston Press Services Ltd for Table 6.2; The Physiological Society and E.F. Evans and R.V. Harrison for Fig. 5.4; Pro-Ed for Fig. 2.1 and Table 5.1; W.B. Saunders Company for Fig. 1.1; John Wright & Sons Limited and J.C.G. Pearson and W. Taylor for Fig. 5.1.

General preface

This series focuses upon disorders of speech language and communication, bringing together the techniques of analysis, assessment and treatment which are pertinent to the area. It aims to cover cognitive, linguistic, social and education aspects of language disability, and therefore has relevance within a number of disciplines. These include speech therapy, the education of children and adults with special needs, teachers of the deaf, teachers of English as a second language and of foreign languages, and educational and clinical psychology. The research and clinical findings from these various areas can usefully inform one another and, therefore, we hope one of the main functions of this series will be to put people within one profession in touch with developments in another. Thus, it is our editorial policy to ask authors to consider the implications of their findings for professions outside of their own and for fields with which they have not been primarily concerned. We hope to engender an integrated approach to theory and practice and to produce a much-needed emphasis on the description and analysis of language as such, as well as on the provision of specific techniques of therapy, remediation and rehabilitation.

Whilst it has been our aim to restrict the series to the study of language disability, its scope goes considerably beyond this. Many previously neglected topics have been included where these seem to benefit from contemporary research in linguistics, psychology, medicine, sociology, education and English studies. Each volume puts its subject matter in perspective and provides an introductory slant to its presentation. In this way we hope to provide specialized studies which can be used as texts for components of teaching courses at undergraduate and postgraduated levels, as well as material directly applicable to the needs of professional workers.

David Crystal
Ruth Lesser
Margaret Snowling

Introduction

'Deaf and dumb' is a term which nowadays, thankfully, one rarely encounters. It is an expression full of misleading implications. It suggests not that there is a large range of degrees and types of hearing impairment, but that a person is either completely deaf or normally hearing. It also implies that if a person is deaf, he or she will also be dumb: 'unable to speak, abnormally . . .', as the *Oxford English Dictionary* puts it. To these misconceptions is inevitably added that which derives from the pejorative meaning of dumb. However, the outdated expression 'deaf and dumb' does underline one broad truth, and that is that our primary language is an oral one, and a functional auditory system is required for the normal acquisition of this language.

For a variety of reasons, about two children in a thousand are born with, or acquire shortly after birth, a hearing loss caused by pathological changes to the cochlea (inner ear) and its innervation of the auditory (VIII) nerve. Such hearing losses may vary from being of a mild degree to being of a severe or profound degree, but in all cases they are likely to have a significant effect upon the development of normal receptive language skills. In turn, the development of expressive language will often be adversely affected. Although the early identification of these hearing losses (which, sadly, is far from guaranteed) and the prescription of suitable hearing aids (likewise) is of great importance, in the majority of cases it is not enough to restore *normal* function: it has been known for a long time that peripheral hearing loss due to damage to the inner ear is characterized not only by a simple loss in sensitivity, but by a whole series of psychoacoustic effects which are as yet only partly understood.

A larger number of children will, in their preschool or early school days, suffer from mild to moderate hearing loss due to middle-ear disorders. Unlike inner-ear impairments, such disorders do not generally involve complex psychoacoustic effects; furthermore, they are usually amenable to medical or surgical treatment and will often resolve without intervention. Nevertheless, the chronic recurrent middle-ear disorders which do not respond easily to treatment, and which occur before linguistic skills are fully developed, can have marked effects upon receptive and expressive language, albeit often somewhat less serious effects than those due to inner-ear impairments.

The purpose of this book is to examine and specify our present knowledge about language disability resulting from impaired hearing in children. It does not cover the rather different set of problems encountered by those who acquire a hearing loss postlingually, after language is fully developed. In terms both of suffering and of resources this type of impairment should be of great concern, but it is not the province of this book, since the effect of such impairments upon language (rather than speech skills) is relatively minor.

Chapters 5, 6, 7 and 8 examine our current knowledge of the effects of hearing impairments upon receptive and expressive language skills and their development, upon auditory perception, and upon reading ability are described. While the book is concerned chiefly with bilateral and largely symmetrical hearing losses, which are more prevalent than monaural or markedly asymmetrical losses, recent figures have suggested that the latter are more common than was once thought. Chapter 9, therefore, is concerned with the effects of monaural impairments. Since one good ear will generally provide adequate input for the development of normal linguistic competence, these effects concern the relationship between certain difficult acoustic environments and receptive language performance. Chapter 10 looks at central auditory dysfunction. Peripheral hearing impairments result from pathology of the end organ, but recent work has identified certain auditory dysfunctions, often language-based, which are thought to reflect problems of structure or function in the central auditory pathways. These pathways, from eighth nerve to brainstem, midbrain and auditory cortex, are extremely complex and our knowledge of their physiology is limited. With peripheral hearing impairments we know a good deal about the pathology and a fair amount about the resulting functional impairment, at least for simple signals. For central auditory impairments, other than those involving gross pathology such as tumours, we know almost nothing about pathology, and little about the functional impairment. Nevertheless, it is an area attracting much recent interest and is an area with educational implications.

In order to understand why and how hearing impairments have their effects upon receptive and expressive language ability, it is necessary to consider in some detail our rather limited knowledge of auditory perception and auditory processing in the hearing-impaired. Chapter 5 deals with this topic, and it is here that we attempt to bridge the gap between complex speech perception and basic sensory processes in the hearing-impaired. This is a crucial interface, and the better it can be mapped, the more we will understand the why and how of the effects of hearing impairment on language ability, and the greater the prospect of alleviating these effects by properly underpinned rehabilitative procedures.

In order to understand auditory perceptual processes and their effects upon language development in the hearing-impaired, it is necessary to be aware of the processes of auditory perception and speech perception in the normally hearing adult, and of the development of auditory perception and language in the normally hearing child. This is a vast area, containing its fair share of controversy, and it is outside the scope of this book to review it in detail. However, the early Chapters (1, 2 and 3) are devoted to a summary of current thoughts on these topics, and the reader may find that it provides a useful foundation for the later sections of the book. Thus, although this book is about language disability, much of the discussion necessarily centres around auditory perception and the processes of speech perception. Some may wish to omit these background chapters and go directly to later sections, but it is hoped that some of the early overviews provide useful summaries. Chapter 4 provides a brief description of the auditory system and of the types, causes, prevalence and treatment of disorders affecting it. This information is available from many other sources, but it is included here to complete the background for the unfamiliar reader.

Hearing loss varies from mild to very severe ('profound'); of those born with a hearing loss the majority will not have a severe impairment. Such children, despite their hearing disabilities, which may be quite significant, will usually develop good oral language skills and will be found integrated in the normal school environment with appropriate support. Many of those with more severe impairments will also develop good oral language skills. Why some hearing-impaired children do not manage so well with oral language is something not yet fully understood; sometimes, of course, it is related to poor service provisions (e.g. late diagnosis, poor or inappropriate amplification). But there are other less obvious reasons in some cases. The ambition of those who work in this area of study is to be able to identify reasons in individual cases, and to be able therefore to plan appropriate rehabilitation procedures which provide good prognosis. In order to reach such a stage there needs to better understanding of the predictive links between hearing impairment, auditory perception and language disability. In addition, however, but beyond the scope of the present book, there is a need to develop appropriate procedures for assessment and remediation. There are those who argue that the provision of optimum services with optimum family support and early language interaction will result in the development of good communicative skills. Hypotheses such as these, not uncommon in the field of education, are virtually untestable; there is certainly some truth in it, and there is little doubt that probably the major facilitative change that could be made would be to provide reliable early diagnosis, early appropriate hearing aid fitting, and good family and educational support. It is frustrating that as we near the end of the twentieth century, with all the technological advances therein the achievement of this relatively simple goal is prevented by lack of adequate resources and planning. Meanwhile, the question of appropriate procedures for assessment and remediation remains. 'Intervention', closely monitored and with clear aims and suitable theoretical underpinning, in order to reduce the disability consequent upon the impairment, is a familiar concept in other areas of communication impairment in children. In hearing impairment, however, structured intervention remains controversial because of the apparent contradition between structure and the natural interactions required for communication to develop. There is a false dichotomy here, and much work needs to be done on the nature of early intervention for hearing-impaired children.

The subject matter of this book is oral language development, and its relationship with hearing impairment and auditory perception. There is widespread interest in non-oral language such as British Sign Language, and the use of such language by hearing-impaired children and the adult deaf community. There is no disagreement that some children will find a non-oral approach appropriate but there is widespread controversy about who such children might be, how they are identified and when such approaches are indicated. Such questions are properly addressed by research, and the literature on and experience of sign language acquisition, bilingualism and so on is growing, with notable efforts by some leadiing centres. That this book limits itself largely to a discussion of aspects of oral language does not indicate any underlying preference, commitment or philosophy of the authors; merely a limitation of size and competence.

1

Auditory and speech perception in the normally hearing adult: an overview

Some basic acoustics

Although the basic acoustics which the hearing scientist needs to understand are largely concerned with the propagation of sound through air, sound energy exists in mechanical, hydraulic and electrical forms as well as in its acoustic form. The hearing process from sound in air, to middle-ear mechanical vibrations, to inner-ear hydraulic effects, to electrical nerve impulses involves all these forms. Sound in its acoustic form is a pressure wave which consists of vibrations of molecules in an elastic medium, which can be a gas, a liquid or even a solid. Thus, sound in air is the disturbance of air particles produced by vibrating objects: for example, the diaphragm of a loudspeaker, a guitar string, or the vibration of the vocal folds.

As the vibrating object is driven backwards and forwards, the air molecules next to it are also driven back and forth, making small to-and-fro motions which are transmitted to adjacent molecules where the action is repeated. The movement of the molecules is purely local, and is directly related to the speed and size of the vibrations of the moving object; this local, to-and-fro motion is not the same as the velocity of the sound travelling through air. Furthermore, the propagation of sound waves in air is three-dimensional, like a rapidly expanding balloon, although not necessarily with equal efficiency in all directions. The velocity of sound, that is the speed at which it travels through the medium, is the speed at which the balloon expands.

The forward movement of the vibrating object compresses the surrounding air molecules, while the rearward movement decompresses the surrounding molecules. The to-and-fro vibratory motion thus creates a series of very small compressions (increase in pressure) and rarefactions (decrease in pressure) of the normal atmospheric pressure. A graph of these fluctuations in pressure at any point in the air as a function of time can be drawn, and this is known as a waveform. The simplest waveform is that produced by sinusoidal vibration, and is known as a sine wave. It so happens that waveforms of this type are heard as pure tones.

The amplitude of the sound wave is directly related to its 'height' – that is to say, it is a measure of the degree of air-pressure change caused by the vibrating object. The intensity of a sound is related to its amplitude, and the sensation of loudness is related to intensity.

A sequence of one compression followed by one rarefaction is known as a cycle,

1

and the number of cycles in one second is known as the frequency of the sound. This is expressed in hertz (Hz). Middle C on the piano has a frequency (F) of 256 Hz. The frequency of a pure tone is closely related to the sensation of pitch, higher frequencies producing sensations of higher pitch. The range of frequencies which can be heard by the normally hearing young adult is from about 20 Hz to 20000 Hz. For most purposes the extreme frequencies are rarely of any importance, and the more crucial frequencies in speech are between about 500 and 4000 Hz. The more extreme frequencies may become important in the hearing-impaired: many hearing losses are worse in the high frequencies, and low-frequency (c. 125 Hz) residual sensitivity may become important for the perception of voice pitch (intonation patterns). Occasionally, high frequency (> 8 kHz) sensitivity is better than that in the low frequencies, and this may be of importance for speech perception (Berlin *et al.* 1976).

The sine wave is the simplest waveform which is periodic; that is, the changes in air pressure repeat regularly in the same fashion. The period of such a wave is the time taken for one cycle (T) and is given, of course, by the reciprocal of the frequency: $T = 1/F$. The distance travelled by a wave in time T (one period) is called the wavelength, and since sound travels through air with a constant velocity, the higher the frequency of the wave, the smaller its wavelength. Thus:

$$\lambda = C/F$$

where

λ = wavelength
F = frequency
C = velocity of sound, which in air is about 343 m/s, depending upon atmospheric conditions

The significance of wavelength for the hearing-impaired in their particular acoustic environments is that sounds with wavelengths larger than an object will tend to bend around it, while those with wavelengths smaller than the object dimensions will tend to be reflected. Simple calculations using the above equation will show that the wavelength of a 500 Hz tone is 69 cm, while the wavelength of a 2000 Hz tone is 17 cm. The size of the head is such, then, that the higher frequencies will tend not to bend around it, while the lower frequencies will.

Apart from the amplitude, frequency and wavelength of a sound wave, there is a fourth descriptor which we should introduce here, and that is phase. If two objects are vibrating in air and producing sound waves of identical frequency, the two waves can be either in phase with each other, in which case the compressions and rarefactions of the two waves will be coincident in time, or out of phase with each other, in which case they will not be coincident. The term 'phase difference' is used to describe the difference between two out-of-phase waves.

A sine wave is not the only kind of sound which is periodic (i.e. which repeats regularly). Many everyday sounds, such as certain speech sounds and the sounds of musical instruments, also show regularity. These complex sounds are not as simple as sine waves, but like sine waves they repeat regularly and they generally exhibit the subjective characteristic of pitch. For sine waves, the number of periods occurring in one second is called the frequency, but for complex periodic sounds the number of periods in one second is called the repetition rate. The pitch of a complex periodic sound is related to its repetition rate.

Objects which are caused to vibrate sinusoidally may produce not only the fundamental sine wave; also, because of properties associated with the thickness of the object and the manner in which it is vibrated, they may produce various amounts of sound energy at frequencies which are multiples of the fundamental frequency. These multiples are known as harmonics or overtones. Thus, with a fundamental frequency of 100 Hz, harmonics may occur at 200 Hz, 300 Hz etc. In physics, the fundamental (F_0) is also regarded as the first harmonic, with $F_0 \times 2$ as the second harmonic; in music, however, $F_0 \times 2$ is called the first harmonic. Middle C on the piano does not sound the same as middle C on the violin, although the pitch of the two sounds appears identical. The subjective difference is known as a difference in quality or timbre, and is related to the different harmonics which are present in the two sounds. In certain circumstances, in hearing aids and pure-tone audiometers, for example, harmonics are undesirable, and great effort is expended in electronic design to minimize these distortions.

A complex sound wave is any wave that consists of more than a simple tone of one frequency. In the early part of the nineteenth century a French mathematician, Fourier, proposed a theorem which says, in effect, that any complex waveform can be decomposed into fundamentals and harmonics (all sine waves) of various frequencies, amplitudes and phase differences. Some years later, Fourier analysis of complex waveforms was demonstrated, and nowadays modern technology enables extremely complex acoustic stimuli to be analysed by Fast Fourier Transform into their 'components'. The distribution of sound energy with frequency is known as a sound spectrum, and spectral or frequency analysis results in graphs of frequency against amplitude. Periodic sounds produce line spectra, with energy at discrete frequencies. Continuous spectra occur when there is a continuous distribution of sound energy over a band of frequencies. Sounds of this kind are usually random – that is to say, they are aperiodic, do not repeat regularly, and therefore lack the sensation of pitch. Figure 1.1 shows some acoustic waveforms and their corresponding spectra.

Some speech sounds, those produced by turbulence in the air being expelled from the vocal tract without voicing (i.e. without vibration of the vocal folds), have continuous spectra (e.g. /s/, /f/). It is possible to have a combination of line and continuous spectra (Fig. 1.1 d), and some of the voiced consonants in speech are such (e.g. /d/, /v/). In contrast, all the vowels and a few consonants (e.g. /l/, /m/, /n/) have periodic waveforms; in fact, for a variety of reasons to do with the nature of voicing, these waveforms are really quasi-periodic, and resolve not into spectra with discrete frequency components so much as into continuous spectra with distinct energy peaks at certain frequencies. These energy peaks are known as formants.

We noted earlier that the intensity of a sound is directly related to pressure

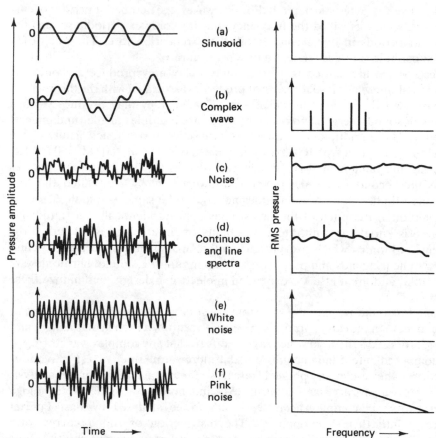

Figure 1.1   Examples of waveforms and their spectra (from Manhart, J.K. Acoustics for the study of hearing; in Gerber 1974, p. 36, Fig. 2.10).

change – that is, to the amplitude of the waveform. The greater the amplitude, the greater the sound intensity. The human ear can deal with a huge range of sound intensities: a whisper is about 1000 times more powerful than a just-audible (i.e. threshold) sound: conversational speech 1000000 times more powerful, and a loud shout 1000000000 times more powerful. This makes it inconvenient to deal with sound power in absolute terms, and we therefore use a logarithmic scale of the ratio between one sound and another (reference) sound. The sound-pressure level (SPL) in decibels (dB) of a sound having pressure P_1 is given by

$$SPL = 20 \log_{10}(P_1/P_0)$$

where P_0 is the reference (zero) pressure; the International Standard reference zero for sound pressure in air is 20 micropascals (μPa). Reference zero was chosen such that 0 dB SPL represented average human absolute threshold for a 1000 Hz tone. In fact, depending upon how it is measured, the average absolute normal threshold for such a tone seems to be at about 7 dB SPL. The above formula may be used to show that a doubling of the sound-pressure level results in an increase in 6 dB.

The inverse square law describes how the intensity of a sound decreases with the increasing distance from the vibrating source. Most sound waves in a space without reflecting surfaces are three-dimensional. The surface area of the sphere is increasing rapidly, then, although the total sound energy remains constant. Thus, as the wavefront area increases, sound energy per unit area decreases, and the intensity therefore decreases. It decreases as the square of the distance from the sound source (intensity is inversely proportional to the area of the sphere, $4\pi r^2$), and it can be shown that in an anechoic (echo-free) or perfectly freefield environment, the SPL decreases by 6 dB for each doubling of distance.

When surfaces of an object lie in the path of the expanding sphere, reflected waves are produced in addition to the direct waves, and the sound level at a given point will be increased, because both waves contribute to it. Thus the degree to which the inverse square law fails (that is, the degree to which the SPL fails to decrease by 6 dB for a doubling of distance from the sound source) can be used as a measure of sound reflection in an environment.

When the number and arrangement of reflecting surfaces is such that they provide a complete or nearly complete enclosure (e.g. a room), the effect is to cause reverberation. If a sound source is suddenly stopped, there is in all but near-perfect anechoic rooms a measurable time taken for the sound field to decay to inaudibility. This time is called the reverberation time. The fact that the sound level does decay in a reverberant environment is due to the absorption of sound energy by the walls and surfaces. Nothing is completely absorptive, and the percentage of sound absorbed varies with the type of material (and other factors, such as the angle of incidence of the sound wave upon the surface) from 0.01 to 100 per cent. Lightweight, fluffy materials such as fibreglass have the best absorptive capacity, whereas heavy dense materials such as steel or concrete reflect most of the sound energy. Carpeting, curtains and soft furnishings absorb the mid to high frequencies quite well, and can be used to reduce the amount of reflection and reverberation in a room. It should be noted, however, that these materials will not decrease the amount of sound transmission through the walls. Thus, to soundproof a room, rather than to make it echo-free, multiple walls with heavy damped materials (e.g. concrete or sand) are required; the heavier the material the less the vibration amplitude and the better the sound insulation.

While such considerations may not seem particularly relevant to the subject matter of this chapter, it is as well to cover them briefly at this early stage, for they provide some of the background to later discussions. The receptive language performance of hearing-impaired people is vulnerable to adverse acoustic conditions. The noise levels and the reverberation times found in many school classrooms are higher than they should be (Wills 1987), and the successful use of hearing aids is greatly constrained by these factors.

The perception of loudness

Loudness is the perceptual correlate of sound intensity and is 'that perceived property of sounds which permits us to order them on a scale extending from very quiet to very loud' (Gerber and Bauer 1974). Although the intensity of a sound is largely responsible for perceived loudness, other factors (frequency, duration etc.) are involved, and the psychoacoustic term 'loudness' should never therefore be used synonymously with the acoustic term 'intensity'.

Stevens (1957) investigated subjects' ability to scale sounds according to their subjective loudness. He arbitrarily defined the loudness of a 1000 Hz pure tone at 40 dB SL (sensation level: referenced to that individual's detection threshold for that tone) as one sone, and then asked his subjects to vary the intensity of a 1000 Hz comparison tone until it sounded twice (three times, half etc.) as loud as the one-sone standard. In this way he was able to construct loudness scales, and he found that a power function best related the sensation of loudness, L, to the physical attribute of intensity, I, thus:

$$L = kI^{0.3}$$

A doubling of loudness, therefore, is brought about by an increase in intensity of 10 dB (whether it be 10 to 20 dB, or 80 to 90 dB). In fact, loudness scales have been much criticized and have turned out to be not very useful. Instead, physical measurement with simple sound-level meters in terms of dB SPL has proved much more usable, coupled with some idea of the subjective loudness of different sound intensities. Thus, if minimum audibility is at 0 dB SPL, 30 dB SPL will be whisper-like, 60 or 70 dB SPL will be represented by the loudness of normal speech, and 100 dB SPL will be like the loudness of a shout at close range, and will be beginning to feel uncomfortable.

The threshold of audibility

Figure 1.2 shows the average normal minimum audible sound-pressure level as a function of frequency. There are a number of methods of measuring minimum audibility curves. They can be measured under headphones, in which case they are called Minimum Audible Pressure curves, or in the sound-field from loudspeakers, in which case they are called Minimum Audible Field curves. Instructions to subjects may vary slightly, and the position at which the SPL is monitored may vary. Biological thresholds are never absolute, going from zero per cent 'no' responses to 100 per cent 'yes' responses in one stimulus increment; rather, there is an increase in the probability of 'yes' responses over a small range of stimulus increments, and the criteria for deciding the exact position of an arbitrarily defined threshold (usually the 50 per cent point) may vary. However, these are fine details, and minimum audibility curves for young, otologically normal adults show the standard U-shape illustrated in Fig. 1.2. This is an average curve, and variability between individuals is considerable (± 10 dB or so). Minimum audibility curves have to be measured in very good acoustic conditions, with a minimum of

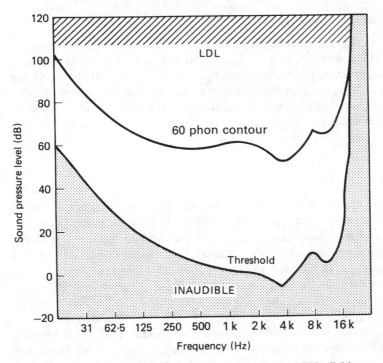

Figure 1.2   The threshold of audibility (minimum audible field curve averaged from a group of otologically normal young adults). Also shown is the 60 phon loudness contour, and loudness discomfort levels (adapted from Davis, H. and Silverman, S.R., *Hearing and Deafness*, 4th edn, New York: Holt, Rinehart and Winston, 1978, 21, Fig. 2.4).

background (ambient) noise. In many everyday listening conditions, thresholds will be raised because of the masking effects (see below) of ambient noise. Maximum sensitivity is found in the mid-frequency range, between 0.5 and 5 kHz, and the system is progressively less sensitive to lower and higher frequencies. It is worth noting that these mid-frequencies include most of those of particular importance for speech perception, and that the sounds of our own blood circulation and of our bodily movements contain much high and low-frequency energy respectively. The outer ear, consisting of the pinna and external ear canal, is partly responsible for the enhancement of the mid-frequencies through resonance effects, and it has been shown (e.g. Wiener and Ross 1946), by comparing SPLs at the canal entrance and at the eardrum, that this enhancement amounts to a maximum of some 10 or 15 dB at 4 kHz. Pascoe (1978) has measured the sensation level for each one-third-octave band of the long-term average speech spectrum in a group of normal listeners. As one would expect from the minimum audibility curves and the external ear enhancement, he found a peak sensation level at about 3000 Hz. Less predictably, he found a second peak at about 600 Hz, with a dip between the two peaks of about 8 dB at 1000 Hz. The reason for this is not clear.

The range of sensitivity

Figure 1.2 also shows the normal range of sensitivity, which lies between the threshold of audibility and the loudness discomfort level (LDL). The latter is more susceptible to slight changes in the instructions given to the listener than are detection thresholds, but reasonable consistency can still be achieved with care. Note that LDL, unlike minimum audibility, changes little with frequency, and the normal range of sensitivity – the 'dynamic range' – is therefore less at the extreme frequencies.

Equal loudness contours

Minimum audibility and LDL represent two curves within each of which loudness is judged to be equal. Equal loudness curves can also be constructed for intermediate intensities. The question is not how loudness changes with intensity for a given frequency (that is, loudness scaling), but how loudness changes as a function of frequency. The listener's task is to adjust the intensity of a comparison tone so that it sounds equally as loud as a standard tone of different frequency. The standard is usually a 1kHz tone, and the loudness contour can be derived at any level. Thus, if the standard is a 1 kHz tone at 60 dB SPL, the intensity of the comparison tone of different frequency is adjusted by the listener to be of equal loudness level; the units of loudness level are called phons, and the equal loudness contour so constructed would be called the 60-phon contour. The 60-phon contour for a sample of normal ears is also shown in Fig. 1.2, and it can be seen that it is much less variable across frequency than is the threshold curve.

The audiogram

The most widely used measure of hearing impairment is that in which an individual's minimum audibility to pure tones is assessed and compared with the normal minimum audibility curve. This is called pure-tone audiometry, and the results are generally recorded on a pure-tone audiogram (Fig. 1.3). In order that the sensitivity of each ear can be measured separately, earphones are used, and pure-tone audiometers are calibrated in such a way that the average minimum audibility curve of a large group of otologically normal young adults is called zero dB Hearing Level (HL); thus 'audiometric zero' or 0 dB HL is a straight line, and does not vary with frequency. This makes the drawing and interpretation of pure-tone audiograms considerably easier than if they were expressed in dB SPL, in which case the 'baseline' would be a U-shaped curve. Care must be taken, however, when comparing, say, speech levels (in dB SPL) with pure-tone thresholds (in dB HL), or when selecting a hearing aid (specified in terms of dB SPL) for a given degree of hearing loss (in db HL). Conversion from one unit to the other is simply a matter of adding or subtracting a constant number of dB; the number varies across frequencies.

Although clinical audiology uses the pure-tone audiogram extensively, it must be

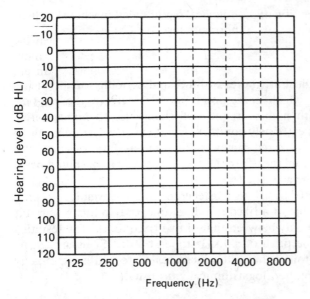

Figure 1.3 Blank pure-tone audiogram form: decibels hearing level by frequency of pure tone (recommended standard form, *British Journal of Audiology*, 1975).

stressed (see Chapter 5) that this is just one measure of hearing loss, and it may not be a particularly good predictor of the hearing for more complex signals such as speech.

Coding of loudness by the nervous system

It was once thought that the outer hair cells of the cochlea had different thresholds from the inner hair cells, and that associated with this were different groups of auditory nerves which responded to different signal intensities (Katsuki *et al.* 1962); with such a system, loudness would be coded in terms of which fibres were active. More recent work has shown this not to be the case; there is a range of thresholds for fibres which are similarly 'tuned' (see below), but that range is relatively small, perhaps about 20 dB for 80 per cent of the fibres (Kiang 1968, Liberman and Kiang 1978). Another way in which loudness can be coded is in terms of the rate of firing of individual neurones. However, the dynamic range of individual fibres (i.e. from threshold to saturation) appears to be of the order of only 40 dB, and therefore other mechanisms have to be sought to account for loudness coding throughout the 120 dB or so intensity range with which normal ears can cope. One possibility which is certainly involved, although it does not answer all the problems (see Moore 1989), is that at higher intensities the fibres which are tuned to the particular stimulus frequency (see below) are saturated, but other fibres with different 'characteristic frequencies' are brought in or 'recruited', and intensity changes are coded by changes in the firing rates of these other fibres. This possibility is consistent with the shape of physiological tuning curves and may provide a physiological explanation of pathological recruitment, in which loudness in ears with cochlear pathology grows abnormally fast (see Chapter 5).

Perception of pitch

Pitch is one of the psychological attributes of tones and periodic sounds; it is a quality of tonal perception which corresponds most closely to the physical dimension of frequency, with higher frequencies giving rise to higher pitch. However, pitch perception is extremely complex, is not entirely dependent upon the stimulus frequency, and is affected somewhat by stimulus durations and even slightly by stimulus intensity; and therefore the psychoacoustic term should never be used synonymously with the acoustic term.

Scales of pitch are constructed by asking a listener to adjust a variable tone until its pitch is half (double etc.) that of a fixed standard tone, or to adjust a variable tone such that its pitch is half-way between that of two fixed tones. The resulting scale is expressed in mels (the pitch of a 1 kHz tone at 40 dB SL is arbitrarily defined as 1000 mels). It is found that pitch increases more and more rapidly with increase in frequency (plotted logarithmically, as usual).

Place theory

The three great names responsible for the development of the place theory of pitch perception are Ohm, Helmholtz and von Békésy. Much of the early work used complex tones, like musical notes, for stimuli. Such stimuli contain a number of harmonics depending upon their source, but we hear only one pitch which appears to correspond to the fundamental frequency. In the mid-nineteenth century Ohm formulated his acoustic law which stated that the pitch of a tone was determined by its fundamental frequency, and that a pitch could only be heard if the stimulus contained energy at the corresponding frequency. Helmholtz (1883) provided Ohm's law with a physiological basis when he proposed that the basilar membrane inside the cochlea contained transversely stretched fibres, with each fibre resonant to a different frequency. Thus, the cochlea would perform a crude Fourier (spectral) analysis on the incoming signal, with place on the basilar membrane providing the basis for this analysis. It was assumed, correctly, that the auditory nerve fibres were able to preserve this place information by way of the organization of their connections with the hair cells on the basilar membrane. In the years between the two world wars, von Békésy (1960) was able actually to observe the movement of the basilar membrane, and although he showed no simple resonance of the type originally envisaged by Helmholtz, he demonstrated that the basilar membrane was excited by a travelling wave, and that the place of maximum vibration of the membrane changed in an orderly way as the stimulus frequency was changed. Thus he provided confirmation that the cochlea performed a spectral analysis based upon place, confirmation which seemed to support the Ohm–Helmholtz theory. This theory is consistent with a number of psychoacoustic phenomena, in particular masking and the critical band, and frequency selectivity.

Masking and the critical band

Masking is the process by which the threshold of audibility of one sound is raised by the presence of another (masking) sound. This is a familiar notion: speech perception can be disrupted by background traffic or aircraft noise; pure-tone audiograms can be invalidated by the presence of ambient noise; and so on. Although it is possible to demonstrate a small amount of central masking, in which masking noise presented to one ear masks a signal presented to the other ear, the important type masking is peripheral, and occurs when signal and masker are presented to the same (ipsilateral) ear. (Presenting the masker to the contralateral ear assumes practical importance in various audiometric situations where prevention of crossover to the non-test ear is required.) Studies of masking have involved the measurement of pure-tone thresholds at different frequencies in the presence of a masking tone or narrow band of noise (to avoid the beats produced by two tones of similar but not identical frequencies) of fixed intensity and frequency. The most striking thing about the resulting 'masked audiograms' (Fig. 1.4) is that the masker has its effect of elevating thresholds only at frequencies corresponding to or close to the frequency of the masker. This is clearly consistent with the place theory, in that both stimulus and masker would be maximally exciting the same place on the basilar membrane. The other important aspect of masked audiograms is that as the level of the masker is increased, its effect (i.e. the amount of masking) not only increases but also spreads outwards to adjacent

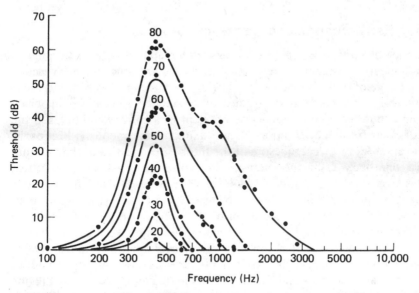

Figure 1.4   Masked thresholds for a narrow band of noise centred at 410 Hz. Each curve shows the elevation in pure-tone threshold as a function of frequency for a particular level of masking noise (20–80 dB SPL). (Adapted from Egan, J.P. and Hake, H.W., On the masking pattern of a simple auditory stimulus. *Journal of the Acoustical Society of America*, 1950, 22, 622–30.)

frequencies. Furthermore, the spread is much more marked upwards (on the frequency dimension) than downwards, and this has become known as the upward spread of masking. It is important in speech perception, since the more intense lower-frequency sounds such as vowels can mask the less intense higher-frequency consonants which are so important for speech intelligibility, particularly if speech is amplified (e.g. by hearing aids).

Fletcher (1940) proposed the concept of the critical band to account for masking. As we have seen, a pure tone presented in the presence of surrounding narrow-band noise will have its threshold raised relative to the tone in isolation. As the width of the noiseband is increased, so the tone threshold will increase until at a certain point – the critical bandwidth – no further increase in threshold occurs. It has been suggested that the critical band be thought of as the effective limit of spatial summation along the basilar membrane, and it is clear from a number of other psychoacoustic demonstrations that we can regard the action of the basilar membrane as reflecting the effects of a bank of overlapping filters (critical bands). The filters do not act like perfect rectangular filters, and if stimuli have enough energy some interactions across critical bandwidths do take place (e.g. upward spread of masking). The filter edges must be sloping, therefore, and considerable interest has been centred on the shape of the auditory filter (e.g. Patterson 1974, 1976, Patterson and Moore 1985) which appears to be that of a rounded exponential function, symmetrical at lower stimulus levels but with a shallower filter skirt on the lower frequency side as the stimulus level increases.

Frequency discrimination and frequency resolution

The frequency difference limen (the smallest detectable change in frequency) for normally hearing listeners is very small; listeners are able, for example, to perceive a change of only about 3 Hz in a 1 kHz pure tone of moderate intensity. Similar findings have come from studies of frequency resolution, in which listeners have to detect one frequency component of a complex stimulus in the presence of other frequency components, presented simultaneously. Frequency resolution represents a direct measure of the filtering properties of the auditory system. In one such task, the intensity of pure-tone maskers of different frequencies just needed to mask a low-level pure tone of fixed frequency is measured. It is assumed that the degree to which one tone just masks another is a measure of the frequency resolution of the two tones, perfect resolution requiring that masking would occur only when the tones were of exactly the same frequency. The curves of necessary masker level against frequency which can be constructed from such experiments are called psychophysical or psychoacoustic tuning curves and Fig. 1.5 shows an example. Normally hearing listeners typically exhibit very fine frequency resolution, although when other auditory cues are properly eliminated (see Patterson and Moore 1985, p. 168) the tuning curve may be rather broader around the tip, and not unlike an inverted version of the auditory filter.

The physiological data tell a similar story. Using microelectrodes, single-cell

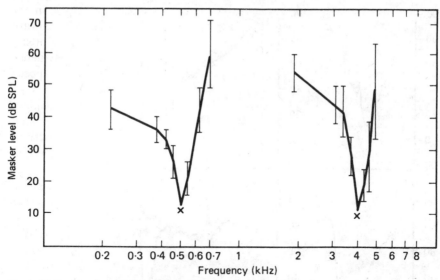

Figure 1.5   Psychoacoustic tuning curves: average curves for test tone frequencies of 500 and 4000 Hz for normally hearing listeners ($n = 28$). Curves show the intensity of maskers of different frequencies needed to just mask the test tone (from Gribben 1981).

recordings have been made of the electrical activity in individual auditory-nerve fibres (e.g. Kiang *et al*. 1965, Evans 1972, Liberman and Kiang 1978). The threshold of activity in such neurones, which has to be arbitrarily defined since there will be activity even in the resting state, can be measured in response to pure tones of differing frequency presented to the ears via loudspeakers. The resulting 'tuning curves' of threshold in dB against frequency are shown in Fig. 1.6, and their steep slopes indicate better frequency resolution than might be expected from basilar membrane mechanics. In general, these physiological tuning curves support the notion of place theory, since the nerve fibres arise from particular places on the basilar membrane, and the so-called characteristic frequencies of the curves vary in an orderly and predictable fashion throughout the nerve bundle. Note in passing that the tuning curves are generally steeper on the higher-frequency side, which is consistent with the shape of the travelling wave on the basilar membrane. The curves are also consistent with the findings from masking studies, in particular the upward spread of masking: the steep slopes on the high-frequency side of the physiological tuning curves will prevent signals of higher frequency than the characteristic frequency from exciting the neurone; on the low frequency side, however, signals of moderate intensity levels will be able to excite the neurone, thus tending to mask a signal presented at the characteristic frequency.

Early studies of basilar membrane mechanics (von Békésy 1960) seemed to indicate that the tuning of the basilar membrane is rather broad. On the other hand, the tuning of individual auditory nerve fibres had been shown to be sharp (e.g. Kiang *et al*. 1965). This discrepancy of an apparently broadly tuned cochlea output with a sharply tuned neural output at the level of auditory nerve fibres

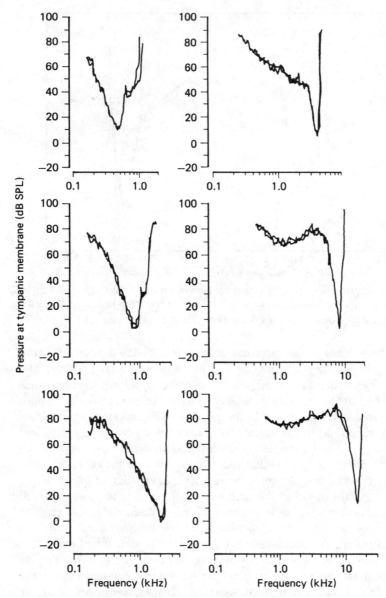

Figure 1.6 Physiological tuning curves of cat auditory nerve fibres for six different frequency regions (from Liberman and Kiang 1978).

led to the notion that the sharp tuning of individual fibres was due to the action of some 'second filter' within the cochlea. Russell and Sellick (1978) were able to demonstrate, however, the sharp tuning of the inner hair cells within the cochlea, and Sellick *et al.* (1982) then showed that the mechanics of the cochlea were also sharply tuned, and that there is no need therefore to postulate further tuning mechanisms. The early experiments of von Békésy had been performed on cadavers, using high sound pressure levels, and the later studies had found great difficulty in measuring cochlear mechanics without causing interfering damage. It is now firmly established, however, that there is no progression of sharper and sharper tuning in the auditory system, but rather the fine tuning of the system is set by the mechanical frequency tuning of the cochlea (see Yates 1986).

There are a number of psychoacoustic phenomena, however, which do underline the inadequacies of the place theory of pitch perception. Perhaps the most important of these is the phenomenon of the missing fundamental.

If a complex tone consisting of, say, three pure tones at 800, 1000 and 1200 Hz is presented to a listener, the perceived pitch corresponds to that associated with the fundamental frequency of the harmonics, namely 200 Hz. This is a major problem for place theory, since the complex tone contains no energy at the fundamental frequency. What it does have, of course, is periodicity, with a repetition rate of 200 Hz. In the early days of place theory, the missing fundamental was accounted for by supposing that nonlinearities in the outer and middle ears introduced energy at the missing frequency. This ad hoc proposal kept place theory alive in its original form until experiments by Schouten (1940) and others forced some rethinking. Schouten presented his listeners with a complex tone consisting of the harmonics of a 200 Hz fundamental, with the fundamental removed. As expected, pitch corresponding to the fundamental frequency was perceived. He then added a tone of 206 Hz to the stimulus, reasoning that if the fundamental was present as a distortion product in the signal arriving at the cochlea, audible beats would be produced. They were not. Licklider (1954) presented listeners with a series of complex tones with the fundamentals removed, so that the series gave a perceived melody of the missing fundamentals. On adding low pass noise to the signal, sufficient to mask any supposed distortion products, the melody did not disappear.

Temporal theory of pitch perception

As early as 1886, Rutherford proposed an extreme version of temporal, or frequency, theory for pitch perception, namely that every hair-cell responded to every tone, and that frequency information was carried only in the frequency of the nerve impulses. Since auditory nerve fibres do not fire at more than about 300 times per second, some form of volleying (Wever 1949), in which different fibres fire on different stimulus cycles, is required for any temporal theory, even if Rutherford's extreme version is discounted. As it turns out, nerve fibres fire with equal probabilities in every part of the cycle for stimuli above 5 kHz. However, below that frequency, fibres tend to fire to a particular part of the stimulus cycle: that is, they are phase-locked (Rose et al. 1967). Volleying is exhibited, in that fibres do not fire on every cycle, but when firing does take place it is in response to a particular part of the cycle. Schouten argued in favour of a version of temporal theory of pitch perception which allowed for some spectral analysis based upon place, and which has been called 'fine structure theory'. He proposed that incoming signals first undergo a crude spectral analysis based upon place of excitation on the basilar membrane. The temporal fine structure of the first stage of analysis would be preserved in the temporal patterns of nerve firings, and pitch would be extracted from this temporal patterning: in particular, the pitch would be determined by the time difference between the stimulus waveform peaks, the reciprocal of the time difference giving the pitch.

While temporal theories can account for the missing fundamental phenomenon, there are a number of studies which have been published in the last decade or so which show psychoacoustic effects incompatible with such theories. For example, Patterson (1973) showed that scrambling the starting phases of the harmonics in a complex tone has little effect on the perceived pitch, although the temporal fine structure is markedly altered. Furthermore, studies (e.g. Houtsma and Goldstein 1972) have shown that presentation of the different harmonics to different ears in a complex tone of only two components does not alter the pitch percept. Central rather than peripheral processes must be at work, and it is difficult to see how the interaction of the components required by fine structure theory could take place. The evidence on mechanisms of pitch perception is conflicting. The change in function at 5 kHz is firmly established, such that spatial (spectral) analysis is quite sharp above this point, and no temporal information is preserved; whereas below 5 kHz electrical recordings clearly show that temporal patterning is preserved. There are those theorists, therefore, who argue in favour of temporal mechanisms at lower frequencies and spatial mechanisms at higher frequencies. Studies of central mediation of pitch using dichotic presentation have led to a new group of theories known as the pattern-recognition theories (Goldstein 1973, Wightman 1973, Terhardt 1974, Wilson 1974). These theories emphasize the complexity of the pitch-extraction process and that it is based upon two stages. In the first stage, a complex tone is analysed into its component harmonics, using place or time information, or both. Frequency selectivity is the crucial feature of this stage. In the second stage the component information is presented to a central pattern recognition device which in various possible ways searches for appropriate harmonic patterns that would correspond to the components.

Binaural hearing

There are a number of psychoacoustic effects which are dependent upon the use of both ears. The hearing-impaired exhibit deficits in binaural psychoacoustic processes as they do in monaural psychoacoustic processes. The monaural changes are the more marked: elevated detection thresholds, poor frequency discrimination and so on (Chapter 5); but the less obvious binaural impairments can have serious effects upon performance, particularly receptive language performance. In a two-dimensional, non-reverberant world, language competence and performance would be unaffected by impaired binaural processes. But in the real world, hearing-impaired people exhibit great difficulties with the localization of sound sources and in listening to speech in noisy or reverberant environments (see Durlach *et al.* 1981 for a review).

Localization

Localization refers to the ability to judge the position in space of a sound source. It is of course a very useful ability for many everyday listening situations, from early development where the infant can learn to identify a voice with a speaker, to identifying a speaker in an area (e.g. classroom) containing many potential speakers, thereby allowing the use of speech-reading cues; orientation responses and the use of localization in the context of warning signals is also important. Basically, the ability to locate sound sources allows us to bring our attention, visual and auditory, fully to bear on the stimulus.

If we consider sinusoidal sounds, it is clear that there are two possible cues to the localization of their source. In the case of a sound source lying to one side of the head, the sound is nearer one ear than the other. It will arrive at the near ear earlier than at the far ear, and the continuing signals will be out of phase with each other at the two ears; in addition, the sound at the near ear will be slightly more intense than that arriving at the far ear (the head-shadow effect). Thus, if the auditory system is able to preserve temporal information at each ear – that is, if auditory nerves fire at particular points in the cycle of a periodic tone – and if it is able to preserve intensity information at each ear, then presumably it can use the interaural differences in these two cues to locate sounds. We have seen that there is good evidence that temporal information is preserved at frequencies below 5 kHz, and we know of course that intensity differences are available to the system.

Experiments have confirmed the use of interaural time and intensity differences as the basis of localization (e.g. Stevens and Newman 1936, Sandel et al. 1955). It turns out that intensity differences are more important for high-frequency signals. This is not unexpected, because tones with long wavelengths will tend to bend well round the head, giving rise to only small intensity differences. High frequencies may differ by as much as 20 dB at the two ears. On the other hand, interaural phase differences will be greatest for low-frequency sounds, and temporal cues seem to predominate in the low frequencies. For a sound source directly to one side of a head, the time-of-arrival difference between the two ears will be of the order of 700 μs, corresponding to a 'path difference' of about 23 cm. When the wavelength of a sound is about double this distance, ambiguities begin to occur, in that the phase difference could be attributed to more than one location of the sound source. Reflections and head movements help to minimize these ambiguities (Hirsh 1971), but the ambiguities increase as signal frequency increases. The result is that localization is poorest for signals of about 1500 Hz, when neither the low-frequency temporal cues nor the high-frequency intensity cues are suitably strong and clear.

Most sounds in nature, including speech, do not consist of pure tones, but are complex signals containing a number of onsets and offsets and containing rapidly changing frequency spectra (transients). The time-of-arrival differences of onsets and offsets, and of transients, at the two ears has been investigated using headphone presentation and manipulating the interaural differences (Klumpp and Eady 1956, Tobias 1972), and it is clear that these differences provide a further cue to the localization of complex signals.

The physiological basis of sound localization has been studied, and it has been found that a large number of neurones at or beyond the superior olivary complex, which is located in the brainstem and is the lowest level to receive inputs from both ears, are responsive to interaural timing or intensity differences. Indeed, it appears that animals with relatively small heads may have more of the neurones which are sensitive to interaural temporal differences than of those which are sensitive to interaural intensity differences. The major problem with the physiological data is that the neurones appear to be sensitive only to time or intensity disparities which are larger than those actually encountered at the ears as a result of the location of sounds in space.

There is some evidence from psychoacoustic studies that monaural localization is possible (Freedman and Fisher 1968, Harris and Sergeant 1971). Monaural localization improves with the complexity of the signal. It is thought to be related to changes in spectral patterning at the ear produced by head movements, or, perhaps more importantly, to the acoustic effects of the pinna on incoming signals (Batteau 1967, Gardner and Gardner 1973).

The precedence effect

Most everyday listening takes place in reverberant environments. We are not normally aware of the echoes of a signal, even though the reflected energy may be as great as the acoustic energy received directly. Wallach *et al.* (1949) investigated this phenomenon, and found that the binaural auditory system was able to fuse echoes into a single percept, within certain limits. The successive sounds have to be close together in time, below about 40 milliseconds (ms); they have to be complex and similar in spectral pattern, and the echoes have not to be markedly more intense than the leading, direct sound. If these conditions are met, then the listener judges the location of the sound to be that of the first, or direct, signal – hence the precedence effect.

The precedence effect is thought to be a binaural phenomenon, and as Moore (1989) points out this can be subjectively demonstrated by occluding one ear and listening to a speaker in a reverberant room. Furthermore, hearing-impaired listeners do have great difficulty with speech perception in reverberant conditions. However, it is not clear that some degree of fusion of echoes is not possible monaurally; Batteau (1967) suggests that the pinna effects can help fusion.

Binaural release from masking

A pure tone with a noise masker presented to both ears simultaneously through headphones will have a certain masked-tone threshold. If the phase of the tone is reversed in one ear only, the masked threshold is decreased, perhaps by as much as 10 dB for lower-frequency tones. This interesting phenomenon is called binaural release from masking, and the difference in thresholds is called the binaural masking level difference (BMLD). Binaural release will occur even if, having presented tone and noise to one ear only, noise alone is added to the other ear. It occurs for complex tones, clicks and speech as well as for pure tones. The conditions under which it occurs seem to be that whenever the phase or intensity differences of the signal at the two ears are not the same as the phase or intensity differences of the masker at the two ears, then the ability to detect and identify signals will be improved. Since these differences occur in real situations only when the signal and masker are at different spatial locations, there is an obvious connection between binaural release from masking and our ability to listen to speech in background noise (the cocktail party problem of Cherry 1953), which we would expect, therefore, to be improved with binaural listening and when signal and noise were spatially separated. This is indeed the case. In this situation the ability to localize the absolute position of sound sources is perhaps less important than the ability to judge the separation of sound sources. Localization and escape from masking may not be mediated by identical processes, however: Carhart *et al.* (1968) investigated BMLD with speech signals and a variety of noise backgrounds in different phase relationships at the two ears; although the general picture was confirmed of high BMLD at phase differences equivalent to large spatial separation, the largest BMLD occurred in the antiphasic condition, where separation is subjectively unclear.

Other binaural effects

Many psychoacoustic effects are enhanced by the use of two ears, but in most cases other than those already discussed, the degree of improvement is of limited practical significance. Auditory threshold is some 3–6 dB better in the binaural condition, and this can be relevant to the decision to prescribe binaural hearing aids.

Not strictly binaural effects, but concerned with two ears and of some interest, are the head-shadow effect and right-ear advantage. Head shadow has already been mentioned: it refers to the fact that the ear nearest a sound source will receive the signal at a greater intensity (and slightly earlier) than the ear furthest away. This is due to diffraction of the sound round the head, and applies particularly to the high frequencies (i.e. short wavelength).

Broadbent (1958), Kimura (1961, 1964) and others studied the processing of dichotically presented signals (in which different signals are presented to the two ears) and noted a right-ear advantage for speech and a left-ear advantage for nonspeech sounds (e.g. melodies). The effect is attributed to the prepotency of the contralateral auditory pathways to the language-specialized left hemisphere. Many infant hearing-screening tests are based upon orientation (localization) in response to sounds presented either to the right or to the left of the child (see Chapter 2). Mature localization responses do not appear in the developing infant before about six months, but it has been reported that in the early stages of localization development there is a significant tendency to turn to the right. This may be related to right-ear advantage.

The right-ear advantage does not apparently depend upon sounds being meaningful. Shankweiler and Studdert-Kennedy (1967) showed right-ear advantage for the recall of initial stop consonants, although, curiously, not for steady-state vowels. Darwin (1971) showed that vowels *can* give a right-ear advantage, but that whether or not they *do* depends upon the complexity of the perceptual discrimination. In Darwin's study, right-ear advantage for vowels was shown when there was uncertainty as to vocal tract size, but not when the vowels came from the same vocal tract. This and other results are consistent with the view expressed by Studdert-Kennedy and Shankweiler (1970) that specialization of the left hemisphere in speech perception is due to its possession of a linguistic device, rather than to specialization in auditory analysis. In other words, whereas either hemisphere can extract acoustic features from a signal, they can be related to phonemic features and a phonemic response only in the left hemisphere.

Speech perception

During breathing, the vocal folds are open, but for phonation (uttering) they are brought together, and air is forced out of the lungs, making the folds oscillate at a freqency partly determined by their tension and mass. The tension of the folds is similar in both sexes, and different fundamental voice pitches in the sexes are occasioned by differences in the mass of the cords and in the length of the windpipe and larynx. The vocal folds control mainly the fundamental frequency and the rise/decay times of the sound signal, which is forced into the oral and nasal cavities above. The sounds produced by the vocal folds are not, of course, pure tones, but are complex periodic sounds containing many varying harmonics. The vocal tract is formed by the pharynx (throat), the nose and nasal cavities, and the mouth and tongue, and the tract applies a 'transfer function' to the complex sound emerging from the vocal folds. Thus, the harmonics of the fundamental are filtered or emphasized by resonance, depending upon the geometry of the vocal tract. The tract does not add any components – it emphasizes or de-emphasizes those already present in the complex sound emitted by the vocal folds. In fact, the vocal tract is analogous to, but much more complicated than, an organ pipe open at one end, for which the resonant frequencies are the fundamental, the third harmonic, the fifth harmonic, and so on. The fundamental is determined mainly by the length of the tract, but also by the 'flare': as the mouth is opened, the frequency increases. The fundamental frequency of the vocal fold signal for males is approximately 125 Hz, and for females 250 Hz, although there is a considerable range across individuals. Detailed descriptions of the acoustics of speech can be found in, for example, Fant (1960).

One way to look at speech acoustics is to examine the waveform. As we have seen, the waveform shows the amplitude of a signal as a function of time, and although the waveform of a pure tone is simple, that of a rapidly varying signal such as speech is very complex. The problem is that the speech signal varies not in two dimensions, but in three, and description in terms of any two may not be very revealing if speech perception is based upon aspects of all three. There is no doubt that temporal, frequency and intensity information is involved in speech perception, and therefore not only the waveform (intensity/time) but frequency spectra (intensity/frequency) are of limited use on their own in our understanding of the speech signal. The most useful way of characterizing the speech signal is by means of the speech spectrogram, which preserves information in all three dimensions of time, intensity and frequency. In the spectrogram the horizontal axis shows time, the vertical axis shows frequency, and the intensity of the signal is shown by the darkness of the trace. An example of a spectrogram is shown in Fig. 1.7. It will be noticed that, as expected, the unvoiced /s/ sound contains energy across many frequencies, particularly the higher frequencies. The vertical striations correspond to the underlying periods of vocal fold vibration (i.e. the fundamental frequency), and are not evident for the unvoiced /s/. They are clearly evident for all the vowel sounds in the figure, however, and for the nasal /m/. Although the complex periodic tones of the vowels are not resolved by the spectrogram into individual harmonics, what is clear is that there are frequency

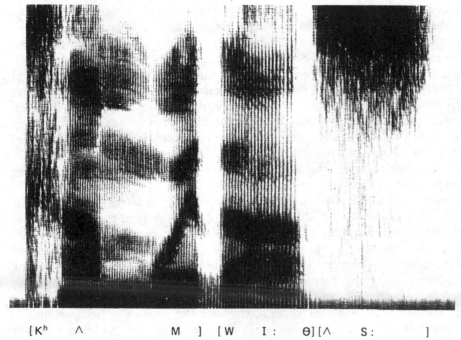

[Kʰ   ʌ   M] [W   I :   ɵ][ʌ   S:]

Figure 1.7 A speech spectrogram of the utterance 'come with us'.

areas in which the acoustic energy is concentrated. The dark bands in Fig. 1.7 are such. These are the formants, and are numbered first, second, third and so on, starting at the formant with the lowest frequency. Formants represent the peaks in the spectral envelope, rather than any individual harmonics of the fundamental frequency. They seem to be of particular utility in speech perception.

Discussions in the field of both auditory and visual perception in the last two decades have tended to concentrate on the rather false dichotomy of whether units are recognized by means of a process of template matching or feature detection (e.g. Neisser 1967). If it is accepted that whatever is involved, it must for reasons of economy be organized in a parallel and hierarchical fashion, and be active in the sense that later analysis stages can alter the state of earlier stages, then at some level 'template matching' and 'feature detection' begin to look conceptually rather similar. The question then arises: with what input units do these processes work? Do we match templates at the level of sentences? Unlikely, because of the infinite number of unique sentences which can be generated. There are fewer words than possible sentences, but there are still around a million English words, and the receptive vocabulary size of adults may be in the region of 100000 words. On the other hand, there are only about 4000 syllables in English, and about 40 or 50 phonemes are enough to describe all English words. For many years, linguists have been aware of the utility of phonemes as descriptors of speech. They are the smallest units of sound which, in any particular language, differentiate between one word and another. There is only one syllable in each of the words *pat* and *bat*, but three phonemes, the first of which differentiates between the two words. Similarly, the middle phoneme differentiates *pat* from *pit*, and the final phoneme differentiates *pat* from *pad*. Some workers argue that the phoneme is merely a linguistic device, and has no perceptual reality for speech perception (Warren 1975) or for reading (Gleitman and Rozin 1973), but there is no doubt that in general the perceptual psychologists have taken the phoneme as their basic unit as have the descriptive linguists before them. With a vocabulary of only 40 or so phonemes (in English) to be recognized, the template-matching process becomes more possible, although at the cost of a faster rate of processing: instead of handling decisions at the rate of two or three words per second, the rate rises to about a dozen or so phonemes per second.

Linguists have developed classification systems for phonemes which are based upon their articulation. Vowels (open vocal tract) are classified by tongue position and degree of constriction. Consonants are classified according to whether they are voiced or unvoiced, by the manner of production (stops, fricatives, nasals) and by the place of production (labial, alveolar, palatal). Linguistic systems of articulatory 'distinctive features' have proved to be powerful descriptive tools. Not surprisingly, therefore, speech scientists looked for acoustic correlates of the linguistic distinctive features which might form the basis of speech perception. Examination of speech spectrograms indicates just such correlates, which experiments have shown to be crucial for perception. We have seen that the spectral energy of vowels is concentrated into bands of frequencies, called formants; in addition, there are often marked and rapid changes ('formant transitions') in the frequency of some of the formants when the vowel is preceded by a consonant. It turns out that these formant transitions provide major cues for the discrimination of certain phonemes (Liberman *et al.* 1959).

For example, the differentiation of /ba/ from /da/ depends largely upon the cues provided by the second formant transitions. A low starting frequency with rising transition will (for most vowels) be heard as /b/, while a higher starting frequency and falling transition will be heard as /d/. The parentheses have to be added, for if the vowel is altered, the same initial phoneme can be cued by different transitions. For example, the first formant transition has been found to provide the cue to the class of voiced stops /b, d, g/. The second formant transition differentiates between the members of this class. But if the sounds /di/ and /du/ are compared, the position of steady-state formants discriminate between /i/ and /u/, and each vowel is preceded by a quite different second formant transition. In the case of /di/ it is rising and of /du/ it is falling. Thus the same phoneme can be cued in different contexts by different acoustic features. Liberman *et al.* (1967) argue that the context-dependent cues for the /d/ phoneme are common in speech, and that invariant cues to phonemes are rare. Even for vowels, which in their steady state have relatively invariant cues, some restructuring takes place at rapid speech rates. Thus, it is argued, there is only rarely a simple one-to-one invariant relationship between acoustic cues and perceived phoneme, and a single acoustic cue can carry information about two successive phonemes. This helps to get over the problem of the rapid rate of decision-making required by a system based on the phoneme as the perceptual unit, but it does make for complex acoustic–perceptual relationships. Nevertheless it is clear from many studies that the formants and their transitions do provide crucial, if complex, perceptual cues. This will prove to be an important consideration for the hearing-impaired, whose frequency and temporal resolving ability may be less than perfect.

A line of discussion which has occupied much of the literature in recent years concerns whether 'speech is special': whether there is a special speech mode in auditory perception. Evidence for such a view comes from studies in which it can be shown that the perception of speech sounds is distinct from the perception of nonspeech sounds. The 'categorical perception' of certain speech sounds has been taken as suitable evidence. It is possible to synthesize the speech sounds /ba/ and /da/, and furthermore to synthesize a number of sounds (e.g. eight) in between. These intermediate stimuli are formed by taking gradual and equal-step increases of the starting point of the second formant transition from the lower frequency appropriate to /b/, to the higher frequency appropriate to /d/. When listeners are asked to identify these sounds, they tend to place them into either the /ba/ or /da/ category, with a rapid switch from one to the other at the 'phoneme boundary'. There is nothing particularly surprising in this outcome, since we have only two labels (two outputs) to use for the identification task. When, however, the listener is asked to discriminate the sounds using an ABX paradigm (the task is to judge whether X was the same as A or B), it is found that discrimination, too, is categorical. Discrimination is good across phoneme boundaries, and poor within phoneme boundaries. For simple nonspeech stimuli varying in one dimension (e.g. pitch) we are normally able to discriminate far more stimuli than we can identify. These findings have been taken to show that speech sounds are *perceived* in terms of distinctive features, and that other acoustic details of speech stimuli are ignored.

Categorical perception applies particularly to consonants; vowels, on the other hand, are perceived more or less continuously (Fry *et al.* 1962). It has been suggested (Crowder and Morton 1969, Pisoni 1973) that a listener has two short-term memory stores for incoming speech signals. One store is for acoustic information (echoic), the other store is for phonetic information. The discrete nature of the latter ensures a longer life for the memory trace. Since consonants are of very short duration, the echoic memory will decay especially rapidly, and the listener may have to rely on the phonetic store (i.e. discrete phoneme labels) for his discrimination.

The classic experiment demonstrating categorical perception (in this case that place of articulation — for /b/, /d/, and /g/ — is perceived categorically) was that of Liberman *et al.* (1975). This and later experiments led to a three-point criterion for the perception of auditory stimuli to be described as categorical:

(i) Stimuli lying along an acoustic continuum can be systematically, reliably categorized by listeners to yield a sharply defined identification function.

(ii) Discrimination function is high at the category boundaries and near to chance level within the categories, giving a picture of peaks and troughs between and within categories.

(iii) There is a correspondence between the peaks and troughs and the shape of the identification function; the discrimination function could be predicted correctly from the identification function (Studdert-Kennedy *et al.* 1970, Burns and Ward 1978).

It has been demonstrated in other experiments that voiced/voiceless contrasts, for example /b/ vs /p/, are perceived in a categorical manner. The categorization in this case is thought to be based on the relative timing of the onset of the voicing of the first formant and the burst of energy resulting from the release of the constriction at the place of articulation. In fact a number of acoustic cues are available in the definition of natural voiced/voiceless contrasts. The principal cues are: the presence of a voiced transition at the onset of voicing, voice-onset time (VOT), and the frequency of the first formant at voicing onset. Voice-onset time has been the subject of many studies. Lisker and Abramson (1964) demonstrated three common types of plosive in a study of voiced–voiceless sounds occurring in 11 different languages: *(i)* those in which the voicing substantially preceded the release of the plosive voice, known as prevoiced; *(ii)* those in which the voicing closely followed the plosive burst, known as short voicing lag (or voiced), *(iii)* those in which the voicing considerably lagged behind the release of the plosive burst, known as long voicing lag (or voiceless).

In different languages, these differences in voice-onset time are preceived as different phonemic contrasts. For example, in English, stops employing VOT of less than about 20 ms are perceived as voiced, and stops employing a longer VOT are identified as voiceless (i.e. /ba/ versus /pa/), the VOT boundary varying with place of articulation. Spanish speakers, on the other hand, use contrasts between the lead and the short lag stop consonants. That is, they perceive prevoiced/voiced sounds as different sounds, although most adult native English speakers would not be able to distinguish these. Hence, if the speechlike sounds /ba/ and /pa/ are synthesized such that the VOT alone is varied on a continuum of milliseconds and all the other features are held constant, then English-speaking listeners tend to label sounds with a VOT of less than 20 ms as /b/. In a discrimination task the same listener will discriminate better between sounds that fall either side of the apparent category boundary than between sounds within the same category. It has been suggested by some authors that the ability to perceive speech contrasts in this way is due to a set of biological linguistic feature detectors that are preset from birth, and that the new infant is equipped to make these acoustic discriminations (see Chapter 2). This raises a number of questions such as whether feature detectors operate in a domain unique to speech sounds; whether other auditory phenomena are categorically perceived; and furthermore, whether speech sounds from languages other than an infant's normal linguistic environment are perceived in a categorical manner.

Some studies have been published which throw doubts on the 'speech is special' view. For one thing, categorical perception has been demonstrated with non-speech sounds (Cutting and Rosner 1974, Cutting 1978); for another, it has been shown that irrelevant acoustic detail is not ignored and is available to the listener of speech sounds. And finally, it is clear, for example, that different cues are used to discriminate voiced from unvoiced stops in the initial position in a word from those used to discriminate voiced from unvoiced stops in the final position. In the former case it is voice onset time, in the latter, the length of the preceding vowel. Nevertheless, the evidence on categorical perception of many speech sounds is compelling: there are areas of the brain which are specialized for dealing with speech; and sounds are either heard as speech or not: 'it is impossible to hear speech in terms of its acoustic characteristics, i.e. as a series of hisses, whistles, buzzes etc. Rather we perceive a unified stream of speech sounds' (Moore 1989, p. 268).

We have seen that phonemes are context-dependent, in that their acoustic pattern depends, among other things, upon neighbouring phonemes. There are many other contextual constraints in running speech which affect speech perception, usually favourably, by providing the listener with statistical probabilities about what is likely, and this can help reduce the load on the system by allowing it to look first for what is likely to be there. There are strong syntactic and semantic constraints which are established in running speech by patterns of stress, pause and intonation. The first two are strongly dependent upon voice intensity and timing, the latter upon perception of the fundamental pitch of the voice. These prosodic features may be processed at the same time as the phonetic features of speech, and prosodic information can help identification if acoustic quality is poor, or vice versa. The prosodic features of speech, particularly intonation, may be relatively more available to hearing-impaired listeners than the high-frequency acoustic phonetic features. The identification of neighbouring phonemes, syllables, words and sentences can also help establish the syntactic and semantic constraints within running speech, which in turn aids perception by making certain events more likely than others.

The context effects of fluent speech must be an important factor in speech perception. It is clear, for example, that we do not perceive speech in terms of discrete phonemes which are 'built up' into larger units, such as words. Studies have shown that listeners respond quicker to words or nonsense words than they do to individual phonemes (e.g. Savin and Bever 1970), and this is difficult to explain on a 'bottom-up' model. Furthermore, the decision rate for speech in which phonemes have to be individually classified must be in the order of 10–15 classifications per second, on top of which order information must be preserved (Huggins 1981). Warren *et al.* (1969) have shown that four nonspeech sounds must each last several hundred ms before their order can be correctly judged by a listener. However, if the sounds are made more similar, by using portions of steady-state vowels for example, the minimum duration for order identification drops. In addition, if transitions are added to make the vowels run smoothly into one another, the rate drops still further. Huggins (1981) argues that the main reason for the results produced by Warren *et al.* (1969) is that the sounds were so disparate that they formed separate auditory streams, and he cites the study of Bregman and Campbell (1971) in support. Using pure tones, Bregman and Campbell created two subsets based on frequency differences, one set of three high-frequency tones, one set of three low-frequency tones. When they played these tones to subjects in a repeating order of mixed high and low tones, subjects were able to report order correctly within subsets but not between subsets. Bregman and Campbell proposed that the auditory system creates substreams of sounds whenever different types occur rapidly in sequence. This 'auditory streaming' was further studied by Bregman and Dannenbring (1973). They pointed out that speech is not constituted of separate segments of sounds, but that phonemes connect, overlap and dissolve into one another (phonetic context effects). They repeated the earlier study, but added two conditions: one in which successive tones were connected by frequency glides, another in which they were connected by partial frequency glides (as in formant transitions in speech). The insertion of full and partial glides made auditory streaming less likely. Thus, it may be that speech sounds form a single stream or group within which order can be followed.

Normally hearing listeners are able to perceive speech in the presence of high levels of background noise. How is this achieved? Broadbent (1958) and Bregman (1978) have argued that low-level processes operate on simple attributes of sounds to group them into streams or channels which share certain properties. These groups are then presented to later processes for phonetic categorization. Studies in selective attention (Cherry 1953, Treisman 1960) and in auditory streaming (Bregman and Campbell 1971) have identified simple physical parameters such as spatial location which can affect grouping. In addition, experiments with synthetic speech have suggested that the fundamental pitch of voice is used to group together consecutive sounds into the voice of one speaker (Darwin and Bethell-Fox 1977), and to group simultaneous harmonics into one voice (Broadbent and Ladefoged 1957). Darwin (1981) argued that these studies do not present direct evidence on the contribution of such grouping to speech perception (phonetic categorization), and he constructed stimuli which would provide a direct test. For example, he asked whether the two formants of a vowel which are synthesized to be on different fundamentals would be perceived as the vowel, or whether the timbre of each formant would be perceived separately. In the event the vowel *was* perceived; the evidence for the fundamental affecting phonetic categorization was weak at best, and in most cases categorization was unaffected by manipulations of the fundamental. Darwin suggested two reasons for this lack of effect. If the input consists of several voices, the acoustic features of one of which have to be grouped for perception, the perception of fundamental pitch would be a poor cue for such grouping, since the individual harmonics from several voices which would have to be resolved out (i.e. analysed and identified) would fall within the critical band. With one voice, or with widely spaced formants, they would tend to fall into separate critical bands and the fundamental might become a usable cue. The wider critical bands of hearing impaired listeners might make the grouping cues from the fundamental relatively less usable, even for a single voice. Darwin's second suggested reason was that in real, as opposed to synthetic speech, there are many occasions where noise is present, especially in the higher formants (because of 'breathy' voice, turbulence etc.), and therefore grouping could not always rely on simple fundamental frequency perception. Darwin concluded that it seems unlikely that a common fundamental exercises a strong constraint in grouping together the frequency components of normal speech. 'Whether there are other general auditory constraints that can do this, or whether all such grouping must be left to phonetic rather than auditory processes is not yet clear' (Darwin 1981).

An interesting correlate of grouping is the effect of substituting a nonspeech sound, such as cough, for a speech sound in running speech. Warren (1970) showed that when this occurred listeners heard the cough as a sound or event quite separate to the speech; they were, however, unable to localize the cough in the speech, and were unaware that any speech sound had been deleted: it was as though the speech perception system filled in the missing portion. If, however, silence was used instead of a cough, it was heard as part of the speech stream, and the missing part was not filled in. This is presumably because silent intervals are a natural part of speech, with an important function; coughs are not. Huggins (1981) points out, however, that silent intervals if used excessively can be employed to destroy the perceptual streaming of speech. Powers and Wilcox (1977) showed that speech intelligibility is improved if noise rather than silence is interspersed in the signal. Plomp (1981) has discussed the perceptual phenomenon whereby a tone burst is perceived as uninterrupted when interspersed with noise bursts, provided the tone frequency falls within the noiseband frequency. Either with single words (Miller and Licklider 1950) or within running speech, the insertion of silent intervals of given duration between speech segments of given duration can destroy intelligibility. Indeed, Huggins states that when continuous speech is broken into 30-ms samples by the insertion of 150-ms silences, it is possible to hear and track the movements of the second formant, especially during vowels. The speech is perceptually reduced to its acoustic elements. We shall see in later chapters the extent of the problems with speech perception and language development encountered by children with hearing losses. The importance of temporal processing, of efficient frequency resolution, of intact perceptual functioning in the context of formants, formant transitions, grouping, streaming, order effects, and so on is becoming apparent. Impairment of these perceptual processes is likely to account for some of the data on language disability in the hearing-impaired.

2

Development of auditory and speech perception: an overview

A parent of a newborn child will talk to the infant without stopping to consider the infant's capacity to discriminate, identify or comprehend the components of the speech message. Even without encouragement or instruction most mothers will provide a rich spoken language environment to their children, confident that comfort, at least, is conveyed by voice and that exposure to sounds is a 'natural' requirement for their baby to develop spoken language. Speech communication is for most mothers a normal and spontaneous component of the mother–infant bond. Few people would stop to question the extent to which their baby can discriminate the speech sounds used, and yet probably even the most naïve reader would think there was some association between the speech sounds the infant hears and the spoken language it goes on to develop. This interdependence of the development of hearing and language is complex and not fully understood, and in practice much of the impetus for the formal studies of the development of auditory and speech perception arises from the study of language development.

Methodological considerations

There is a large gulf between the evaluation of auditory capabilities in adults and the same evaluation in infants and young children. Infants demonstrate a variety of spontaneous behaviours which successfully compete with event-related behaviour and confuse the assessment of underlying capabilities. The deductions made from the observations must allow for the distance between the response and the auditory parameters under test.

The data from studies of auditory development, and in particular from studies of infants' perception of speech contrasts, are generally used for comparison with the auditory capabilities of adults. These comparisons provide the basis for descriptions of the development of speech perception. Thus, we are comparing data about the auditory capabilities of infants and adults when the experimental techniques and responses modes used may be very different. In obtaining psycho-acoustic measures from adults, particular attention is paid to the experimental paradigm, since the technique used may have some bearing on the results. Particular caution should be taken in comparing the data derived from the very different procedures used in infant auditory perception studies.

Eisenberg (1965) suggests that we think of the infant as a 'response organism'. Into this system we introduce an auditory signal which may inadvertently be in conjunction with nonauditory signals, dependent upon the infant's state, which she describes as intrinsic signals. The observed behaviour of the infant then comprises spontaneous nonauditory behaviour and auditory behaviour, which are differentiated by the observer. The two main areas of difficulty which Eisenberg identifies as arising from this model are, first, that a given signal may not exert constant effects within a test period and that changes in state and effects of environmental changes may occur; and secondly, that the sensitivity of the different physiological and behavioural measures varies – that is, the apparent sensitivity to a particular auditory contrast depends in part on the measure used. Observer skill and judgement introduces a further variable.

Studies of infant auditory behaviour use age appropriate physiological and behavioural measures, each of which are subject to Eisenberg's cautions on interpretation. The review of auditory development presented in this chapter is based on data derived from experiments using a range of measures which are described in the following paragraphs. The reader may find it necessary to refer back to this collective review of experimental techniques, since most of the inconsistencies in the data on auditory development can be attributed to methodological differences.

The behavioural measures used to assess auditory function in neonates and infants of less than 5 months depend upon observer recognition of a change in the resting activity of the infant. The infant's basal or pre-stimulus state is monitored by trained observers, who identify a response as a change in state following stimulus presentation. It is inferred that this change has been caused by the change in the auditory background, which may take the form of introduction of a stimulus or modification of a background stimulus.

In the early months, auditory behaviour studies primarily use stimuli of the order of 80–90 dB SPL to elicit primitive reflex responses such as a head turn, generalized body movement, eye blinks or eye movement. The basal state of the infant affects the infant's response, and there is an interaction between response type and basal state. The observer may have some difficulty in distinguishing behaviour due to the auditory stimulus from nonstimulus behaviour or from perception of nonauditory stimuli. In general, the infant is more likely to show a quietening of behaviour if it is fully awake and alert, and more likely to show an arousal, motor-reflex or eye-reflex response if it is in any other state between deep sleep and being quietly awake. Infants give more recognizable responses when they are lightly sleeping or just awake (Bench *et al.* 1976a, b and c).

There is also an interdependence between the type of stimuli used, the state of the infant and the response behaviour, including the percentage of identifiable responses which may be found (Fig. 2.1). High-frequency and brief-duration stimuli are less effective in eliciting responses in sleeping or wakeful newborn infants than lower-frequency or longer-duration stimuli. Responses to low-frequency stimuli are best elicited as the infant dozes. Stimuli of frequencies above 4000 Hz elicit a high proportion of arousal and eye-reflex responses and are more effective when the infant is fully awake. Similar reports have been made of older infants. For example, Kearsley (1973) found that infants responded differentially

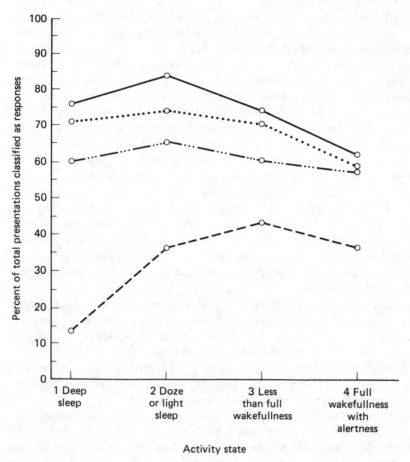

Figure 2.1   Response ratios as a function of pre-stimulus activity state. State, graded on four-point continuum, is shown on the abscissa. The functions graphed refer, in descending order, to onionskin paper (——), drum (. . . .), sticks (—···—) and whistle (----). (From Eisenberg 1976, p. 58.)

to short and long rise-time stimuli. With 70 dB SPL white noise and a rapid rise-time, the newborn closed its eyes, startled and showed an increase in heart rate. Kearsley interpreted this as defensive behaviour. If the same sound reached maximal intensity over a 2-second period, the infant typically looked around, opened its eyes, and showed a decreased heart rate. Kearsley interpreted this as the infant showing interest in the latter stimulus.

Infants of 4–6 months begin to localize towards the sound source, and this capability has been utilized in the observation of auditory behaviour. A formalized audiological test procedure for assessment of sensitivity was described by Ewing and Ewing (1944) and is described as a 'distraction test' of hearing. This is designed for infants from about 7 months of age. Convention-ally, the infant is held by a parent on his or her knee, supported as necessary by allowing free head movement of the infant. Auditory stimuli are presented at ear level, out of the child's visual field, and a response to the sound is reported when the infant turns its head towards the sound source. In clinical practice, where conventional stimuli such as hand-held warblers (i.e. warble tone generators) are presented, the tester and warbler provide the child with visual 'reward' on turning. More recently, in some clinics, the technique has been brought under greater control, giving acoustic signals which are better calibrated. The stimuli are presented through loudspeakers and the visual reward is a toy which is illuminated or animated if the child correctly turns to the stimulus. In that case, the toy acts as a reinforcer which will tend to increase response rate. The basic, less controlled version of the distraction technique if interpreted literally has been shown, with normal-hearing 6-month-old children, to have only a 35 per cent response rate with pure-tone stimuli. This rises to a response rate of 55 per cent with more 'familiar' stimuli, such as a spoon scraped against a cup, crumpling of tissue paper or low- and high-frequency rattles (Boothman and Orr 1978). Bench and Mentz (1975) presented data which indicate that it is the complexity of the stimulus — in particular, its bandwidth — which is the crucial factor, rather than its 'familiarity' or 'meaningfulness'. The response rate increases with the age of the child. Boothman and Orr (1978) also found a marked difference in response rate depending on whether a positive response was described strictly as a clear head turn or as one of a list of less definitive responses.

On the other hand, when a reinforcement paradigm is introduced to condition the infant, not only may pure tones and other stimuli be used with equal efficacy, but there is a significant increase in response rate. The method of visual reinforcement was developed by Suzuki and Ogiba (1960), who used the illumination of dolls sited beneath the sound source as their reinforcer for children aged 1–3 years. Auditory stimuli well above presumed threshold were generated from one of two loudspeakers, followed immediately by illumination of the appropriate doll. Once conditioning was effected, the visual stimulus was used only to reinforce a correct turning response. Suzuki and Ogiba found this method to be very successful in eliciting responses in this age group but had less success with younger infants. Other authors have found it, or variations of it, useful with infants down to 6 months of age. Thus, for example, a higher response rate was obtained by Moore *et al.* (1977), using an animated toy as a reinforcer, with children of even 5 months, but they were not able to increase the response rate of younger infants.

The effect of reinforcement on infants 11–12 months of age was evaluated by Trehub *et al.* (1981). They recorded a higher psychometric function in the reinforced condition than in the unreinforced condition for both low and high-frequency stimuli. The infants also turned their heads less frequently in the unreinforced condition. These data support the notion that an unreinforced localization procedure yields a relatively low response rate, rendering it a less effective technique for the assessment of auditory sensitivity (Fig. 2.2).

It should be noted in passing that although we have mentioned the use of pure

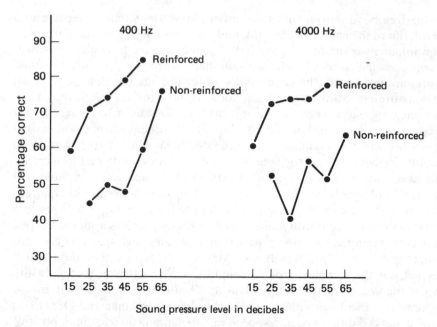

Figure 2.2 Percentage of correct head turns as a function of decibel level of two test frequencies and of reinforcement or nonreinforcement. (Reinforcement conditions included unlimited response intervals; nonreinforcement conditions included limited response intervals.) (From Trehub *et al.* 1981.)

tones in soundfield conditions, acoustic considerations make the use of such stimuli questionable. If frequency-specific stimuli are required narrow-band noise or, better, warbled tones are recommended.

Development of localization ability

In a number of the techniques described, an ability to localize sound is assumed. During checks on normal development in infancy, hearing ability is frequently assessed via attempts to elicit a localizing response. But how well can infants localize sounds, and at what age is there sufficiently high reliability to warrant the use of this procedure?

Most of the experimentation in this area is concerned with the origins of auditory–visual coordination and the conditions under which infants will flick their eyes in the direction of an off-centre sound source. The theoretical debate on the origins of a common audiovisual perceptual space has evolved between the empiricists and the naturists. The former hold that the various perceptual systems are separate at birth and that the role of experience which enables the systems to become coordinated must be established (Piaget 1952). Coincident eye movement to a sound stimulus is described as a simultaneous event of seeing with hearing — not as a seeking event. The naturists, on the other hand, hold that the coordination between the senses is present at birth (Bower 1974) and that no learning process is required for the coordination of perceptual space.

The first apparent evidence of neonatal intermodal functioning was provided by Wertheimer (1961). Following observations made at the birth of his own child, Wertheimer began a series of localization trials within the first 10 minutes of life of an infant girl. He presented clicks with a toy 'cricket' next to the right or left ear of the subject as she lay on her back. Fifty-two trials were carried out in the first few minutes after delivery, before habituation occurred. In that period, two independent observers substantially agreed that there was a significant number of eye turns in the direction of the click. This was only a single case and replications using more subjects followed from other authors. Butterworth and Castillo (1976) presented sounds to the infant whilst continuously recording eye movements by video. Infants were held in their mother's lap as test stimuli consisting of 450 Hz tones of 500 ms duration and short-duration clicks were presented at 85 dB through two loudspeakers 15 cm from each ear. Butterworth and Castillo found that newborns reliably turned their eyes away from the sound. They showed a higher rate of response to the tone stimulus, which is perhaps surprising since adults more readily localize clicks than tones because of the spectral cues in the click (Stevens and Newman 1936). McGurk et al. (1977) investigated Wertheimer's claim of early intermodal functioning. They tested infants of four days on a visual tracking task and then observed the influence of an added sound to the visual target. The auditory stimulus was, like Wertheimer's, a toy cricket, producing a complex noise in the range 250–8000 Hz, with a maximum intensity of 90 dB at 4000 Hz. The addition of the auditory stimulus did not enhance the visual tracking, and the authors did not find a convincing level of eye movements in response to the sound. McGurk et al. concluded that neonatal visual behaviour is relatively independent of auditory stimulation.

Some of these experimental discrepancies may be explained by the influence and interaction of infant state, stimulus duration and stimulus intensities on the response. In 1966, Turkewitz et al. tested 2-day-old infants in states of high and low arousal (pre- and postprandially) and with sounds of comparatively weak intensity (white noise burst of 66 dB) and a higher intensity (white noise burst of 87 dB). They demonstrated a complex interaction between the state of the infant, the direction of the eye movement and the objective intensity of the stimulus, such that it appeared that it was the effective intensity of the stimulus (i.e. with reference to the infant's state) rather than the actual intensity which is the principal determinant of directional responding. The infants in this study turned their eyes towards the sound source for the weak effective stimuli and away from the sound for the strong effective stimuli. Thus, when the state of arousal is low the effect of the stimulus is the same as when the objective stimulus is of low intensity. When the level of arousal is high, then the effect of the stimulus is the same as when the objective stimulus is high. Alegria and Noirot (1978), in a study of neonatal orientation to a male human voice, also suggest that low intensities produce an ipsilateral visual response and high intensities produce a contralateral visual response.

While these studies may provide some evidence for neonatal audiovisual coordination, they do not provide information on the infant's ability to locate sounds in space. A number of authors report reliable neonatal head turns towards the sound source; and where responses are not obtained, Muir *et al.* (1979) suggest that this is due to unsuitable positioning of the infants, to too short a stimulus duration, or to competition from a visual stimulus. Convincing evidence that newborn infants do orient to sounds was provided by Muir and Field (1979). The infants in their study were tested in an alert state and the sound stimulus was generated from one of two rattles at 20 cm from each ear, at an angle of 90 degrees from the infants midline and at 90 dB SPL. The stimulus length was variable up to 20 seconds. One of the rattles was a 'dummy' silent rattle. Both were shaken so that equal peripheral visual stimulus was given. Using this long stimulus presentation, Muir and Field found that the infants turned their heads towards the sound source significantly more than towards the silent rattle; furthermore this turn was through the full 90 degrees. The median latency of the response was 8 seconds, and some infants did not respond until the stimulus had been present for 20 seconds. This emphasizes the importance of using adequate stimulus duration in assessing this function.

Data from the literature on the use of localization as a guide to hearing integrity dates the emergence of localization responses at about 4 months (e.g. Northern and Downs 1978). There are several experimental studies on localization in infants between 1 week and 16 weeks which seem to indicate that the neonatal localization pattern is not maintained during this period, and in which attempts to elicit head turns from infants in response to sound give results at less than chance levels. However, Field *et al.* (1980) tested infants at 3 days and 1, 2 and 3 months with the procedure described above (Muir and Field 1979) and found their subjects turned their heads through an average of 67 degrees towards the sound. The number of correct responses was significantly greater than incorrect responses for all the ages excluding 2 months. At this age there was a slight increase in the latency of the response and a considerable decrement in performance.

Field *et al.* tested at more frequent age intervals than other authors and used a more sensitive test paradigm. In general there is agreement that localization responses are stronger in the neonatal period and after 3 months than in the intervening period. The most appealing explanation for this categorizes the auditory localization response in infancy with the primitive reflexes, such as the palmar and the stepping reflex. These reflexes decline and are replaced in the second or third month with more sophisticated, cortically mediated voluntary behaviour.

Muir *et al.* (1979) speculate that the early decrement in performance may mark a change from simple processes to a perceptual–cognitive process which may by 3–4 months demonstrate the ability to associate visual and auditory characteristics. Some support for this is found in the work of Kuhl and Miller (1982), who investigated the correspondence between aurally and visually perceived speech for 18- and 20-week-old infants. Each infant looked at a screen which had two filmed faces projected side by side, one face saying /i/ and the other /a/. When an audible signal was presented with one of the vowels, a significant number of the infants looked towards the appropriate face. Kuhl and Miller suggest that this interesting result may imply that infants relate specific articulatory postures to the concomitant speech sounds.

Auditory sensitivity in infancy

The procedural difficulties inherent in the assessment of auditory sensitivity in infancy by behavioural methods have been described. Behavioural assessment of neonatal auditory sensitivity has been limited to elicitation of autonomic responses to relatively intense auditory stimuli. The infant is several months old before reinforced behavioural responses to near-threshold stimuli can be obtained, and consequently before criteria of normal behaviour to suprathreshold signals are available. Measures of auditory threshold may be obtained by various physiological and more objective techniques. These techniques also reflect a developmental process, and it is important to separate the two emergent developmental processes: one, the underlying capability to detect sound stimuli (i.e. the physiological threshold) and the other, the development of the infant's behavioural response to sound.

Objective measures of auditory sensitivity may be made by recording from the scalp the infant's electrophysiological response to sound stimuli. This overcomes the difficulties of carrying out a signal-detection task with an infant where the motor functions and integrative functions are rapidly changing. Auditory electro-physiological responses from neonates and young infants have most satisfactorily been recorded from the afferent structures in the eighth nerve and brainstem in newborn infants, and it has been shown that auditory sensitivity is only slightly raised above adult values in infancy. For example, Starr et al. (1977) reported that responses could be recorded with stimuli only 25 dB above normal adult thresholds. There may be slight elevation of thresholds relative to normal adults because of possible reduced transmission through the middle ear: Robertson et al. (1968) suggest a middle-ear hearing loss of 5–10 dB, based on measurements of middle-ear function. To some extent, the waveform recorded in auditory electrophysiological assessment gives an indication of the area of the cochlea which has been stimulated by the click-sound stimulus. The data suggest that the slightly reduced sensitivity of infants' hearing may perhaps be attributed to incomplete maturation of the outermost row of hair cells and the basal portion of the cochlea. The auditory electrophysiological measures recorded from the eighth nerve and brainstem enable a study of the maturation processes of the lower central auditory pathways by observation of central transmission times. It seems that some features of central auditory processing may continue to develop through the first 18 months of life, and this may reflect the maturation of the more complex auditory processing capabilities. Thus, Hecox and Galambos (1974) noted that the latency values of waves originating from activity in the higher brainstem are increased with respect to adult values until 18 months. Central transmission times decrease rapidly in the first 6 weeks of life, but then decrease more gradually (Salamy et al. 1982).

The development of the behavioural thresholds to sound stimuli follows a different course. The behavioural thresholds are response thresholds where the relationship to the underlying absolute sensitivity is indirect, and these thresholds are better regarded as attentional thresholds. In general, infants tend to respond more readily to sounds of lower intensity with increasing maturity. Most success in the behavioural estimation of sensitivity at different frequencies has been obtained using a conditioned head-turn response. Pure-tone and noiseband stimuli have been used with equal efficacy to determine the developmental sequence of the auditory curve. The infant and adult external and middle ear show some structural differences, so it might be expected that maturational processes may result in relative changes in sensitivity at different frequencies. For example, the adult ear canal is longer and less distensible than the infant's. The dimensions of the ear canal and pinna cause specific acoustic effects; the ear canal is essentially a tube closed at one end with a broad resonance peak at 2600 Hz. The small size of the infant's ear canal tends to shift this resonance to higher frequencies, and we might expect the infant's auditory sensitivity to be reduced in the mid-frequency range in comparison to the adult.

The conditioned head-turn response was used by Trehub et al. (1980) to investigate sensitivity at various frequencies. These authors presented stimuli in a two-alternative forced-choice procedure from one of two loudspeakers at 45 degrees either side of the child. If the infant turned from the midline towards the stimulus, he or she was rewarded by the illumination of an animated toy. The signal remained on until a turning response occurred, giving the 'forced choice' aspect of the procedure. Octave bands of noise from 200 to 10000 Hz were presented. Results showed that response thresholds at 10000 Hz approached the threshold of two normal adult control subjects (+ 10–15 dB). To low frequency stimuli, the infants showed thresholds raised by 20–30 dB in comparison with adult data, and this difference decreased during the 6- to 12-month period. Clifton et al. (1981) suggested that the results reflect the development of the infant's ability to localize sound. This task load is reduced by the single-speaker design used by Moore and Wilson (1978): using a conditioned head-turn method, these authors found thresholds to approach adult values more closely in the low frequencies. Berg and Smith (1983) used a similar method but incorporated an up–down tracking procedure. They found the auditory sensitivity of infants of 10, 14 and 18 months to tone bursts of 500, 2000 and 8000 Hz to differ from adult thresholds by 5–15 dB with the greatest difference at 2000 Hz. These data satisfy the predictions based on shifting ear-canal resonances.

Since it is not clear to what extent the sensitivity of the response measure at different frequencies confounds the results, auditory electrophysiological studies become particularly important in identifying the relative degrees of sensitivity across frequencies. For example, Hecox (1975) found that low-frequency masking noise presented simultaneously with the click presentation eliminated the brainstem response. High-frequency masking presented in this way did not affect the response, suggesting that the more apical areas of the infant cochlea respond preferentially to click stimulation. This pattern of results is not found in normal hearing adults, where the response has a more basal origin. It is not a surprising result, since a more apical location for the response also explains the relatively long latency of the first wave. The data are also supported by electrophysiological studies in animals; Atkin and Moore (1975) (reported by Starr *et al*. 1977) reveal that sensitivity develops first in the lower frequencies and extends with maturation.

Frequency discrimination

In addition to describing infants' sensitivity to sounds of various frequencies, it is also of interest to examine their ability to discriminate between frequencies. Again, to some extent, the difference threshold for frequency seems to depend in part on the technique used. Leventhal and Lipsitt (1964) used stimuli that were as much as 300–400 Hz apart, but were unable to demonstrate discriminability. Olsho *et al*. (1982) used an operant head-turn design in which the infant was trained to make a head-turn whenever a repeated tone-burst changed frequency. With infants of four to eight months they obtained very variable results of 7 to 57 Hz, with the average frequency discrimination threshold being 17.6 Hz. This value is more than twice as large as the average adult threshold, which is found to be 7.4 Hz using the same technique.

Detection of signals in noise

Most of the time, an infant will be listening to signals in the presence of background noise, so the effect that background masking has on the infant's detection of a signal has been of interest. Trehub *et al*. (1980) found that the effect of masking on the infant's perception of octave-band noise centred at 4000 Hz appeared to be as for adults. They found that an increase in the level of the masking noise required equal rises in the signal intensity for detection. The only remarkable developmental changes that these authors noted was that infants of 6 months (the youngest they tested) required a signal to noise ratio seven to eight dB more favourable than the infants of 12 months and above. This raises the question of how masking noise affects signal detection in infants of less than 6 months. It also suggests that, in practical terms, infants of 6 months and less are more severely impaired by background noise than are older children. Schneider *et al*. (1979) discuss this issue further and suggest that, in a typically noisy urban environment, some signals which are readily perceptible by adults may be inaudible to young infants.

Infant speech perception

In the preceding paragraphs, some developmental trends in infants' response to sound stimuli have been described, and it appears that some auditory skills continue to develop during infancy. In the following section the infant's ability to carry out the fundamental yet complex task of processing speech sounds will be examined. The task is not simply a composite of increasingly fine auditory discriminations. The phonetic segments of speech are not invariant, and the infant perceives a waveform which does not bear a simple relation to the sounds of speech. Yet it is accepted that there is some relation between infants' perception of speech sounds and their acquisition of spoken language. Perhaps then the infant is specifically equipped to discriminate speech sounds. If this is so, then it becomes important to determine how and to what extent, if any, this process is developed and modified by auditory experience or to what extent it is innate.

It is clear that this question is of interest not just to students of infant development, but also to students of speech perception. The mature listener processes linguistically relevant acoustic contrasts to recover the relevant phonetic segments from speech. One issue that has been central to debates on speech perception is whether this retrieval takes place in a categorical manner (see Chapters 1 and 5). Similarly, a considerable body of the work on the development of auditory perception is devoted to determining whether or not infants perceive speech in a categorical manner, or in a manner approximating to this.

In the remainder of this chapter, the infant's capabilities to process speech sounds will be discussed. A fuller discussion of the data and the issues may be found in Aslin et al. (1983) and Kuhl (1986). The development of the infant's perception of voicing contrasts is discussed in some detail in order to examine the evidence for infant categorical perception and its development. The development of perception of some other speech contrasts is examined more briefly to give the reader an outline of the apparent changing ability to discriminate these various contrasts. In the discussion, studies demonstrating evidence of sensitivity to a variety of speech contrasts in infancy are presented, along with studies across different native language groups, since cross-language studies can be used to assess the role of language experience on the development of speech perception.

The experiments carried out with adults to investigate the phenomenon of categorical perception have been described in some detail in Chapter 1. The design of a satisfactory procedure to obtain behavioural measures of infant auditory threshold is not without some difficulties, and clearly, in a discrimination task the difficulties are compounded. Because of the dominant effect of methodology on the data obtained in these experiments, we will first discuss the principal methods used in studies of infant speech perception.

Methods used with infants

High amplitude sucking techniques (HAS)

The majority of demonstrations of speech-discrimination abilities in infants have been made using the high-amplitude sucking (HAS) technique (e.g. Eimas 1975a). This is an operant conditioning paradigm in which infants suck on an artificial non-nutritive (blind) pacifier, or nipple, which is attached to a pressure transducer.

A baseline period of high-amplitude sucking is determined for each infant individually. Individual baselines are essential, as each infant sucks with different degrees of strength and enthusiasm. From this point, a speech stimulus is presented every time the infant produces a high-amplitude suck, such that presentation of a stimulus is made contingent upon the infant's non-nutritive sucking behaviour.

As the infant learns that it is the high amplitude sucks which determine the stimulus event, the rate of HAS (per minute) increases above the baseline. The observed increase is then attributed to the reinforcing properties of the speech stimulus. As the same stimulus is continually presented, the rate of HAS begins to decrease. When the subject has habituated in this way to a criterion amount, a new stimulus is introduced. Typically, this occurs after 7–12 minutes of sucking. The stimulus trials are then of the form:

```
Experimental:   AAA ..............................A /BBB ..............................B
Control:        AAA ..............................A /AAA ..............................A
and             BBB ..............................B /BBB ..............................B
```

If the rate of HAS increases relative to that of the control group which continues to receive the same stimulus, then it is inferred that the infant has discriminated a stimulus change. The increase in HAS which occurs is called 'the shift', and the experimental condition is referred to as the 'shift condition'. The control condition is referred to as the 'no-shift' condition. The conventional representation of the data is shown in Fig. 2.3.

The technique appears at first sight to yield repeatable evidence for speech discrimination, which may account for its popularity. However, the technique is subject to a number of criticisms. Firstly, less than half the subjects generally complete the experiment because of distress, fatigue, rejection of the nipple or other reasons. A second concern is the occurrence of habituation as the infant's responsiveness declines. Response recovery at the introduction of a new stimulus is interpreted as discrimination of the two stimuli, and the infant is assumed to have 'remembered' something about the familiar stimulus. Adaptation and memory effects are therefore implicit in this paradigm.

Eimas (1975b) suggests that feature detectors, sensitive to acoustic and phonetic features of speech-sound contrasts, may adapt as a result of repeated stimulation. General adaptation of all receptors is discounted, since recovery would be unlikely with the introduction of the new stimulus; thus it is supposed that the new stimulus is activating a different feature detector. However, adaptation effects may differentially modify the strength of the HAS procedure depending on the phonemic contrast under investigation, giving a contribution to studies of categorical perception not present in adult studies (Miller and Morse 1979).

Memory factors may also affect measures of infant speech-perception using the HAS procedure. Research on adult vowel-perception indicates the presence of short-term memory constraints on discrimination paradigms (see Chap. 1, p. 23); Pisoni (1973) indicated that differences between categorical and continuous modes of perception of different speech stimuli are primarily due to a failure to retrieve information from short-term memory. Pisoni and other authors have proposed

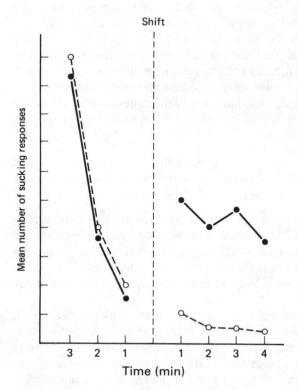

Figure 2.3 Schematic diagram of high amplitude sucking responses as a function of time, for different stimulating conditions.

that phonetic category information is retained in a phonetic short-term memory, and if the experimental paradigm is such as to force the subject to rely primarily on this, then within-category discrimination becomes more difficult. The duration of the stimuli and the intervals between the stimuli are the main factors which influence the discrimination task, and this seems to be true for infants too. Pisoni found that an increase in the delay intervals between test trials reduced discrimination both between and within categories, independent of vowel length. The same negative correlation between delay interval and discrimination was found for infants by Swoboda *et al.* (1976). Although in experiments using the HAS procedure the stimuli can be carefully controlled, the paradigm is not very similar to studies of adult speech-perception. Because of individual variation in any operant conditioning design, the interstimulus intervals will vary between and within subjects. Trehub (1979) notes a range of 500 ms to around 30 s or greater in HAS studies. The memory task at the extremes of this range is very different, and hence the degree of categorical perception described will vary.

In order to reduce the memory load, Spring and Dale (1977) modified the stimulus presentation. They compared an alternating stimulus, post-shift, with no change in the stimulus, post-shift:

Experiment AAA ....A /ABABAB ....AB
Control   AAA ....A /AAA ....AA

They then compared the results from this paradigm with those from a conventional paradigm, and found that the post-shift increase was significantly higher for the alternating paradigm. This improvement may be due to a reduction in memory load, but may alternatively be due to the use of a stimulus which the infants find more interesting, in that it changes more frequently. Kuhl and Miller (1982) note that a longer period is required for habituation to be reached using an alternating type of presentation. They suggest a relationship between habituation, memory and recognition of similarity by the infants.

Heart-rate dishabituation procedure

The other major procedure in use is the heart-rate (HR) habituation/dishabituation paradigm. A change in heart-rate level or variability occurs when a sound is presented to an infant at a comfortable listening level. In studies of infant perception, a connection between the direction of the HR response and cognitive processes was proposed by Sokolov (1963). He determined that measures of heart-rate response yield a reliable index of the orienting response (OR), and it is this unconditioned response to a sound stimulus which facilitates subsequent processing. According to Sokolov, continued presentation of the stimulus causes a 'critical model' or memory of the stimulus to develop; and when this is achieved, such that the incoming stimulus matches the critical model, the response habituates. If a new stimulus is presented it will not match the critical model and the OR is re-elicited; in other words, the response is dishabituated. The change of heart-rate is thus a physiological measure reflecting the infant's attention to a novel event. The heart-rate response correlates with behavioural responses, but precedes behavioural changes. The change in heart-rate in infants of less than 3 or 4 months of age takes the form of acceleration, while in older infants and adults, deceleration occurs.

In this technique, the heart-rate data are recorded via a three-electrode array on the infant's chest. The heart-rate is calculated from the interval between spikes (nerve discharges). As with other measures, there is some evidence that the amount of change after stimulation is related to prestimulus values (von Bergen 1983), although this may be restricted to the extremes of the stimulus intensity range and the arousal-state continuum.

The heart-rate orienting response has been used successfully in auditory discrimination paradigms using infants older than 4 months. Moffitt (1972), an early and successful investigator in this area, presented subjects of 5–6 months with synthetic speech stimuli, to which the infant habituated, followed by contrasting dishabituation stimuli. Each trial, separated by 40 seconds, consisted of 10 syllables: either /ba/ or /ga/. Eight trials were presented, comprising the habituation stimuli (six or seven depending on the experimental group to which the infant was assigned) and the dishabituation stimuli. A control group received the habituation stimuli through all eight trials. By varying the amount of stimulus change from habituation to dishabituation between groups in this way, Moffitt was able to identify that infants could discriminate between the two stimuli, /ba/ and /ga/. The rate of habituation increase varies with age up to 52 weeks (Lewis 1971). The dishabituation is affected by subject-state and stimulus factors, but it is possible to recognize the response under most conditions (Eisenberg 1976). It has proved more difficult to obtain reliable, valid heart-rate orienting in newborns and young infants (Berg 1972). Part of the problem is that state seems crucial: orienting is most likely in awake states and neonates are awake and alert for only about 10 per cent of the time. Stimulus factors also affect the probability of obtaining an orienting heart-rate response.

Kearsley (1973) demonstrated the heart-rate orienting response in young infants. He recorded it simultaneously with eye opening and closure and head movement, from infants as they received stimuli of different rise-time, frequency and intensity. Kearsley found that orienting behaviour, as recorded by eye opening and reduced head movement, was associated with cardiac deceleration, and that the classically defensive behaviour of eye closure and increased head movement was associated with cardiac acceleration. Kearsley also showed that the magnitude of the cardiac response depended on an interaction of the various dimensions of the stimulus.

Of the criticisms applied to this technique, memory factors are clearly again important. The conventional paradigm was reduced by Leavitt et al. (1976) by removal of the intertrial period, in order to reduce the processing and memory tasks for the infant; with this modification they were still able to demonstrate discrimination of place of articulation cues by infants. However, discrimination of other cues has not been shown using this method.

Both the HAS and the HR paradigms depend on a habituated response to a familiar stimulus before discrimination may be demonstrated. Unlike the HAS paradigm, a learning conditioning period is not required in the HR method, and it is suitable for a wide age range, from infants of 4 months to adult. In this way, data are more directly comparable across age groups, although the role of adaptation, attention and memory is still poorly understood. Both the techniques have a number of difficulties, and the precise extent to which these influence the results is not known.

Visually reinforced infant speech-discrimination (VRISD)

Although a number of difficulties associated with HAS and HR techniques have been presented, it is these two techniques which are most commonly used. To overcome some of the problems Eilers *et al.* (1977) successfully used a visually reinforced infant speech-discrimination (VRISD) paradigm. This is a modification of the visual reinforcement paradigm described earlier for sensitivity assessment, and provides a behavioural response in which infants gain feedback on their performance. It is a technique suitable for infants mature enough to make a controlled head-turn response (5–6 months) and may be successfully used with children up to 2 years. In this procedure the infant is seated on his parent's lap and faces an observer, who is usually not visible to the infant (by use of a one-way observation window). A loudspeaker and a reinforcer is positioned at 45 degrees to the child. A distractor uses interesting toy material to keep the child's head in the midline. A background sound is continuously presented (Eilers *et al.* used one syllable at 50 dB SPL). This is interrupted after a stabilizing period, and a second stimulus is introduced. It is this change of stimulus that is reinforced if the infant makes a well defined turn in the direction of the stimulus. If the infant does not turn, the visual reinforcer is still initiated and the child given encouragement to look, in the manner of training trials. Evidence of discrimination of two speech sounds is provided by more frequent turns on change trials compared to no change trials.

There are a number of advantages to this procedure. First, the reinforcement is not the test stimulus itself, as it is in the HAS paradigm. In HAS, a contrast which is 'uninteresting' reduces the sensitivity of the procedure. A visual reinforcer that is unchanged throughout the test procedure, coupled with different test stimuli, can be more interesting and is more constant across tests. Secondly, the task is less dependent on memory than the other tasks. Thirdly, the technique is quick and a number of different stimulus pairs may be investigated in one session. A fourth and very important point is that the identical paradigm can be presented to adults for comparison studies, and although the two populations may employ different response mechanisms, there is a more acceptable similarity than in the other techniques.

In the following sections the application of these techniques to the investigation of infant perception of speech contrasts, especially voicing, is discussed.

Voicing

It is clear that opinion is divided on the ontogenesis of speech perception. Some authors favour an innateness model of speech perception. This model predicts that the infant should be able to discriminate phonemic contrasts from any language, and that the infant is equipped with a mechanism for this from birth. As adults cannot discriminate between contrasts which are not phonemic in their own language as easily as they can distinguish phonemic contrasts in their own language, then a role for language experience as reinforcement emerges. Perception of contrasts which are not reinforced disappear, it is argued, as the infant matures in a particular language environment. The alternative model proposes that infants are able to discriminate some speech contrasts more easily than others. The underlying acoustic properties of some contrasts are more easily discriminated by the auditory system than others, and indeed it is this which may form the basis for their inclusion in the productive repertoire. The infant's language environment provides the necessary range of discriminable contrasts with which the infant gradually becomes familiar.

In order to examine these theories, contrasts across the voice-onset continuum have often been used as the test stimuli. Three categories of voicing are delineated across the world's languages: voicing lead, short voicing lag, and long voicing lag. Native speakers of English label the latter two categories 'voiced' and 'voiceless' respectively. The voicing lead/short voicing lag contrast is not phonemic in English, but it is in some of the other languages of the world, for example Spanish. These differences may be capitalized on to examine the debate surrounding an innateness theory of speech perception. The abilities of infants of several native language groups to discriminate contrasts which are phonemic either in their own or in other languages, or are not known to be phonemic in any language, may be examined. These investigations have been carried out on infants of various ages. This approach is, at first sight, appealingly simple in its logic. By collecting data on the contrasts which infants can and cannot discriminate, and examining these in relation to the contrasts which occur in their own language, it should be possible to gain insight into the developmental processes of speech perception. An examination of the available evidence does not, unfortunately, provide such clear insight.

Systematic investigation into this area began with a study by Eimas *et al.* (1971). These authors demonstrated, using the HAS paradigm, that infants of one to four months could discriminate between the synthetic bilabial stops /b/ and /p/ on the basis of voice-onset time (VOT) differences. In this experiment, three variations of the voiced stop and three variations of the voiceless counterpart, as defined by adult identification functions, were presented to the experimental group of infants. Each stimulus consisted of the first three formants, and they differed only in the onset time of the first formant relative to the second and third formant. The second and third formants were excited by a noise burst. VOT values from − 20 ms to + 80 ms in 20-ms incremental steps were used. A negative VOT indicates that the noise burst follows the onset of voicing. The adult voice/voiceless category boundary for the bilabial stop occurs at 25 ms. Eimas *et al.* divided the infants into three groups, each of whom received different paired contrasts to discriminate. Group D received stimuli from two different adult phonetic categories VOTs of + 20 and + 40 ms; Group S received stimuli from the same adult phonetic category, either − 20 and 0 ms or + 60 and + 80 ms; Group O served as a control, and received a single stimulus randomly selected from the six possible stimuli. In each case, the first of the paired stimuli acted as the reinforcer. The rate of high-amplitude sucking decreased as the reinforcing properties of the limited novel stimulus decreased. When the decrease from the minute immediately preceding the first decrement exceeded 20 per cent for two consecutive minutes, then the second stimulus was introduced. After four further minutes the experiment was ended. Results of this study are shown in Fig. 2.4.

When the mean response rate for the first two minutes before shift is subtracted from the mean response rate for the two minutes immediately after shift, Group D show a significantly greater change than Group S. That is, the infants in the group receiving stimuli from the same adult phonetic category were less sensitive to the stimulus change than the infants receiving stimuli from two different adult phonetic categories. Within the limits of the shortcomings of the HAS paradigm already discussed, the results indicate that infants of as young as one month can discriminate between synthetic speech contrasts with differing voice-onset times, when the sounds correspond to the adult between-category pairs.

On the basis of these results, Eimas and his colleagues made a number of claims which precipitated several experiments in other laboratories and fuelled the debate over the following years. Their least controversial observation was that the infant is equipped from birth with the ability to make fine acoustic discriminations. However, more controversial is the claim that infants perceived sound 'in a manner approximating categorical perception, the manner in which adults perceive the same sounds'. In the discussion of categorical perception in Chapter 1, it was

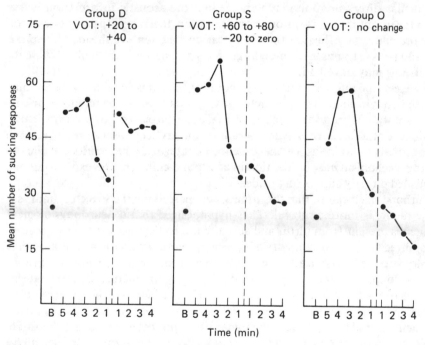

Figure 2.4 Mean number of sucking responses for 4-month-old infants, as a function of time and experimental condition. The dashed line indicates the occurrence of the stimulus shift, or in the case of the control group the time at which the shift would have occurred. The letter B stands for the baseline rate. Time is measured with reference to the moment of stimulus shift and indicates the 5 minutes prior to and the 4 minutes after shift. (From Eimas *at al.* 1971.)

suggested that a three-point criterion must be met for the phenomenon of categorical perception to be said to exist. This criterion may be summarized as a correspondence between a sharply defined identification function and the peaks and troughs of the discrimination function. However, in this experiment, only a measure of between-category versus within-category discrimination has been shown. Neither the discrimination function nor the labelling data with which that would be compared have been established. Indeed, when assessing infants and using an HAS paradigm the logistics of obtaining an identification function across the voice onset time continuum are perplexing.

In order to have an experimental paradigm that is practically viable, the assumption was made that if the phenomenon of categorical perception exists, then any VOT difference that crosses the category boundary will be discriminated. This assumption is derived from a somewhat idealized view of categorical perception, since adults rarely achieve more than 90 per cent correct near the category boundary, even for contrasts as large as 20 ms. The techniques available for the assessment of infants are less sensitive to discriminability than the techniques used with adults. It is not reasonable, therefore, to expect comparable performance from infants. Whilst a positive discrimination is a positive result, lack of evidence of a particular discrimination may indicate that the acoustic information is less salient to the infant than it is for other contrasts. Furthermore, the step size of the stimulus presentation influences the identification function and the location of the troughs and peaks. Eimas et al. used large step sizes, and it is difficult to evaluate the effects this may have had.

Nevertheless, the authors' first claim about the results is reasonable. The claim that perception is in a manner approaching categorical is also reasonable, provided the approximation is broad and the negative results interpreted with caution. Thus, while evidence of a categorical-type discrimination has been shown (Jusczyk 1980) this is not strictly the same as the phenomenon of categorical perception. While the underlying mechanism may be identical in adults and children, this experiment has not furnished directly supporting evidence.

The authors' third claim, that the infants were perceiving the speech sounds in a linguistic mode, is more doubtful. They hypothesized that a neurophysiological mechanism is present from birth, and acts as a linguistic feature detector: that is, they supported an innateness theory of speech perception with the assumption that infants do perceive categorically. The presence of linguistic preprogramming goes some way to providing an explanation for early phonemic discrimination, although it overlooks the complexity of the relation between the perception of phonemes and the acoustic signal. For example, the effects of phonetic environment, speaker effects, and the signalling of phonetic contrasts by multiple cues are sidestepped (Eilers 1977, Jusczyk 1977). In some respects, these experiments are dealing with a very artificial situation, since there is no evidence that a particular VOT represents a natural boundary. Rather than a particular acoustic parameter taking a range of values, it appears that distinctively different properties characterize minimal pairs of phonemes in particular phonetic environments (Stevens and Klatt, 1974). For example, voicing contrast may be signalled either by voice-onset differences or by the absence of the first formant transition. This does not undermine the claim that the infant has an innate ability to make fine acoustic discriminations.

In summary, then, Eimas *et al.* initiated the debate by proposing that there is some evidence for the phenomenon of categorical perception in infants, and that this is part of an innate mechanism for linguistic processing. Theoretical objections of the type outlined above were raised. The work was extended to evaluate the ability of American English-speaking infants to discriminate contrasts which were not phonemic in their own language environment (see Eimas 1975a). They again used an HAS sucking paradigm to present to two groups of 2- to 3-month-old infants VOT contrasts of +10/−70 ms and −70/−150 ms respectively. Following a pilot experiment, it was assumed that the former pair consist of a voiced/ prevoiced contrast and that the latter pair both fall in the prevoiced category. The results were rather equivocal, in that the infants did show an ability to distinguish a prevoiced–voiced contrast, but the HAS recovery did not differ significantly from the group receiving the two prevoiced sounds. It is possible that a step size of 80 ms was too large to demonstrate a difference between the groups. The data may be used to support either the innateness theory or the learning theory. On the one hand it is argued that the sensitivity of the infants to the prevoiced contrast had become attenuated during 2 or 3 months of exposure to a language where this contrast is not phonetic. The alternative explanation is that the contrasts have been differentially learnt in the first 2 or 3 months because of the prevailing language environment.

Further contributions towards an understanding of the development of speech perception are provided by Lasky *et al.* (1975) and Streeter (1976a and b). Both studies supply data which are interpreted as evidence supporting the notion of an innate mechanism for the discrimination of speech contrasts. Lasky *et al.* and Streeter carried out cross-language studies; they investigated infants' ability to discriminate between VOT contrasts either side of category boundaries known to be present or absent in their native language environment. Lasky *et al.* tested 30 Guatemalan infants aged 4–6 months. The infants were from monolingual Spanish homes. The authors used the cardiac-orienting habituation/ dihabituation paradigm to evaluate the infants' abilities to discriminate VOT contrasts. Three pairs of synthetic stop stimuli were presented to the infants: −60 vs −20 ms, −20 vs +20 ms and +20 vs +60 ms. The infants were found to be sensitive to the −60 vs −20 ms VOT contrast and to the +20 vs +60 ms VOT contrast. Both of these discriminations are within category, as judged by adult Spanish speakers, who distinguish only two categories, bounded at approximately 0 ms. Thus the infants did not discriminate the sounds spanning the adult category of their own language. Lasky *et al.* interpret this as evidence that the infant may be 'innately predisposed to perceive three categories of stops differing in VOT, having phonetic boundaries which are not coincident with adult Spanish speakers.'

Streeter (1976a) was similarly unable to demonstrate a strong effect of linguistic bias in the first two months of life. The language environment of the infants in her sample was Kikuyu, a Bantu language spoken in Kenya, which contains only one labial stop, a prevoiced /b/ in which the voice lead is on average 64 ms. Streeter used the HAS paradigm and showed these infants to be sensitive to VOT contrasts of −30 vs 0 ms and 10 vs 40 ms, but not to 50 vs 80 ms. Streeter notes that the former contrast is made by adult speakers of Kikuyu, even though it is not a phonemic contrast. The voiced/voiceless distinction is not present in Kikuyu and yet it is discriminated by the infants, which is taken as evidence of a natural inherent ability to discriminate this contrast. The evidence of these studies together show that Spanish and Kikuyu infants can apparently distinguish prevoiced–voiced contrasts, while American infants cannot, thus implicating some role for linguistic experience in this particular contrast. On the other hand, all the infants could discriminate the voiced/voiceless contrast, suggesting that ability to perceive this contrast is innate or that infants have a greater sensitivity to this contrast and hence discrimination is more easily measured.

Aslin *et al.* (1981) suggested that infants are 'extra sensitive' to the acoustic information in the positive region of the VOT continuum, and systematically investigated differential sensitivity to various contrasts. In a series of experiments on infants aged five to eleven months, employing an adaptive staircase technique and a reinforced head-turn paradigm, Aslin *et al.* set out to quantify the smallest VOT difference which the infant could discriminate. These authors prescribed a background stimulus of synthetic stops with VOTs from − 70 to + 70 ms. When the infants correctly discriminated the target stimulus from the background, the VOT was decreased and when they failed to make the discrimination the VOT was increased. The adaptive staircase procedure was used in this way to determine the smallest difference of VOT which could be discriminated. The authors found that the size of the smallest discrimination the infant could make varied according to the initial location of the VOT contrast. For example, in the 0 to + 70 ms target series, the mean VOT threshold was found to be 29.6 ms; for the − 20 to + 50 ms series the mean value was significantly less ($P<0.05$) at 12.4 ms.

Aslin *et al.* argue that infants do not simply parse the VOT contrasts into discrete perceptual categories. Of the 11 infants who successfully completed the trials, Aslin *et al.* noted that smaller steps in VOT could be identified in the series that straddled the English adult voicing boundary than in the series which did not; in addition, they noted greater sensitivity in the plus region of the VOT continuum. However, the infants did consistently discriminate contrasts which were within the adult categories. Aslin *et al.* argued that the trends in their data support the notion of an innate mechanism for discrimination of VOT contrasts, but such that natural sensitivity is greatest in the positive region of the continuum (the voiced/voiceless region). Adults tested with the same paradigm showed a heightened sensitivity in the region of the English category boundary. Infants, however, did not show this. Aslin *et al.* suggest that there is an acoustic basis for infants' increased sensitivity in the positive region of the VOT continuum, and that later heightened sensitivity at the boundary is a result of increased language experience. The theory that infants are better at discriminating contrasts which signal the voiced/voiceless distinction is said to be due to the presence of a rapid spectral transition for VOTs of less than, say, 40 ms, which acts as an additional cue.

The question of the role of experience has been examined by Eilers and colleagues (Eilers *et al*. 1977, Eilers, Gavin and Wilson 1979, Eilers *et al*. 1982). These authors evaluated the ability of 6-month-old English and Spanish infants to discriminate contrasts using a visually reinforced head-turning procedure. In the first study, they showed that while the English infants discriminated the English lag-boundary only (+40 vs +10 ms), the Spanish infants could discriminate across both the English lag-boundary and the Spanish lead-boundary (+10 vs −20 ms). In their discussion they too suggest that the prevoiced/voiced contrast is less easily perceived naturally, but can be acquired depending on the linguistic environment. These experiments indicate that infants may be innately sensitive to three modes of voicing along the VOT continuum. However, sensitivity is not equivalent along the continuum, and the category boundaries are not equivalent to the adult boundaries. In an innateness theory one might expect all contrasts to be discriminated with equal facility, and this is not the case. In the 1982 study, Eilers *et al*. examined the discriminative capacity of English and Spanish infants on English, Spanish and Czech phonetic contrasts. They reported evidence for the superiority of the Spanish children for Spanish contrasts, though not the English children for English contrasts. Most surprisingly, both groups of infants provided evidence of discrimination of the Czech contrast, despite the apparent absence of linguistic experience with the contrast. This result has prompted Jusczyk *et al*. (1984) to question the design and statistical treatment of the Eilers *et al*. 1982 study, but Eilers *et al*. (1984) have refuted these criticisms. No one denies the effect of experience on discrimination ability (since the results from cross-linguistic studies on adults – e.g. Lisker and Abramson 1970 – are clear); but how and when experience has its effects on infant speech perception remains unclear.

With regard to the data on discrimination of prevoicing, MacKain (1982) notes that prevoiced stops *are* present in American English speech. Drawing from the work of Lisker and Abramson (1964), she demonstrates that a proportion of speakers produce initial prevocalic voiced stops with some voicing lead, and that prevoicing in non-initial positions is actually very common. Zlatin and Koenigsknecht (1976) too showed that for 18 of 20 subjects, about 33 per cent of each speaker's voiced productions occurred with voicing lead. It should be stressed that the prevoicing is not phonemic; in English, it occurs in contextual or free variation and does not occur as often as in a language where it is phonemic. Thus, comparative studies involving infants who are said not to have been exposed to voiced lead stops are in fact studies of infants who have not been exposed to contrastive phonemic prevoiced stops. They have certainly been exposed to voiced lead stops. MacKain suggests that the effect of this linguistic exposure has been discussed only within the context of some very sweeping assumptions. She rightly points out that the literature equates exposure to speech–sound contrasts with experience. MacKain argues that to discuss the role of linguistic experience on a discrimination task involves a paradox, since the infants are assumed to be able to carry out higher-level speech perception tasks in order to be able to benefit from the experience. Essentially these studies are not easily interpretable in linguistic terms, even though speech-like stimuli have been used.

Simon and Fourcin (1978) investigated the effect of language environment, and examined the ability of French and English-speaking children, aged 2 to 14 years, on a labelling task. These authors covaried voice-onset time and the F1 (first formant) transition cue, and by presenting familiar paired words to their subjects they obtained labelling data and not, as in the other studies, discrimination data. In the context of the development of speech perception, it is of interest to note that labelling occurred in a categorical manner in British children by about 4 years of age. However, French children did not label in a categorical manner until age 9 years. The authors attribute the difference to differences in language environment. At about 4 years of age, English children made use of the F_1 transition. This cue is less important in French, and it seems that the availability of a second cue to the British children enables them to label speech contrasts more readily.

It was commented earlier that infants in the previous studies may have been responding to cues other than VOT. Stevens and Klatt (1974) for example, suggested that the Eimas *et al.* (1971) findings may be due to the infants' use of alternative cues. A significant F_1 transition after voicing onset creates a rapid spectral change. With long voicing times (perhaps 40 ms or more) there is a negligible transition and hence a negligible spectrum change. Stevens and Klatt proposed that infants may readily discriminate the VOT of + 20 ms from the VOT of + 40 ms on the basis of the absence versus presence of a rapid spectral change. Simon and Fourcin suggested that this interpretation is modified somewhat. Their data show that infants acquire the ability to make use of the F_1 transition at an age dependent upon language environment, and they note it is unlikely that this ability would be lost only to be relearned. Thus, they argue, the data obtained in the studies of Eimas and others reflect the infants' ability to discriminate differences in the respective spectra of the speech sounds. Limitations to low-level auditory mechanisms are then responsible for the differential sensitivity to various contrasts, and children's perception of consonant sounds are acquired as a result of exposure to a particular language environment.

Perception of voicing cues in infancy has been at the forefront of the debate on theories of speech perception. It is clear that infants do discriminate differences in voiced contrasts in early infancy, but whether this is on any greater basis than differences in the acoustic spectra is uncertain. Further insight may be obtained by examination of the other contrasts which infants can discriminate.

Perception of place cues

Place cues are predominantly distinguished by the frequency of the components of the sound. The constriction of the vocal tract at any point will be reflected in the front and back cavity resonances. In the production of vowel sounds, in general the first formant (F_1) decreases in frequency for increases in tongue height and as the pharynx increases in volume. The second formant (F_2) relates primarily to the front cavity space, and increases with decreases in the size of this cavity. Place information associated with vowel production is thus cued by the formant frequencies: F_1 indicates the tongue height or mouth opening, and F_2 represents the place of the maximum constriction of the tract caused by the tongue. The second formant transitions are important cues to perception of place of articulation of stops, fricatives and affricates; and, particularly for the brief articulations, the frequency of the noise conveys information on place.

The perception of place of articulation cues by infants has been studied both by students of infant development and by students of theories of speech perception. To those investigating the possible basis for an innate mechanism of speech perception, the area has appeal, since the cues to place of articulation have long been thought not to be constant. Liberman et al. (1952) illustrate this by the syllables /di/ and /du/, where they demonstrate that the acoustic cues to the sound identified as /d/ in both cases are quite different, depending on the vowel environment. However, more recent studies suggest that invariant cues to place of articulation exist, and this has further fuelled interest in this area.

Moffitt (1977) was one of the first experimenters in this area; he used a cardiac orienting procedure, and obtained data that suggested that infants of 20 and 24 weeks could discriminate between the syllables /ba/ and /ga/. These synthetic speech stimuli had identical first and third formants. The second formant which cued the speech sound /ga/ to adult listeners had a falling characteristic over the first 55 ms of the 250 ms stimulus; the /ba/ sound had a second formant which had a small rising characteristic over the first 55 ms.

Eimas (1974) investigated the perception of place cues in infants. He hypothesized that it is the process of feature extraction that is categorical; and that the continuous variation in the acoustics of speech sounds is divided by the auditory system and its feature extractors into discrete categories. This mechanism would then be present for different features in speech. Eimas presented synthetic speech sounds that differed in the starting frequency and direction of the second and third formant transitions, to infants of 2 and 3 months. He compared discrimination of two classes of stimuli; those where the acoustic variation signifies a change in place of articulation as measured by adult identification functions, and those where the signals are perceived as the same speech sounds by adults. That is he presented either between-category or within-category pairs. Eimas used an HAS paradigm. Three groups of infants were tested; Group D was presented with stimuli from the adult category /d/, and after habituation the stimulus changed to the /g/ category. Group S also received two stimuli, but they were acoustic variations of the same category. The infants in Group C received only one of the four stimuli. The infants in Group D, receiving the sounds from different adult categories, showed a marked difference in post-shift sucking response to Group S and the controls. In a further experiment, Eimas presented the same acoustic cues in a nonspeech context. Adults perceive these stimuli, which consisted of second-formant transitions, as bird-like chirps. Eimas obtained results from this experiment which were used to support his claim that infants have a built-in biological mechanism for the perception of speech sounds, in that the infants, like adults, responded differently to the speech and nonspeech stimuli. Whatever the implications for theories of speech perception, it does appear that by four months of age infants can discriminate rapid formant transitions.

Studies have also been carried out to study the development of perception of fricatives. Eilers and Minifie (1975) used a high-amplitude sucking paradigm and showed that infants of 4–17 weeks could discriminate /sa/ vs /va/ and /sa/ vs /ʃa/. They did not find any evidence that the infants could discriminate a /sa/ vs /za/ contrast. Eilers *et al.* used a VRISD paradigm on 6 to 14-month-old infants, and demonstrated that by 8 months infants were able to make this discrimination. Examination of their data shows that some contrasts seem to become easier with increasing age. /sa/ vs /ʃa/, /sa/ vs /va/, /as/ vs /az/, and /at/ vs /ad/ are discriminated by all including the youngest age group; /as/ vs /az/ and /sa/ vs /za/ were consistently discriminated only by the oldest age group. The authors and Eilers and Oller (1976) found that the infants could not discriminate the /f/ vs /θ/ contrast. Although attempts have been made to find an acoustic auditory basis for the apparent difficulty of discriminating this contrast, later studies using more trial presentations *have* found evidence for this discrimination (see Jusczyk 1981). This contrast is poorly labelled in adult listeners, and a greater number of observations may be necessary in order to find evidence of the discrimination.

Jusczyk *et al.* (1979) used an HAS paradigm on 2-month-old infants and presented synthetic speech stimuli from two continua: /da/ to /ba/ and /θa/ to /fa/. The two continua differed only in the presence of 130 ms of neutral frication at the beginning of each of the stimuli in the /θa/ to /fa/ continuum. Jusczyk *et al.* found that the infants discriminated between stimuli either side of a single boundary which is not dependent to manner of articulation. There is some evidence that perception of place information by adults is partly dependent on manner. Jusczyk *et al.* therefore suggested that the place boundary for stops and fricatives may initially be coincident, but that there is an effect of linguistic experience which results in a slight shifting of the boundary for fricatives.

Vowel perception

Vowel discrimination for adults is partly cued by the frequency relationship between formants. An early study by Trehub (1973) showed, using an HAS procedure, that infants of 1–4 months of age can detect certain vowel changes, when these follow a common consonant or occur alone. Interestingly, evidence could not be found of discrimination of similar tonal nonspeech contrasts. Although such studies demonstrate vowel discrimination, they do not examine whether infants discriminate vowels categorically. In the earlier discussion on categorical perception (see also Chapter 1) it was noted that, due largely to short-term memory effects, the extent to which the phenomenon could be demonstrated for vowels depended upon the discrimination paradigm. Typically, if the listener is able to make use of auditory short-term memory, then relatively good within-category (i.e. continuous) discrimination may be observed. Swoboda *et al.* (1976) investigated vowel discrimination in 8-week-old infants, using the HAS paradigm. They presented three-formant vowel stimuli in the /i/ to /ɪ/

continuum. They demonstrated that the infants discriminated the vowels more continuously than categorically. In a later study (Swoboda *et al*. 1978), the role which may have been played by short-term memory was investigated. They used brief (60-ms) versions of the 240-ms stimuli used in the earlier experiment. Extrapolating from adult work, more categorical perception would be expected and this was indeed the case. They further investigated the role of short-term memory by examining the relationship between each infant's discrimination score and the duration of the silent interval which occurred for each infant between the last preshift stimulus and the first novel stimulus. A negative correlation was found between these factors, suggesting that memory factors do affect the discrimination task.

Summary

In this chapter, the difficulties of assessing the auditory capabilities and speech-perception abilities of infants have been described, and the principal methods devised to minimize these difficulties have been presented. Using these techniques, it has been found that, while infants have near-normal auditory sensitivity at birth, their ability to make fine discriminations and to localize sounds continues to develop during the first year of life.

Some studies of the development of infant speech-perception have been described and discussed, although methodological problems abound. From the studies, it is inferred that infants are able to discriminate many speech sounds from as early as one month of age. However, it is one thing to show early auditory discrimination, quite another to demonstrate that the discriminations are being used linguistically. Children have to learn to categorize speech sounds and to cope with the variability of particular phonemes, so that different phonemes are treated as signalling different meanings. The evidence points to very early discrimination abilities in infants, but to the use of these discriminations in a linguistic mode developing somewhat later. It is clear from these studies that infants are sensitive to a wide range of speech contrasts; furthermore, cross-language studies suggest that early auditory–linguistic experience influences the infant's perceptual development. In practical terms, it is probable that the normal experience of speech sounds in infancy is of positive benefit to the child who becomes deafened even as early as the end of the first year of life. Conversely, we should be aware that early fluctuating hearing loss may disadvantage the child by causing variations in the available speech contrasts. In theoretical terms, the fact that infants may have early access to at least part of the speech code has implications for theories of speech perception and language development.

3

Development of language in the normally hearing child: an overview

In contrast to the two previous chapters, the subject-matter of this chapter – normal language development – has not only received a great deal of attention over the past two decades, but more particularly has benefited from the fact that the consequent wealth of essays, articles and research papers has been ably reviewed and summarized by several authors within the last few years (Dale 1976, de Villiers and de Villiers 1978, Cruttenden 1979, Fletcher and Garman 1979, Mogford and Bishop 1988). It is not the purpose of this chapter, therefore, to undertake a comprehensive review of normal language development. Instead, the aim is to provide a brief overview of current thinking on the subject, in order that the reader approaching Chapter 6, in which the language of the hearing-impaired child is discussed, may have some normal baselines against which to compare hearing-impaired development. We are concerned to describe, where possible, the broad chronological profiles of the various aspects of language development. The fine detail of chronological development and the 'how' of language acquisition, topics of particular interest to the linguist, will not be dealt with here.

It has been pointed out frequently that 25 years ago language development theory and research was dominated by the study of grammar. The legacy of this approach is still to be found in the study of hearing-impaired language where, as we shall see in later chapters, it is only recently and rarely that other aspects of language have been considered. The advantage of the grammar-dominated approach was that it made the reviewer's task relatively simple, but at the heavy price of an unrealistic, static and oversimple account of language development. More recently, interest has been directed not only towards grammar but towards phonology and towards the more 'psychological' fields of semantics and the contextual aspects of language development. There has been much more work than before on the very early ('prelinguistic') stages of development, and it is now not uncommon to take a starting-point of age 3 months or so. It is now possible, therefore, to give a reasonably coherent picture of language development from the first few months of life to 5 years and beyond; although it is accepted now that the process is far from complete at age 5, nevertheless this age represents a convenient point beyond which complex constructions such as subordination of clauses, the use of the passive voice and the expanding lexicon are of prime concern (but see Karmiloff-Smith 1979).

The description of language development in its various areas – grammatical,

54

phonological, semantic, contextual – would still be reasonably simple if the areas could be regarded as discrete separate aspects of development. Of course they cannot. The modern view is of a dynamic *interactive* system in which development in one area interacts in complex ways with developments in other areas. For the sake of simplicity this chapter will deal with each of the areas in turn, but their interactive relationship should not be forgotten.

The earliest stages

Obvious as it may seem, the emergence of first words at 12 months or so provides the first irrefutable proof of the influence of language perception on the child's output, for the first words are very closely related both semantically and phonetically to the adult language with which the child is surrounded. Earlier evidence of the role of perceptual processes on development is available however, despite the difficulties of designing experimental techniques to investigate it. The early development of auditory perception and attention has been discussed in Chapter 2. It is now widely accepted that the child is capable, perhaps as early as 3 months, of distinguishing speech sounds from nonspeech sounds. Recognition of particular phonetic forms may follow at 5 months or so. What the important features for these early linguistic–perceptual processes are is not clear, although it has been shown that 1- to 4-month-old infants can discriminate for example /ra/ from /la/ (Eimas 1975a). Karzon (1980) has investigated the receptive aspects of prosody in 1 to 4 month olds who have to discriminate a pair of syllables which are discriminable in isolation (e.g. /ra/ vs /la/) but not in a sequence (e.g. /ma-ra-na/ vs /ma-la-na/) unless prosodic features (stress, duration, loudness) are added to the middle syllable. Crystal (1979a) notes that prosodic contrasts can be discriminated as early as 2–3 months. Such prosodic discrimination may be of particular utility to the hearing-impaired child, as we shall see in later discussion. On the question of discriminating phonemic contrasts in general, it appears that the normally hearing child can discriminate most if not all adult contrasts by the age of 3 years.

However, it is commonly argued that in the very early days of a child's life the perception and production systems are relatively independent; the child then 'rapidly develops structural constraints which process what he perceives, and which also therefore increasingly affect the nature of his vocalizations. It is in this way that the production and perception systems start to merge and what the child utters has increasingly to be described in terms of input as well as of output' (Fletcher and Garman 1979, 4). The significance of this statement for the hearing-impaired child is clear. On the very early independence of the two systems it is interesting to note that Ewing and Ewing (1947) claimed that the severely hearing-impaired child typically develops apparently normal babble at 5 or 6 months, only to have it fade away shortly after. However, Myklebust (1954) noted that clinical experience suggested that babbling in such children tended to be absent. Smith (1982) reported on differences in the early linguistic vocalizations of severely hearing-impaired and normally hearing children of age

15 months or so; and Martin (1983) reported an analysis of babbling which indicated the emergence of different patterns between hearing-impaired and normally hearing children by at least 8 months of age. Mogford (1988) re-examines the evidence for early vocalizations in deaf children, and concludes that there are differences between them and the early vocalizations of hearing children, although the differences are affected by age and by how we define babble.

It was once thought that there was little connection between the apparently random early vocalizations and the phonetic characteristics of first words. It is now recognized, however, that there is a relationship or at least a phonetic continuity, between babbling and later speech (Oller *et al.* 1976) and between the prosodic characteristics of early vocalization and these characteristics in the spoken language of the child's environment (Crystal 1979a). Oller *et al.* (1976) define babbling as an 'utterance consisting of at least one syllable wherein a consonantal element (i.e. syllable margin) could be identified, and wherein the child was not crying, laughing, etc'. Thus babbling is syllabic in structure. The syllables tend to be repetitive, particularly of the CVCVCV type (i.e. simple strings of consonants and vowels). Plosives are much more common than fricatives, at least in initial positions, and glides are much more common than liquids (approximants). This reflects the order of emergence of these sounds in meaningful speech, and it seems therefore that the phonetic content of babbling is strongly governed by the structure of the speech-producing mechanisms; it is only later, as 'real' words emerge, that the output is constrained by the speaker's language-specific phonlogy. The early vocalizations are essentially meaningless – although adults may react to them as though they have meaning or at least attention-getting properties – and yet, as first words emerge towards the end of the first year, meaning is clearly evident. Several workers have suggested the existence of transitional forms which bridge the cognitive gap between early meaningless vocalizations (babbling) and first words. These forms have been called 'prewords' by Ferguson (1978), 'phonetically consistent forms' by Dore *et al.* (1976), and 'protowords' by Menyuk and Menn (1979). Unlike the first words, these transitional forms do not resemble any particular adult words; but they do show some phonetic consistency, they appear to have a linguistic function, and they are used by the child in certain particular situations, affective states, and so on.

The first words emerge towards the end of year one, and for the next 9 months or so (0;9–1;6) productive language tends to be word-based. Word-strings, or, in the beginning, two-word utterances do not begin to emerge until about 1;6–2;0. Thus the first stage of productive language development (so called Stage I) is lexically based and it is not until a vocabulary of 50 words or so has been acquired that two-word utterances appear, possibly because the simple lexical approach becomes impractical with a rapidly expanding vocabulary or possibly because the child now has sequences of notions to convey. First words show considerable phonetic variability both within and across speakers (Leonard *et al.* 1980) and have a wide semantic reference. Grunwell (1981) argues that the segmental phonology (i.e. the vowel, consonant, syllable system of sounds) to be found in first words contains many of the basic adult contrastive features, yet exhibits such variability that it is appropriate to regard it as the 'protosystem'. In this view, the development of a full-blown segmental phonological system begins at Crystal *et al.*'s (1976) Stage II - the emergence of two-word utterances at age 1;6–2;0 years.

Phonological development – segmental

In attempting to trace the course of phonological development, the researcher faces four fundamental problems (Ferguson 1978). First, there is great individual variation. Secondly, phonological development involves the gradual extension and regularization of the child's pronunciation; this is therefore a shifting and dynamic process, difficult to describe. Thirdly, as we have seen, the starting point of phonological development is difficult to define. And finally, phonology is applicable to both input (receptive language) and output (expressive language). For phonological *development* we tend to study output phonology, since tapping the input phonology of very young children raises formidable problems. Phonological coding (input) has been heavily researched in adults, and has assumed some importance in the study of the reading ability of older hearing-impaired children (see Chapter 8).

The traditional method of studying output phonological development has been to attempt to answer the question 'when are speech sounds learned?' by performing articulation tests (based on picture-naming tasks) on a large number of children. Menyuk and Menn (1979), Grunwell (1981) and others have argued that this is a bad question, partly because of the four problems cited above, partly because it is often not clear what is the 'correct model' against which the emerging phonology is to be compared (e.g. average adult or average mother), and partly because it does not take linguistic factors into account when assessing so-called 'errors'. Thus, for example, a sound may be in error in adult terms as a substitution, yet it could be providing for the child at that time a useful phonemic contrast. This point may be particularly important in the older but severely hearing-impaired child, who is being helped to improve his pronunciation/ articulation. For example, if such a child were to say /b/ for /p/ in *pin* this would be a substitution error. If he were also to use the bilabial voiced implosive /ɓ/ for /b/ as in *bin*, this would be regarded as a (more serious) distortion error. However, the child might be using /ɓ/ and /b/ as contrastive, and in one sense therefore has developed a phonological rule which is appropriate.

Considerations such as this have led to a more recent approach to phonological development in which the speech is described in terms of the changing relationships between the child and adult forms. The relationships are expressed not as errors, but as rules or phonological simplifying processes (Ingram 1976). They have the advantage over errors in that they can be described so as to take account of context. Ingram has argued that there is an innate tendency consistently to simplify in similar ways adult pronunciation. In this light, phonological development can be seen as a gradual modification and finally disappearance of these simplifying processes.

Grunwell (1981) has reviewed the literature and presented a profile of (segmental) phonological development taking into account the two approaches outlined above. She presents the profile in terms of chronological Stages I–VII which correspond to the Crystal *et al.* (1976) stages of grammatical development (see below). The chart, which is shown in Fig. 3.1, shows the development of the child's own phonemic contrasts, not the acquisition of correct adult pronunciation. It deals with consonants and not vowels: there have been few studies on vowel development, although it is widely accepted that by three years of age the vowel system is complete; for example, a longitudinal study by Bond *et al.* (1982) confirmed the considerable vowel overlap of early speech which is replaced by relatively distinct vowel formants by 29 months; much of this change is accounted for by anatomical maturation of the vocal tract. The left half of Fig. 3.1 shows the development of the phonemic system, and the right the relationships of the child's system to the adult's in terms of the phonological simplifying processes: these are subdivided into structural simplifications (on the left) and systemic simplifications. Processes that are almost always present at a particular stage are shown in upper-case letters, and the gradual disappearance of processes is represented by the use of lower-case letters. Optional processes are in parentheses.

Stage	Labial	Lingual	Structural	Systemic
Stage I (0;9–1;6)	Nasal Plosive Fricative Approximant		*'First Words'* tend to show: —individual variation in consonants used; —phonetic variability in pronunciations; —all simplifying processes applicable.	
Stage II (1;6–2;0)	m p b w	n t d	Reduplication Consonant harmony FINAL CONSONANT DELETION CLUSTER REDUCTION	FRONTING of velars STOPPING GLIDING /r/→[w] CONTEXT SENSITIVE VOICING
Stage III (2;0–2;6)	m p b w	n (ŋ) t d (k g) h	Final consonant deletion CLUSTER REDUCTION	(FRONTING of velars) STOPPING GLIDING /r/→[w] CONTEXT SENSITIVE VOICING
Stage IV (2;6–3;0)	m p b	n ŋ t d k g	Final Consonant Deletion CLUSTER REDUCTION	STOPPING /v ð z ʃ ʤ/ /θ/→[f] FRONTING /ʃ/→~/[s] GLIDING /r/→[w] Context Sensitive Voicing
Stage V (3;0–3;6)	f w	s (l) j h	Clusters appear: obs. + approx. used /s/ clusters may occur	STOPPING /vð/(/z/) /θ/→[f] FRONTING of /ʃ ʤ ʃ/ GLIDING /r/→[w]
Stage VI (4;0–4;6)(3;6–4;0)	m p b f v w	n ŋ t d ʃ ʤ k g s z ʃ l (r) j h	Clusters established: obs. + approx. 'immature' /s/ clusters: /s/→ Fricative obs. + approx. acceptable /s/ clusters: '[s] type' fricative	/θ/→[f] /ð/→[d] or [v] (PALATALIZATION of /ʃ ʤ/) GLIDING /r/→[w]
Stage VII (4;6 <)	m p b f v w	n ŋ t d ʃ ʤ k g θ ð s z ʃ ʒ l r j h		(/θ/→[f]) (/ð/→[d] or [v]) (/r/→[w] or [ʋ])

Figure 3.1   Profile of phonological development. (From Grunwell 1981, Table 4.)

Phonological development – nonsegmental

Segmental phonology, in which the descriptors are typically articulatory, is distinguished from nonsegmental phonology, in which the descriptors are typically auditory. Nonsegmental phonology consists of 'paralanguage' (e.g. whispered vocal effects) and prosody. The latter refers to linguistic variations in the pitch, loudness, speed and rhythm of vocalizations, and has only recently been given more than passing interest. As it turns out, prosodic features may be particularly important in the early discrimination of speech from nonspeech sounds and, as we have noted already, may be particularly useful for the hearing-impaired child attempting to acquire and interpret language input.

In broad terms one can say that prosody functions to expound the linguistic signal, and thereby to give it dimensions which will aid the listener in his interpretation. Crystal (1979a) distinguishes five such roles: *(i)* the grammatical function, to signal a contrast; *(ii)* the semantic function, in which the speaker signals which parts of the message are most important, parenthetic etc.; *(iii)* the attitudinal function, to signal anger, encouragement etc.; *(iv)* the psychological function, in which psychological processes such as later recall can be facilitated by prosodic features in the utterance; and *(v)* the social function, in which information about the speaker's sex, age, class and so on are signalled.

Although there are other prosodic features which, in the first 2 years of life, may be more important than intonation, it is the latter which has generally received most attention. Intonation is the linguistic use of voice pitch, and the interesting aspect of this is that such information will be available to the listener from the relative pitch not only of the formants (the acoustic correlates of articulatory features which seem to be used for the perception of phonemes – see Chapter 1), but from the pitch of the underlying complex signal generated by the vocal folds. Much of this information is carried by low frequencies, corresponding to the vocal-fold vibrations, and it is therefore available to those who can only hear low frequencies (i.e. some hearing-impaired listeners) for whom phonetic information, being of a higher frequency, is not available. Intonation may vary in terms of pitch direction – falling, rising, level, or some combination – and pitch range – high or low, widening or narrowing.

Intonational features combined with features of rhythm and pause are organized into 'tone-units' (Crystal) which provide the most general level of prosodic organization, and can be likened to the notion of sentences in grammatical analysis. Such tone-units are often used to separate clauses from one another.

Another important prosodic feature is the placement of maximum prominence on a given syllable or word. This is primarily a matter of pitch movement, but extra loudness can also be involved with duration and pause.

Crystal points out that the research literature is thin when it comes to prosodic acquisition, but nevertheless he is able to distinguish five stages of development. Stage I may be from birth to six months or less, and concerns the prelinguistic antecedents of prosodic features to be found in the basic cry pattern and in some other vocalizations associated with particular attitudes (e.g. pleasure). Stage II concerns the emerging perceptual system and the awareness of adult prosodic contrasts (perhaps at 3 months; Kaplan 1970, Karzon 1980). Stage III, from about 6 months, involves the gradual focusing of nonsegmental phonological features which are present in early babbling into features which are language-specific, and which resemble in certain important respects the features in the mother-tongue. When this occurs, the contextual aspects of the child's linguistic environment may take on a new significance: adults will 'perceive' the word-like quality of babbled utterances that have adult-like prosodic features, and that are phonetically relatively stable and short in length, and will respond accordingly. As Crystal points out, however, such utterances are still largely phonetically based, and the boundary between the phonetic use of pitch at 6 months and the phonological use at 1 year is quite uncharted. Stages IV and V are regarded by Crystal to be of particular importance. Towards the end of the first year phonological patterns emerge, and it is clear that learned patterns of prosody are becoming characteristic in the child's output. The primitive units (protowords etc.) have a segmental dimension, but the important point for Crystal is that they have a prosodic dimension which is actually more stable than the segmental phonology.

Several possible functions of these prosodic units have been proposed. One popular possibility is the 'social' view that these prosodic units serve to signal joint participation in an action sequence shared by parent and child as part of their general communication activity. This view ascribes much weight to an underlying drive to communicate, a biologically based, perhaps species-specific 'communicative intention'. The emergence of speech is part of a broader pattern of communication – sign of a change from nonverbal to verbal communication, rather than simply the beginning of language. The nonverbal activities that are important are eye contact, shared attention, turn-taking of one kind or another, reaching, peekaboo games, and so on. In support of this view of the function of early prosodic units, Crystal (1979a) points out that in peekaboo games, for example, the adult lexical input may be quite variable, whereas the prosodic features are stable. Crystal goes on to propose a tentative sequence of tonal development within Stage IV based upon his work and that of others. Initially only falling patterns are used. Then falling versus level tones, followed by falling versus high rising tones (age range 1;1–1;4), falling versus high falling (1;1–1;3), rising versus high rising (1;3–1;4), falling versus high rising–falling (1;4), and rising versus falling–rising (1;4–1;6). In Crystal's final Stage V, around 1;6 years, two-word utterances emerge, and the lexical items which have appeared independently as one-word utterances, marked so by pitch and pause, are brought together for semantic, grammatical and/or cognitive reasons. At first the independent prosodic characteristics of each word are maintained, but gradually the pause between them is reduced and a single prosodic contour emerges for the two associated with nonrandom tonic prominence.

Crystal concludes by pointing out how little research has been done on prosodic development beyond two years, although 'once the grammatical patterns and lexical sets develop, then tracing of prosodic patterns becomes a much more straightforward task'. He argues the importance of prosodic features in adult language (in coordination, relative clauses etc.), and suggests that the process of acquisition of such patterns continues well into puberty.

Vocabulary

The study of vocabulary has always occupied a significant corner of language research. In language acquisition, semantics (or meaning) has come recently to occupy an increasingly important theoretical and explanatory role. However, the study of meaning in children is extremely difficult (see Springer 1981 for a summary) and research therefore has had to make do with the one tangible index of semantic development – vocabulary – despite its limitations. Unfortunately, study of vocabulary items tells us little about what the child is actually doing, and therefore gives little scope for therapeutic intervention. Individual vocabulary items are not acquired once-and-for-all (Bloom 1973); furthermore, individual words at the early stages have to be looked at in the contexts of their use. Nevertheless, vocabulary and its size has an appeal as a broad measure of progress (rather like mean length of utterance in grammatical assessment), the importance of which can be easily over-emphasized by parents and others, but which does have a limited usefulness. The often-quoted 'target' of 50 items in productive vocabulary does perhaps have some significance, since it is with a lexicon of about this size, as we have suggested, that single-word utterances become impractical for the verbal communicative requirements of the child, and two-word structures begin to emerge. It is also at this point, at Stage II from 1;6–2;0 years, that there is a sudden increase in the size of the child's vocabulary for reasons which may be related to cognitive development (see below).

Studies of vocabulary in children have a long history (e.g. Doran 1907, Nice 1915, Horn 1925, Burroughs 1957, Goldin-Meadow *et al*. 1976, Benedict 1979). Goldin-Meadow *et al*. found that young children understood more words than they could produce, and that this discrepancy between comprehension and production was greater for verbs than for nouns. As production increased the discrepancy decreased, until the two vocabularies move into alignment around 2 years of age. Benedict (1979) extended this study to a longitudinal examination of the vocabulary of eight infants, starting at 0;9 and following through to 1;8. She found that comprehension development began at about 0;9, while production of words began about 1;0. The 50 word level was reached for comprehension about 5 months earlier than for production (1;1 vs 1;6), and prior to the 50 word level, rate of word acquisition for comprehension was twice that for production. Examination of the word classes of the children's lexicons showed not only that there was temporal difference between comprehension and production, as had been widely supposed, but that there was a different incidence and role of action words in the two vocabularies. This suggests that there are important differences in the two processes of comprehension and production, and that extrapolating from the latter to the former at early ages, before the two systems have grown together, may be inappropriate.

Fletcher and Garman (1979) recognize three basic stages in the encoding of meaning into early vocabulary. The earliest stage, which we have mentioned previously, is when the child has no productive vocabulary but 'will turn to gaze at a familiar object in his environment when that object is suitably named' (p.8). At the next stage, comprehension vocabulary begins to increase rapidly, though underextension of 'meaning' is often evident, and control of vocalization becomes more apparent. This stage is very plastic, naming forms are employed very widely, and the word-form the child responds to may be quite different from that which he produces. The third stage consists of 'building up an intermediate level of representation (the semantic level) between the level of the sound schema and that of the related object/event schema . . . . The progressive detachment of the "meaning" of a word from its . . . schema allows for extension of word use.'

However interesting the early vocabulary as a partial descriptor of early language performance (even if it does little to explain it), we should not lose sight of the fact that vocabulary continues to grow throughout childhood and into adulthood. At a year and a half a child may have several hundred words. At these early stages the words acquired are very much related to the 'here and now'; early vocabularies are surprisingly similar across children of different cultures. Beyond the first three years, however, forces other than parental word selection come into play, and the lexicon loses this communality and grows rapidly. It has been estimated that by the age of 12 the average child will have a receptive aural vocabulary of some 10 000 words.

Grammar

Grammar refers to all matters of structural organization exclusive of pronunciation and semantics (Crystal *et al.* 1976). It encompasses two aspects, morphology and syntax. Morphology is concerned with word-structure, in particular prefixes, compounds and word-endings. Syntax refers to the ways in which sequences of words constitute larger patterns, i.e. phrases, clauses and sentences.

The study of the acquisition of English morphology has not been extensive, partly because English does not make use of morphological items to the same extent as some other languages. Early studies examined the morphology to be found in spontaneous speech, others have used to good effect the techniques invented by Berko (1958) in which morphological items are elicited (e.g. Derwing and Baker 1979).

Syntax research, on the other hand, flourished greatly in the 1960s and early 1970s (Brown 1973). Gradually this enthusiasm has receded to leave syntax in its more appropriate place, alongside and interacting with the other aspects of language, but we have been left with a considerable body of knowledge about syntax acquisition, and with the influential view that the acquisition of syntax structures takes place in a similar manner in all children. The move away from syntax as the dominant aspect of language has been partly due to a switch of interest to the more psychological aspects, in which meaning, intention and cognition are important, and partly a reflection of problems with the notion of grammar in infants. Thus on the one hand context (both external – e.g. conversational structure – and internal – e.g. cognition) has become more important as the key to the acquisition of language, and grammar has therefore become a useful but limited descriptive tool; and on the other hand, we are more aware that the adult model of what is 'grammatical' does not necessarily apply to the child's 'language'; fitting child data to an adult grammar may not only be difficult, it may be inappropriate.

Despite these reservations, the syntax and morhphology of produced language do provide us with a useful descriptive profile which has been used in recent years with some success as a guide to remediation in certain groups (Crystal 1979b). To what extent the normal adult model is appropriate to hearing-impaired children and to what extent it provides a reasonable guide to remediation is by no means agreed, and is a question to which we shall return in Chapter 6.

There are a number of procedures in the literature which are designed to provide a quantitative description of the stage of grammatical development in a particular child. Perhaps the most comprehensive – since at this stage of our 'limited knowledge' as to precisely which structures are important or predictive the authors preferred to adopt the tactic of including almost everything – is that presented by Crystal *et al.* (1976, revised 1981). This Language Assessment Remediation and Screening Procedure (LARSP) has received widespread use in the UK. It is essentially a checklist of syntactic and morphological items arranged in what is thought to be a normal order of emergence, from Stage I to Stage VII (Fig. 3.2). The analyser works through a transcription of a spoken-language sample of the subject, usually elicited by two-way conversation, and records the occurrence of each grammatical item on the profile as it occurs. The first task, not necessarily easy, is to divide the sample into consecutive sentences, which can be as short as one word and with (theoretically) no upper limit to length. The analyser then decides if a particular sentence is unanalysable, in which case an entry is made in Section A. Responses (e.g. to questions) are categorized in Section B, the number of spontaneous utterances are noted in Section C, and some of the tester's reactions (i.e. conversational strategies) are categorized in Section D.

Given an acceptable sentence (i.e. not entered in Section A, unanalysed), the analyser decides whether it is a Minor Sentence or a Major Sentence. Examples of the former are '*Yes, Oh!*, and such sentences are noted under Minor and analysed no further. If it is a Major Sentence, the analyser decides whether it is a command (Comm.), a question (Quest.) or a Statement. The analysis of the latter (i.e. Major Sentence Statements) forms an important part of the profile. Crystal *et al.* have identified a set of syntactic stages through which normal children pass in their progress towards adult language, and these Stages are labelled I–VII in order of advancement. The arrangement of the profile is such that, as one goes down it from top to bottom, the Stages and structures become more advanced. It must be stressed, however, that Stages are not 'discrete entities, periods of ability which switch off and on, like a sequence of relays. Syntactic development is a continuous process, and our Stages are arbitrary divisions along it' (p. 61). They are, however, divisions which have theoretical validity, since each Stage corresponds to some general linguistic process which it is possible to identify in formal terms. The figures associated with each Stage, on the left-hand side of the profile, refer to the age range, in years, in which those structures associated with that Stage tend to first appear in normal children. Note that Grunwell (1981) has designed her profile of segmental phonological development (see Fig. 3.1) to correspond to the LARSP Stages. Strong caveats are of course expressed by both Crystal *et al.* and Grunwell about the specifications of the ages at which structures appear. These ranges will be

| Name | | Age | | Sample date | | Type | |

A **Unanalysed**				**Problematic**		
1 Unintelligible	2 Symbolic Noise	3 Deviant		1 Incomplete	2 Ambiguous	3 Stereotypes

B **Responses**

				Normal Response							Abnormal	
				Major								
Stimulus Type		Totals	Repetitions	Elliptical			Reduced	Full	Minor	Structural	∅	Problems
				1	2	3+						
☐	Questions											
	Others											

C **Spontaneous**

D **Reactions** | | General | Structural | ∅ | Other | Problems |

Stage I (0;9–1;6)	**Minor**	*Responses*			*Vocatives*	*Other*	*Problems*
	Major	Comm.	Quest.	*Statement*			
		'V'	'Q'	'V'	'N'	Other	Problems

Stage II (1;6–2;0)	Conn.		Clause			Phrase		Word
		VX	QX	SV	AX	DN	VV	
				SO	VO	Adj N	V part	-ing
				SC	VC	NN	Int X	
				Neg X	Other	PrN	Other	pl

Stage III (2;0–2;6)	X + S:NP	X + V:VP	X + C:NP	X + O:NP	X + A:AP			-ed
	VXY	QXY	SVC	VCA	D Adj N	Cop		-en
	let XY		SVO	VOA	Adj Adj N	Aux$_O^M$		
		VS(X)	SVA	VO$_d$O$_i$	Pr DN			3s
	do XY		Neg XY	Other	Pron$_O^P$	Other		gen

Stage IV (2;6–3;0)	XY + S:NP	XY + V:VP	XY + C:NP	XY + O:NP	XY + A:AP			n't
	+ S	QVS	SVOA	AAXY	NP Pr NP	Neg V		'cop
		QXY +	SVCA	Other	Pr D Adj N	Neg X		
	VXY +	VS(X+)	SVO$_d$O$_i$		cX	2 Aux		'aux
		tag	SVOC		XcX	Other		

Stage V (3;0–3;6)	and	Coord.	Coord.	Coord.	1	1+	Postmod. 1	1+	-est
	c	Other	Other	Subord. A	1	1+	clause		
	s			S	C	O			-er
	Other			Comparative			Postmod. 1+ phrase		-ly

| | (+) | | | | | (−) | | |

Stage VI (3;6–4;6)	NP	VP	Clause	Conn.	Clause		Phrase			Word	
					Element		NP		VP	N	V
	Initiator	Complex	Passive	and	∅	D	Pr	Pron^P	Aux^M Aux^O Cop	irreg	
	Coord.		Complement.	c	⇄ →	D∅	Pr∅		‿		
			how what	s	Concord	D ⇄	Pr ⇄		∅	reg	
	Other								Ambiguous		

Stage VII (4;6+)	*Discourse*			*Syntactic Comprehension*	
	A Connectivity	it			
	Comment Clause	there		*Style*	
	Emphatic Order	Other			

Total No. Sentences	Mean No. Sentences Per Turn	Mean Sentence Length

© D. Crystal, P. Fletcher, M. Garman, 1981 revision, University of Reading

Figure 3.2 Profile of grammatical development (from Crystal *et al.* 1976).

very variable across individuals, and a difference of 6 months between a child's emerging Stage and the suggested age range for that Stage may well be perfectly normal. Figure 3.3 shows the model of Stages, and illustrates that normal adult language contains many Stage 2 and Stage 3 structures, for example, along with Stage 4 structures.

Stage 1 Statements consist simply of one element, verb-like ('V'), or noun-like ('N'). *Daddy, Car, Shoe* might be recorded as Stage I entries. On a theoretical rather than a descriptive level, there is much interest as to whether one-element utterances are holophrases (i.e. single-element sentences, much · reduced for developmental reasons) or whether they are radically different in kind from the two- and three-word utterances which follow later (e.g. Rodgon 1979). The inverted commas around N and V in Stage I of the profile are there to acknowledge the doubt about the theoretical status of single-word sentences. From Stages II to V on the profile, Statements are analysed at three distinct levels: *(i)* clause level, concerned with the number and arrangement of subject, verb, object, complement and adverbial elements (S, V, O, C, A respectively) and their possible expansion (transitional to the following Stage) into noun phrase, verb phrase and adverbial phrase (NP, VP, AP); *(ii)* phrase level, concerned with occurrence and development of phrase structures within clause elements; and *(iii)* word level, concerned mainly with the occurrence of particular word endings. The latter therfore provides morphological data, while the rest is syntactic data. Information in the literature about the order of emergence of morphological structures is somewhat scant, and Crystal *et al.* have not attempted, therefore, to divide the word structures into

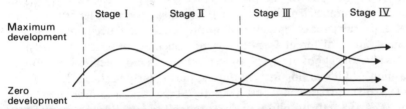

Figure 3.3 Grammatical development: the model of stages (from Crystal *et al.* 1976, 61).

Stages of development, although the order in which they appear on the profile is thought to be a reasonable approximation to the order of emergence: *–ing* ending on verbs (–ing); plurals (pl); past tense (–ed); past participle (–en); 3rd person singular (3s); genitive (gen); contracted negative (n't); contracted copula ('cop); contacted auxiliary ('aux); superlative (–est); comparative (–er); and adverbial suffix (–ly).

Stage II clauses contain two elements such as SV, SO or VC (subject-verb, subject-object, verb-complement). Stage II phrases are such constructions as Determiner-Noun, DN (e.g. *the shoe*) or Adjective-Noun, AdjN (e.g. *red car*). Stage III includes the transitional expansion stage for Stage II clause elements, in which such elements are expanded into phrases. Thus, the subject element from a

Stage II clause (SV: 'car go') might be expanded into a noun phrase ('red car go'), in which case this is noted not only at Stage II phrase level (AdjN) but at the transition to Stage III in which expansions of single-word elements into phrases are noted – in this case subject into a noun phrase: X + S: NP. In Stage III the clauses are three-element (SVO, SVA, etc.) and the phrases are similarly more developed (e.g. DAdjN: *the red car*). There is a transitional expansion area into Stage IV, in which the expansion of any of the Stage III clause elements into noun, verb, or adverbial phrases is noted. For example *the red car is going up the hill* is an SVA (subject–verb–abverbial) clause, with each element expanded into noun phrase, verb phrase, and adverbial phrase respectively. Stage IV clauses contain four elements (SVOA etc.) and the phrase-level entries are similarly developed.

Stage V sees the emergence of multiple sentences which consist of more than one clause. Such sentences can be long and complex, involving coordinated clauses (coord.) linked with a coordinator such as *and*, or subordinated clauses in which one or more of the elements of a clause is expanded itself into a full-blown clause. Any clause element (S C O A) except a verb itself can be expanded into a clause: *she woke up because she was hungry* is an SVA sentence with the A expanded into a (subordinate) clause – which can then be analysed itself onto Stages II–IV.

By the time language structure has developed through to Stage V, it is clear to the listener that the bulk of the grammatical development has taken place and that the spoken language is highly intelligible. Children are getting so much 'right' that in Stage VI it becomes more informative to note some of the syntactic errors that remain. Stage VII notes the emergence of several other advanced linguistic features such as sentence-connecting devices (*actually* etc.) and comment clauses (e.g. *you know*). Finally, at the foot of the profile there are spaces for recording, for example, the mean sentence length (in words). The mean sentence length has been found to be a useful overall measure of grammatical advancement, and was introduced in a rather different form (using morphemes rather than words) by Brown (1973). The concept of mean length of utterance in morphemes was thought to provide a simple index of linguistic maturity, particularly in the early stages of development. Brown questioned its use for later Stages and a number of studies (e.g. Chabon *et al.* 1982) throw doubt upon its reliability in children beyond Stage IV.

Garman (1979) discusses early grammatical development in some detail. He notes that 'there appears to be a trading relationship between the development of syntax and vocabulary. The first, leisurely period of vocabulary growth (Stage I) leads into the first constructions (early Stage II), and vocabulary then develops rather rapidly. By contrast, early constructions develop only slowly until near the end of Stage II when there seems to be rapid development (coinciding with the appearance of verb forms), which is maintained throughout Stage III. Vocabulary growth is again relaxed during this stage, and enters its second (and major) growth period only after the syntactic achievements of Stage III have been accomplished' (pp. 207–8). This interdependence of grammar and vocabulary is one reason why the use of grammar-structure analysis (as in LARSP) should not proceed without due attention being paid to vocabulary. To give a simple example: LARSP analysis on two children might have scored each with 6 SVO clauses; for one of them the actual verbs might be different from each other, while for the other the verbs used might consist only of *got* and *want*. Reliance solely on grammar structure can be misleading.

Contextual aspects of language development

Along with the new interest in nongrammatical aspects of language, such as phonology and semantics and their interactions, has come an interest in the contextual determinants of language acquisition. This refers both to external context – social and environmental surroundings, nonverbal communication, conversational structures, and so on – and to what might be called internal context, which concerns the psychological/cognitive development of the child and the interactive effect this has upon language.

Early contextual antecedents of language development are important, and may be the earliest point at which the hearing-impaired begin to perform differently from normally hearing children. Trevarthen (1974) showed that infants respond differentially to people versus other entities. Stern (1977) has shown that in mother–child interaction eye-contact reciprocity is established within the first few months of life. Somewhat later, the child follows the adult's line of regard (Scaife and Bruner 1975) and this leads to the use of gaze direction (Beattie 1979) and to joint shared attention of other objects. (Wales (1979) has noted that there is no evidence for such mother–child joint attention in species other than humans.) Eye contact clearly helps to bind joint enterprise, and around the time that following an adult's line of regard develops (3 months) Snow (1977) shows that mothers treat the smiles, burps and other noises made by their infants as intentional communicative acts to which they respond, thus establishing an early basis for dialogue. Turn-taking and 'peekaboo' games become important for facilitating the to-and-fro nature of the mother–child interaction (Bruner 1975, Snow 1977). Snow reports that when the child is 6 months old or so, the parent begins to build nearby objects and actions into the now established to-and-fro language 'game', relying heavily on shared attention and eye contact to associate words with things.

Wells (1979) argues for the importance of paying attention to the meaning-intentions of the child, and this is something that may be difficult and slow for the mother of the hearing-impaired child. Data indicate that this can account for individual differences in rate of language development better than can variations in grammatical feedback. As time passes and the child's language emerges into Stage I, so there is an increasing reliance upon vocalization rather than gesture, and object-naming becomes more evident. The context of development beyond this will begin to involve conversation, which will become very obvious and possibly very important during Stages II–V and beyond.

The study of this later conversation is in its infancy. McTear (1981) has pointed out that many apects of conversational interaction and how it develops are still quite unknown. He studied the use of clarification requests, the ways in which children initiate conversational exchanges, and the development of connected discourse. His subjects were two girls, aged about 4 years for one session and 6 years for a follow-up session. Children have generally acquired the ability to make and respond to clarification requests by about 3 years of age. The data on initiations (and reinitiations) indicated that these children had both communicative intent, as evidenced by various nonlinguistic attention-getting and attention-drawing devices, and communicative ability, as evidenced by the ways in which conversation is initiated by reordering, paraphrasing and restructing the linguistic structures that have gone before. Interestingly, unsatisfactory responses tended to have an effect on the forms the children used and the ways in which they used them, pushing the children towards more efficient communications: 'Thus a child can be motivated towards developing a more successful means of communication simply by being confronted, in natural situations, with less familiar persons, objects, events and circumstances' (McTear 1981, 126). Presumably there must be some balance between success and failure for each child which achieves optimum development, and of course the communicative failure met by many hearing-impaired children will clearly not help their conversational development. On the subject of connected discourse, it appears that despite theoretical positions in the past which have emphasized the private or egocentric nature of their speech, children *do* respond to each other's utterances, and discourse can be reasonably connected. Garvey and Hogan (1973) showed that their older children (4;6–5;0) were capable of sustaining connected discourse beyond a simple two-utterance exchange. The nonlinguistic antecedents of conversational discourse which we mentioned earlier are of great importance, and it may be that, as McTear suggests, a more conscious effort to respond to and elaborate a child's talk would aid those children whose conversational ability is less well developed.

On the subject of the internal context for language acquisition one can think of a number of psychological and neurological factors of importance. Greatest interest, however, has always been directed towards the relationship of language and cognition (or language and 'thought'), and it is an area, as we shall see in later chapters, in which studies of the hearing-impaired have been much quoted.

Early work on the explanation (rather than the description) of language acquisition was dominated by the behaviourist tradition of the psychology of learning, in which associations between stimuli and responses were accounted for wherever possible, not by recourse to internal processes, but in terms of the operant conditioning paradigm, in which temporal contiguity of stimulus and response, and reinforcement (by reward) of responses, were important. This approach culminated in Skinner's (1957) learning theory of language which placed language firmly within the context of animal learning in general. By the late 1950s deficiences in this view of learning were widely recognized, particularly with regard to the demonstration of examples of unique and creative performance by the subjects (whether rats in mazes or humans learning a language). In his famous critique of the learning theory approach, Chomsky (1959) emphasized the formal and universal properties of language and postulated innate species-specific bases of linguistic ability. This view was widely influential until in time it too began to fall foul of research findings.

Gradually the view emerged (e.g. Bever 1970) that linguistic abilities are not specific, independent of other aspects of cognition; instead, the child possesses powerful cognitive skills that enable nonlinguistic structuring and interpretation of experiences to take place before language develops, and when language starts to come in it is mapped onto the already developed cognitive structures. Thus semantics, or meaning, has become important, and language acquisition was seen as a process of mapping linguistic forms onto meanings already worked out on a non-linguistic basis. According to this view, which is the antithesis of Whorf's notion (1956) that language determines the nature of thought, the child develops notions of agency, permanence, causality and so on, to which linguistic forms are later matched. The impetus for this mapping process is supplied by the desire or intention to communicate meaning: 'communicative intention'. The idea is that 'the development of new or more differentiated meanings is always in advance of the child's knowledge of conventional linguistic devices for expressing them. Communicative intentions lead her to seek and master ever more elaborate linguistic devices that will allow her to express these intentions more satisfactorily' (Bowerman 1981, p. 5).

With this view of language acquisition, models of cognitive development became of much greater interest to the linguist than previously, and one of the most comprehensive account of children's cognitive development was that of Piaget (Piaget 1959, Flavell 1963). Piaget's sophisticated theory of cognitive development provided a framework for the view in which language was seen as a product of intellectual growth. The general relationship between language and cognition in Piaget's terms is illustrated by studies like that of Corrigan (1978). She studied the development of Piaget's concept of object permanence (i.e. the notion that objects still exist even when removed from view) in relation to linguistic development, and she concluded that the onset of search for displaced objects coincided with the emergence of first words, and the attaintment of the full concept of object permanence was coincident with a spurt in vocabulary growth around 1;6 years. This spurt is thus seen as a result of an intellectual transition to mental representations. Other cognitive theories of language development (Bruner 1975, Vygotsky 1978) have emphasized the crucial role of early social interactions, especially those between mother and child. Mutual gaze, turntaking and shared reference are examples of such early interactions upon which communicative development is based.

There are however a series of problems with this cognitive view of language development (e.g. Donaldson 1978). For one thing, Piaget's theory suggests that little sophisticated cognitive development takes place in the early months of life – yet there is little doubt that some pretty complex language processes are beginning to emerge. Furthermore, Bowerman (1981) points out that cross-language and cross-cultural differences in the selection of meanings and in the make-up of the categories to which forms are attached raises serious problems for the straight cognitive theories. Bowerman argues that in the old view meaning is sacrificed to form: the child is granted meaning via nonlinguistic cognitive processes. She suggests an interactive model, in which meaning is 'promoted out of cognition into the domain of language, what is to be learned' (p. 11). New forms can still be mapped onto meaning derived from cognition; but meaning can also develop through attention to linguistic forms, presumably using cognitions (discriminating, categorizing etc.) as a vehicle. This interactionist view of cognition and language is now popular. Language skills are not isolated from the rest of cognitive development; level of intelligence is not independent of language level (Wells 1979); what children are doing is attending to both linguistic form and perceptible properties of the situation in order to understand the meaning. We shall return to this topic again, when we consider language development and cognition in hearing-impaired children.

4

Hearing disorders in children: an overview

Structure

Although most of this book is concerned with function, auditory or linguistic, it is necessary for the reader to be at least superficially cognisant of the anatomical structures which mediate these functions. Figure 4.1 shows a diagram of the ear, which for descriptive purposes is generally divided into three parts – the outer ear, the middle ear and the inner ear. The outer ear consists of the pinna (or auricle) and the external auditory canal. These structures are relatively unimportant in humans, but they do nevertheless have certain minor perceptual effects (e.g. in the localization of sound sources and the enhancement of certain frequencies) which were mentioned in Chapter 1. The middle-ear cavity, which forms part of the middle ear cleft, is separated from the outer ear by the tympanic membrane, while the medial wall of the cavity is the bony wall of the inner ear. The cavity contains the three ossicles known as the malleus, incus and stapes. These transmit sound vibrations from the tympanic membrane, to which the handle of the malleus is attached, to the oval window of the inner ear, to which is attached the footplate of the stapes. The tympanic membrane, ossicular chain and oval window structures act partly as an amplifier for incoming vibrations and partly as an impedance-matching device between the air in the external ear canal and the fluids in the inner ear. The middle-ear cavity is joined to the nasopharynx by means of the eustachian tube. This tube is about three or four centimetres long in the adult, but in children is shorter, wider and more horizontal than in adults. The eustachian tube is the chief route by which infections enter the middle-ear cavity, and its size and shape in children give rise to the increased incidence of middle-ear infections in infants and young children.

The inner ear consists of the cochlea, concerned with hearing, and the utricle and three semicircular canals, which are concerned with balance. All these structures consist of a complex arrangement of membranous fluid-filled cavities, contained within bony cavities situated in the petrous part of the temporal bone. The cochlea resembles a snailshell of two and a half turns (in humans). The soft membranous inner tube of the cochlea is known as the scala media (or cochlear partition) and contains endolymph fluid. Separating the scala media from the outer bony tissue is the scala vestibuli, at one end of which is the footplate of the stapes, and the scala tympani, which ends in the round window in the medial wall of the middle-ear cavity. The scala vestibuli and the scala tympani contain perilymph fluid

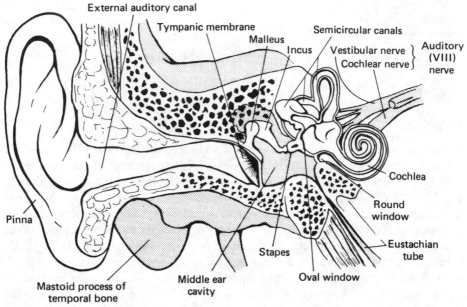

Figure 4.1   The structure of the ear. (From Crystal, D., *Introduction to Language Pathology*, London: Edward Arnold, 1980.)

(identical with cerebrospinal fluid), and are joined at the apex of the cochlea through a small opening called the helicotrema.

The soft membranous scala media is triangular in cross-section, and contains the sensory end-organ of hearing. Its base is formed by the basilar membrane, the outer wall by the stria vascularis consisting of a network of fine blood vessels, and the upper wall by Reissner's membrane. The organ of Corti runs along the whole length of the basilar membrane, from basal turn to apex, and includes a single row of inner hair-cells and three rows of outer hair-cells. The basilar membrane is covered by a gelatinous flap, known as the tectorial membrane, into which the hairs of the underlying hair-cells are embedded to a greater or lesser extent.

When a sound vibrates the tympanic membrane, the vibrations are transmitted to the oval window via the middle-ear ossicles. The vibrations then cause movement of the cochlear fluids and the cochlear partition, displacing fluid to the round window. The movements cause a wave of displacement to travel along the basilar membrane, from base to apex. When the basilar membrane moves up and down, relative movements will occur between the organ of Corti and the tectorial membrane, causing the hairs of the hair-cells to bend in various complex ways and action potentials to be generated. The cochlea is innervated by about 30000 sensory neurones in humans, which transmit the auditory information from the cochlea to the central nervous system. The nerve fibres are bipolar, and run from the hair-cells in the cochlea to the cells of the cochlear nucleus in the brainstem. The great majority of auditory fibres connect with the inner hair-cells, while a few fibres pass to the outer hair-cells after running basally for about 0.6 mm. The afferent nerve fibres together form the auditory or eighth cranial nerve, which passes through the internal auditory meatus on its way to the brainstem. The central auditory pathways, from the brainstem to the auditory cortex, are extremely complex and only partly understood. Pickles (1982) discusses our current state of knowledge in some detail, but Fig. 4.2 shows in diagrammatic form the most important interconnections and nuclei.

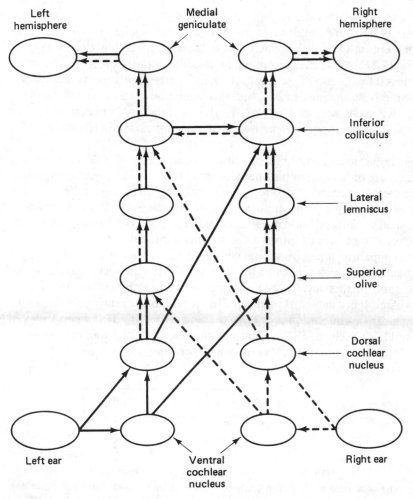

Figure 4.2 The most important of the interconnections and nuclei from ear to auditory cortex. The nuclei illustrated are located in the brainstem. (From Moore 1989, Fig.1.20.)

Types of hearing disorder

When discussing typology and prevalence rates, it is important to be quite clear about the relationships between terms such as pathology, impairment, disability and handicap. Haggard *et al.* (1981) have illustrated these relationships within the pattern recommended by the World Health Organization, and this is shown in Fig. 4.3. It is appropriate to consider pure-tone threshold measurements as a measure of impairment, but since the anatomical bases of pure-tone hearing impairment are several, it cannot be taken as a reliable indicator of pathology. Similarly, since the detection of pure tones is not in itself a particularly life-relevant task, pure-tone audiometry is not generally considered to provide a very valid measure of disability. 'A disability is present when the whole person, including the automatic compensation within his body and his behaviour, cannot perform the various general and basic functions that underlie the broad range of particular behaviours required by the physical and social environment; the auditory perception of speech is such a basic psychological function' (Haggard *et al.* 1981, p. 242). The measurement of disability, therefore, may be more validly achieved by the use of speech itself than by attempting to predict speech-hearing from pure-tone audiometry, the most common measure of impairment. Indeed, as we shall see in Chapter 5, the correlation between pure-tone thresholds and some important measures of speech-hearing is not particularly high.

Of course, impairment in the ability to detect pure-tone thresholds is not the only plausible measure of hearing impairment, despite its very widespread clinical use. Impairments of frequency resolution, temporal resolution and other psycho-acoustic functions may also be important in determining disability. In the next chapter we shall see how possible it is to predict the disability of hearing for speech when these other measures of impairment are taken into account.

Finally, an impairment (e.g. in speech perception) may lead to a greater or lesser degree of handicap, which relates to the individual within a social environment. Depending upon factors such as age, occupation and family circumstances, the disability will result in a degree of handicap. In the domain of hearing this is usually assessed by means of questionnaires (e.g. the Social Hearing Handicap Index of Ewertsen and Birk Nielson, 1973). Hearing handicap is not the subject matter of this book, which is primarily concerned with hearing impairment and speech perception–language disability.

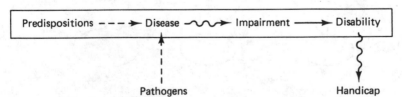

Figure 4.3   The relationships between pathology, impairment, disability and handicap. Wavy lines convey a variable link and the box conveys the boundary of the individual. (From Haggard, Gatehouse and Davis 1981, Fig. 1.)

Since there are many gaps in our knowledge of the physiological changes underlying hearing impairment, and since in any case such fine distinctions may be as yet of little clinical value, it is customary to distinguish only three or four broad types of hearing disorder. Thus, *conductive* hearing impairment is applied to a hearing loss due to conditions affecting the external or middle ears; *sensorineural* hearing impairment is applied to a hearing loss due to conditions affecting the cochlea and the eighth nerve as far as the brainstem (sensorineural impairment can be subdivided into sensory problems, affecting the cochlea, and neural problems, affecting the eighth nerve); and *mixed* hearing impairment, in which both conductive and sensorineural types are involved.

This is the extent of the usual typology, but to it we would add *central auditory dysfunction*. To many clinicians this is a much less familiar (though not necessarily rare in its occurrence) type of hearing disorder. Sensitivity thresholds as reflected by the pure-tone audiogram may be within normal limits, but nevertheless certain higher complex perceptual and interactive processes are disrupted, causing problems with speech-hearing under unfavourable listening conditions (e.g. in excessive background noise). The impairment/disability distinction is somewhat blurred for this type, since assessment of the disorder is often made entirely with the use of speech materials in various difficult acoustic situations – hence the term 'central auditory *dysfunction*' rather than 'central auditory impairment'. Development of our knowledge of this type of disorder may allow us in time to identify certain component perceptual processes which might underlie the linguistic disability – poor localization or poor binaural release from masking, for example – in which case the impairment/disability distinction may become more usable for this type of hearing disorder. Theoretically there is no reason why central dysfunction should not occur in conjunction with the other categories of hearing impairment – indeed, it is even possible that the other, peripheral, types of impairment could lead to a degree of central dysfunction. Central auditory dysfunction is somewhat controversial in its prevalence, cause, measurement and treatment, and further discussion of it will be deferred until Chapter 5 and, particularly, Chapter 10, where it is dealt with as a separate topic.

Causes of hearing impairment in children

Conductive impairment

Conductive impairments are caused by factors, congenital or acquired, which obstruct the progress of acoustic energy through the outer and middle ears. The external ear canal may be blocked by wax or by foreign bodies; or it may be occluded by bony out-growths from the canal wall. In all cases the occlusion has to be complete to cause a significant degree of hearing loss. In addition, atresia (closure) of the canal can occur because of congenital malformation. The tympanic membrane may be sclerotic, scarred or even perforated, either by trauma or as part of the sequelae to disease, and this may cause some degree of hearing loss.

Hearing impairments caused by conditions of the middle ear may be due to trauma causing ossicular fracture or discontinuity, or to acute or chronic inflammations of the middle-ear cleft. The latter are of particular importance in children because of their relative prevalence. The most frequent cause of acute inflammation in the middle-ear cleft is the common cold, but any infection of the upper respiratory tract can spread to the middle ear. When the inflammation spreads to the eustachian tube the middle ear cavity ceases to be aerated adequately. Negative middle-ear pressure may ensue, with retracted tympanic membrane, followed by swelling of the mucous linings and exudation of fluid. The fluid may be clear at first (acute serous otitis media) and may gradually fill the middle-ear space. If the condition continues, the clear fluid changes to pus (acute suppurative otitis media) and the tympanic membrane may perforate, releasing the pus. Chronic otitis media is a recurrent form of this disease. The tissues of the middle ear intermittently undergo destruction, healing and scarring following recurrent infections. The fluid to be found in the middle ear is frequently purulent; often, perhaps due to the incorrect use of antibiotics, it reverts to a thick non-infected mucoid state which is an ideal culture for future infection. This thick mucus is known as glue, and 'glue ear' can result in quite marked degrees of conductive hearing loss. Various complications (ossicular fixation, monomeric tympanic membrane, polyps and so on) may be associated with chronic suppurative otitis media.

Thus, conductive hearing loss results from a reduction in the efficiency of the transmission characteristics of the middle ear, and in children this is most commonly caused by an increase in the stiffness of the middle-ear system as a result of effusion behind the eardrum. It is this increased stiffness which impedes the transmission of sound energy to the inner ear and results in a hearing loss. The suspected presence of middle-ear effusion is the most common reason for referral to an ENT department, but it often escapes detection, as the hearing loss is usually mild and transitory.

In general, otitis media may be described as an accumulation of fluid in the middle ear as a result of a failure of the ventilating function of the eustachian tube. Attacks of otitis media may occur frequently. The simple schematic shown in Fig. 4.4 indicates the predominant forms of otitis media. The difference between the chronic and acute forms is generally taken to relate to the time course of the condition, the acute stage sometimes developing into the chronic condition, which may then persist. It is not the presence or absence of bacteria which distinguishes between the acute and chronic forms. Because of the possible effects of repeated episodes, several investigators have attempted to establish the epidemiological features of the condition and to look for improved methods for its detection. However, considerable confusion arises from the literature on these studies, because of the lack of agreement on the definitions of otitis media, on the distinctions between the various pathologies, and on criteria used for diagnosis of a particular form of the middle-ear disease. As a result, it is often not possible to make direct comparison between many studies which purport to

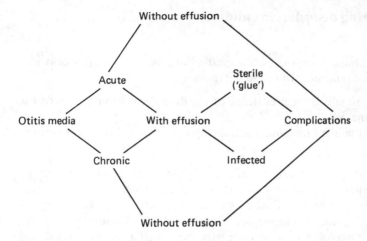

Figure 4.4 The predominant forms of otitis media.

be studying the same condition. A detailed consideration of the consequences of a lack of a consensus of a working definition, and some proposals towards formulation of a solution, have been provided by Bluestone and Cantekin (1980).

In many cases of otitis media in childhood, the condition clears spontaneously over a period of 1–3 months, and does not recur, but in a number of cases variously estimated at between 20 and 40 per cent of all cases, the condition is persistent. Treatment of otitis media depends not only upon its particular form (i.e. pathological considerations), but also upon its severity and persistence (i.e. the disability associated with it). Treatment may involve the use of antibiotics (to clear infection), decongestants (less popular now than previously), surgery (removal of fluid and insertion of a ventilating tube or grommet), and/or the use of hearing aids.

Sensorineural impairments

Sensorineural hearing loss, which involves damage to the fine structures in the inner ear and/or eighth nerve, is not amenable to surgical treatment. It may be genetic in origin, or caused by prenatal, perinatal or postnatal complications. Prenatal problems include rubella infection, cytomegalovirus, herpes infection, maternal ototoxicity; perinatal problems include prematurity and/or low birth weight, anoxia and respiratory complications, toxaemia of pregnancy; and postnatal problems include measles, meningitis, mumps, severe jaundice and ototoxic drugs. Because of the relatively restricted range of options for treatments there is less interest in various types of sensorineural disorders than there is with conductive disorders.

Prevalence of hearing disorders in children

Otitis media

The epidemiological characteristics of otitis media have been the subject of many investigations. Studies fall into two broad categories:

(i) cross-sectional, in which the prevalence of the disorder is estimated across a sample at any one time, and

(ii) longitudinal, in which one population group is monitored over a period of time.

Within these categories, the population under study varies from random samples to high-risk groups, such as symptomatic children attending a general practitioner or hospital clinic. For example, estimates based on a cross-sectional survey to detect all children with a middle-ear pressure of worse than $-150\,mmH_2O$ would suggest a much lower prevalence for otitis media than such a survey carried out among children attending a general practice. The former group would contain many asymptomatic children. The latter group would contain only those children with symptoms and whose parents have sought medical intervention. Another parameter which is not consistent across studies is the description and definition of the disease. There is confusion in reporting serous and purulent infections, and in the identification criteria.

In general, the available data indicate that otitis media is a very common disorder, with the risk being highest in the preschool and early school years. American (Eagles 1972) and British (MRC 1957) studies of school-age children found evidence of either active or recent middle-ear disease in 20 per cent of children, with the highest attack rate occurring in the first school year, and rarely occurring in children over 10 years.

Lowe et al. (1963) and Kersley and Wickham (1966) also find the average age for the highest prevalence of otitis media to be 5–6 years. The estimate from Sade (1979), which is based on children attending an ENT clinic, is higher at 7–9 years. The children reported all have middle-ear disease such that they need to seek help; and the higher age of the children in Sade's study may reflect a longer time course leading to referral to the ENT department, the majority of children being treated by their general practitioner. Studies of this same type carried out on preschool children suggest that the condition is also very common in children of less than 2 years, and probably most frequently occurs from the ages of 6 to 12 months (Lowe et al. 1963, Task Force 1978). Estimates of a prevalence rate of up to 60 per cent in the first year have been made (Klein 1978). Other studies support this figure, suggesting that improvement occurs in the third or fourth year (Renvall et al. 1975, Tos and Poulsen 1976, Fiellau-Nikolaysen 1981). Thus episodes of otitis media often occur early in infancy, and it is thought that the occurrence of more than one bout of otitis media within the first year may indicate later development of the chronic condition (Howie et al. 1979): the children who had persistently recurring attacks of otitis media during childhood had their first two attacks before 12 months of age.

When cross-sectional studies are carried out using impedance measurements, it appears that a true picture of the population is seen to be dominated by subclinical cases. A study by Fiellau-Nikolaysen (1981) revealed a prevalence rate of 37 per cent of suspected middle-ear problems in 3 year olds, and that 35–95 per cent of children suffer an attack of SOM at some time in the first 10 years. He suggests that up to 75 per cent of these cases recuperate leaving no sequelae. These results lead to concern about the possible effects of previous underestimates. It has been suggested that the prevalence of otitis media in childhood is related to socioeconomic factors; in addition studies have reported high incidence of SOM in Eskimo and American Indian groups. However, the socioeconomic and racial factors are difficult to isolate. The striking contrasts in poulation are paralleled by high-risk environmental conditions and difficulties in access to medical care. These particular groups correspond to areas of poverty in Alaska and Appalachia. It is not possible to relate prevalence of SOM to socioeconomic factors on the evidence available.

It appears therefore that most children suffer an attack of otitis media at least once before the age of 10. In the majority of cases this resolves, but in 20–40 per cent of children the condition recurs, and in these cases the first attack is frequently within the first year.

Some groups of children are more susceptible to middle-ear effusions than others. Two such groups are those with Down's syndrome and those with overt or submucous cleft palate. Children with Down's syndrome very often exhibit small pinnae and narrow external ear canals; the latter can make otological observation of the tympanic membrane and treatment by surgery very difficult, as well as making the external ear prone to wax blockage. As well as a strong tendency to repeated bouts of otitis media (e.g. Brooks *et al.* 1972), anomalies of middle-ear ossicles occur and sensorineural hearing loss is not uncommon. The prevalence of recurrent otitis media in children with overt cleft palate has been reported to be from 50 to 90 per cent, with hearing loss occurring in perhaps 90 per cent of this affected population (Northern and Downs 1978); submucous cleft-palate children also show a high prevalence, with one study (Bergstrom and Hemenway 1971, reported in Northern and Downs 1978) finding a 39 per cent rate of chronic middle-ear disease. The source of the problem for cleft-palate children is probably the deficiency in palate musculature, which causes poor eustachian tube function. This often results in poor aeration of the middle-ear cavity, tympanic membrane retraction, effusion of fluid, and hearing loss.

Sensorineural impairments: prevalence and aetiology

The prevalence of sensorineural hearing loss in children is, thankfully, considerably less than for conductive hearing loss. While most middle-ear disorders will respond to medicine or surgery, or will recover spontaneously, treatment for childhood sensorineural hearing loss is more problematic. The cornerstone of treatment has to be the early provision of appropriate hearing aids, backed up by assessment and facilitation of early communication, family support, auditory training and so on. Upfold and Isepy (1982) reported a retrospective study of Australian children born between 1949 and 1980 and fitted with hearing aids. This revealed a ratio of 2.6 cases for every 1000 live births. Mild to moderate hearing losses (averaged thresholds at 0.5, 1 and 2 kHz: the three frequency pure tone average) were present in 58.8 per cent of the children (1.5 per 1000), severe losses in 23.7 per cent (0.6 per 1000), and profound losses in 17.5 per cent (0.5 per 1000). Upfold and Isepy were interested particularly in the prevalence of reported maternal rubella during the pregnancy of the hearing-impaired child, and it appeared that a history of rubella was reported in 11 per cent of the cases. These cases tended to be prior to 1976, rather than more recent, and there was little doubt that they were associated with the more severe and profound degrees of hearing loss.

A smaller but nonetheless thorough study by Parving (1983) evaluated 117 children (median age 8 years) with known permanent hearing loss (three frequency average of 35 dB HL or more) for prevalence rates and aetiology. Children with acute or chronic otitis media were excluded from the study. Parving found a prevalence rate of 1.4 per 1000; in 91 per cent the impairment was sensorineural, in 4 per cent conductive and in 5 per cent mixed. Congenital or 'early acquired' hearing loss was thought to have occurred in 85 per cent of the cases, and in 63 per cent the impairment had been confirmed by the age of 3 years. The ratio of moderate to severe or profound hearing loss was approximately 2:1. Progression of the severity of the hearing impairment was noted in only 4 per cent of cases, and in 16 per cent additional handicaps were noted.

Aetiology of the hearing loss was unknown in 27 per cent of cases. A further 27 per cent suffered from hereditary hearing loss (without associated abnormalities), largely dominant with high penetrance, 16 per cent from hearing loss caused by maternal rubella infection, and 14 per cent from neonatal causes. Finally, 16 per cent were ascribed to different factors or inherited syndromes known to be associated with hearing impairment (e.g. meningitis, $n = 3$; ototoxic drugs, $n = 2$; Waardenburg's syndrome, $n = 2$). The relatively high proportion of unknown aetiologies has been confirmed by other studies (e.g. Taylor 1980). A survey of children with permanent hearing loss in the European Community indicated that cause was unknown in 42 per cent of cases (Martin 1982). This study concerned itself specifically with 8-year-old children with hearing losses of 50 dB or more in the better ear. The survey found an overall prevalence rate of nearly 1 per 1000, with only 6.8 per cent of the cases being conductive impairments. Of the congenital cases, rubella was the most common cause (17 per cent of total sample), followed by genetic factors (10 per cent); the most frequent cause of acquired hearing impairment was meningitis, accounting for 6 per cent of the total. The common finding of high prevalence rate for impairment caused by maternal rubella underlines the gains to be made by preventative immunization.

Data from Bergstrom (1974, reported by Northern and Downs 1978) show unknown cause in some 28 per cent of 423 prelingually impaired patients. Of this sample, 40 per cent were judged to have impairment due to hereditary factors, including syndromes and other abnormalities. Interestingly, in this study the ratio of dominant to recessive was roughly equal. The remaining 32 per cent of nongenetic causes were made up of 15 per cent prenatal factors (almost entirely maternal rubella), 7 per cent perinatal factors, and 1 per cent postnatal factors; 9 per cent were listed as 'deafness with associated defects of uncertain aetiology'. A study by Newton (1985) examined a sample of 111 children with bilateral sensorineural hearing loss. The aetiology of the hearing losses fell into six main categories: congenital rubella ($n = 12$), congenital cytomegalovirus ($n = 3$), perinatal causes ($n = 15$), postnatal causes ($n = 5$), genetic (mendelian $n = 28$, chromosomal $n = 5$) and unknown ($n = 40$, plus $n = 3$ congenital defect). The overall prevalence rate was estimated at 1 per 1000 live births. However, it is likely that figures such as these are subject to relatively rapid change as new practices in neonatal care, immunization and so on are effected.

Data on prevalence rates and aetiologies from different developed countries have therefore been broadly in agreement. For some years the 'accepted' approximate figure for severe congenital sensorineural impairment was in the order of 1 per 1000, rising perhaps towards 2 or 3 per 1000 if milder impairments are included, and perhaps 4 per 1000 if postnatal childhood hearing impairment is included. As rubella immunization programmes improve, and as more births take place in well-serviced facilities, one might expect a fall-off in the number of congenital hearing impairments of nongenetic origin. However, this may well be offset by an increase due to changes in neonatal paediatrics, and the ability of paediatricians to save very low-birth-weight premature babies. There is some evidence for this shift; McCormick et al. (1984), for example, report prevalence rates of 0.7 per 1000 for normal births and 7 per 1000 for babies admitted to a neonatal intensive care unit. Davis (1990) presents data which indicate an overall prevalence of between 0.75 and 1.5 per 1000 for moderate and greater congenital loss; but an increased risk for ICU neonates of about 12.2:1 for such impairments. These relative prevalence rates have prompted renewed interest in the use of high-risk registers for automated neonatal screening (Shepard 1983) and in the automated screening of all ICU neonates (Galambos et al. 1982, Sancho et al. 1988, Stevens et al. 1989).

5

Auditory perception in sensorineural hearing loss

The motor theory of speech perception has been highly influential in determining the direction of speech research. The motor theory points out that the decisive factor in the evolution of human speech was not the development of the ear but the development of the vocal organs and the speech area of the motor cortex. Many years ago Paget (quoted by Richardson, 1981) stated that 'in recognizing speech sounds the human ear is . . . listening . . . to indications, due to resonance, of the positions and gestures of the organs of articulation.' Speech is said to be perceived by reference to articulation, in that articulatory movements (or their sensory or neural representations) mediate between acoustic stimulus and speech percept. Studdert-Kennedy (1976) has summarized this view of the special nature of speech perception:

> The sounds of speech constitute a distinctive class, drawn from the set of sounds that can be produced by the human vocal mechanism. Speech does not lie at one end of an auditory (psychological) continuum which we can approach by closer and closer acoustic (physical) approximation. The sounds of speech are distinctive. A signal is heard as either speech or nonspeech, and once heard as speech, elicits characteristic perceptual functions.

The phenomenon of categorical perception of certain speech sounds (see Chap. 1) has been quoted in support of the motor theory of speech perception, since articulation is itself categorical: 'With /b,d,g/ we can vary the acoustic cue along a continuum, which corresponds . . . to closing the vocal tract at various points along its length. But in actual speech the closing is accomplished by . . . categorically different gestures: by the lips for /b/, the tip of the tongue for /d/, and the back of the tongue for /g/' (Liberman et al. 1967). As we saw in Chapter 1, there are reasons to doubt that the motor theory provides the appropriate explanation for categorical perception of certain speech sounds. For one thing, certain nonspeech sounds have been shown to exhibit categorical perception; for another, alternative explanations, in terms of the length of time an input is available in precategorical acoustic storage, may account for categorical perception.

Nevertheless, the view that the processing of speech sounds is essentially a linguistic skill, distinct from more general auditory and nonlinguistic skills, has been a powerful one, and because of the influence of the motor theory of speech perception there has been a tendency to look at speech and language in terms of phonetic, grammatical and semantic variables, with little regard to the acoustic aspects. 'Insufficient attention has been paid to . . . the mechanisms of coding and analysis of the speech signal' (Evans *et al*. 1977, 368). It may indeed be true that listeners learn speech perception as they learn their language, and that speech perception does not precede language acquisition. But it also seems reasonable to suppose that the adequate development of 'perception in the speech mode' (Studdert-Kennedy 1976) depends upon adequate peripheral perceptual processes of a more general (auditory) nature. Hearing impairment is, at least primarily, an auditory perceptual deficit, and it is particularly relevant, therefore, to look closely at the perceptual end of the chain in order to understand the linguistic deficits which appear later. The later linguistic consequences are partly a direct result of the peripheral perceptual deficits; but other important factors which are secondary to the perceptual impairment can also intrude with devastating effects. In this chapter we are concerned with the peripheral perceptual processes only. Consideration of the other, contextual, factors will be included in Chapter 6.

The more the interface between acoustic analysis and subsequent phonetic and semantic analysis is mapped for the hearing-impaired, the more opportunity there will be to direct rehabilitative effort into potentially successful channels. If impaired perception of phonetic features can be accounted for in terms of reduced performance with specific acoustic cues, then this would eventually enable individual deficits in speech discrimination to be described in more detail and perhaps, therefore, remediated more successfully. That in many verbal language situations the hearing-impaired do attempt to use similar perceptual cues to those used by the normally hearing is not in doubt at the acoustic end of the chain (Pickett *et al*. 1972, Franks and Daniloff 1973, Busby *et al*. 1982). Thus in this chapter we feel justified in examining the details of the peripheral perceptual deficits of the hearing-impaired by comparison with those peripheral processes in the normally hearing, some of which were reviewed in Chapter 1.

This normative comparison applied to peripheral processes should not mislead the reader into an uncritical acceptance of the view that such normative comparisons are necessarily appropriate later in the chain. Development of spoken language skills and reading skills in hearing-impaired children have traditionally been treated by normative comparison (see Chapters 6 and 8), but more recent studies have aimed to investigate not *how* poorly the hearing-impaired compare with their normally hearing peers, but *why* this is so and what are the cognitive processes involved. These differing approaches will be revisited in the following chapters; meanwhile the dichotomy, if it is such, does not apply to the subject of this chapter. The problem for this chapter is that unfortunately we are nowhere near yet being able to identify all the stages of normal analysis of speech signals, and consequently we are unable to isolate fully the defective peripheral mechanisms in the hearing-impaired. What we are left to do is to make plausible guesses as to which perceptual aspects are important and then examine these processes in the hearing-impaired. The current plausible guesses include detection, frequency discrimination and resolution, temporal discrimination and resolution, intensity coding, and pattern recognition (central analysis) processes.

Two further points should be made before we consider each of these topics in detail: firstly, in our discussions of the hearing-impaired child in this and all subsequent chapters except Chapter 9, we are concerned with bilateral and (broadly speaking) equal hearing loss across the ears; discussion of the rather special case of unilateral (monaural) hearing loss is reserved for Chapter 9. Secondly, this chapter deals with the complex question of auditory perception in those with sensorineural hearing loss, and omits discussion of auditory perception in those with conductive hearing loss. Pure conductive losses tend to be mild or moderate in degree of pure-tone threshold elevation; they often give flat rather than sloping pure-tone audiograms, with perhaps slightly greater loss of sensitivity in the lower-frequency regions; and they act essentially as sources of straightforward attenuation of sound travelling to the inner ear. The disordered perceptual processes which seem to be associated with sensorineural losses are therefore not to be found in conductive losses; one consequence is that amplification with hearing aids is likely to be more successful with the latter, since hearing aids are amplifiers which can overcome the effects of straight attenuation, but can do little to compensate for more complex perceptual dysfunctions. This view of conductive hearing loss is probably over-simple, and certainly there is evidence for the assertion that the attenuation produced by conductive losses is not linear, and that some distortions are introduced into the input signal. However, further discussion of the perceptual effects of this type of hearing impairment will be postponed until Chapter 7.

Detection

Elevation of detection thresholds for pure tones is the most common sign of, and the most commonly used test for, hearing impairment. Thresholds for pure tones are expressed in dB HL (decibels hearing level) and are calibrated such that the average thresholds for all frequencies (at least from 0.25–10 kHz) for normally hearing persons are at zero (see Fig. 1.3). Variability of normal sensitivity and less than perfect test conditions usually means that pure-tone thresholds up to, say, 15 dB HL are regarded as normal. School screening audiometry generally uses 20 or 25 dB HL as the pass/fail point.

Non-normal pure-tone audiograms come in a variety of forms. The degree of hearing loss may vary from slight, through moderate and severe, to profound. These categories correspond to average pure-tone hearing loss of up to 40 dB (slight), 41–70 dB (moderate), 71–95 dB (severe) and 96 dB or more (profound). The notion of such arbitrary categorization (these particular categories have been recommended by the British Association of Teachers of the Deaf, 1981), has some face validity, since, broadly speaking, the greater the pure-tone hearing loss the greater the effect upon language and the greater the disability. However, pure-tone audiometry is a measure of impairment; disability and then handicap come later in the chain, and are not directly predictable from the degree of impairment.

Apart from the degree of the loss, pure-tone audiograms can vary in their configuration. That is to say, detection thresholds may be elevated by the same amount at all frequencies, or by different amounts at different frequencies. Although U-shaped audiograms and audiograms with greater loss in the low frequencies are not rare, by far the largest number of hearing impairments of sensorineural origin exhibit greatest loss in the high-frequency regions. The relationship between frequency and vulnerability to elevated threshold is neatly illustrated by Pearson (1977) for an adult population (Fig. 5.1). The reasons for the greater vulnerability of the high frequencies are not fully understood; it may reflect the fact that the basal turns of the basilar membrane are involved in the perception of higher frequencies, and that there is tonotopic organization of the eighth nerve such that neurones carrying information about the high frequencies tend to be on the outside of the bundle.

It is an unfortunate quirk of nature that sensorineural hearing losses are likely to be worse in the higher frequencies, since it is the consonants which are the major

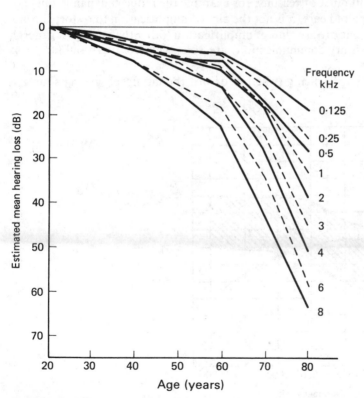

Figure 5.1   Relationship of presbyacusis to age in 262 females from a rural environment. Hearing loss is estimated as difference from 15- to 24-year-old age group. Different lines are simply to aid reading. (From Pearson 1977.)

source of intelligibility in the English language, and these have most of their acoustic energy in the higher frequencies. In fact this is something of an oversimplification, since we know that the acoustic properties of consonants depend upon the vowel(s) with which they are conjoined. As expected, it is the vowels with relatively high-frequency second formants which are most sensitive to elevated high-frequency thresholds (Egolf *et al.* 1970). In addition to their generally high-frequency characteristics, consonants tend to be spoken at lower intensities than vowels, and the frequency spectrum of speech does indeed show a decrease of intensity in the higher frequencies. Thus, if we plot the pure-tone detection thresholds for an imaginary hearing loss of moderate degree, worse in the high frequencies, and superimpose the speech spectrum onto the audiogram (Fig. 5.2) it can be seen that the lower-frequency components of speech are detectable, but the higher-frequency components are not. Note in passing that in order to make this comparison the pure-tone hearing loss, which is usually expressed in terms of dB HL, has to be converted to dB SPL. The aim of amplification with hearing aids is to increase selectively the sound-pressure level of the speech at the eardrum such that it is at least detectable in the important frequencies. For a number of reasons, for example the reduced dynamic range of sensorineurally impaired ears, it is not the aim of amplification to restore normal thresholds. Indeed, the precise aims of amplification (other than the most general, i.e. to improve auditory communication) are somewhat controversial (see, e.g. Byrne 1979).

The three features of voicing (whether or not the laryngeal voicing source is

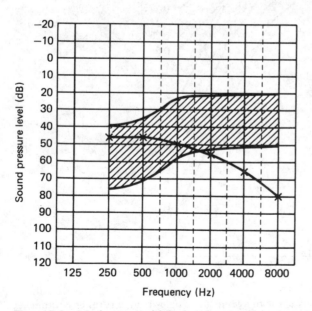

Figure 5.2 Moderate sensitivity loss for pure tones superimposed on the long-term average speech spectrum.

active during consonant production), manner of articulation (the type of vocal-tract gesture made) and place of articulation (the point in the vocal tract of maximum constriction during production) enables the unique classification of all English consonants. Miller and Nicely (1955) used the classical method of studying feature recognition by examining the recognition-errors of phonemes under different conditions of filtering (with normally hearing listeners). Amongst other things, they showed that as more and more high-frequency information is filtered out of the speech signal, the number of place errors increases markedly, while perception of voicing was largely unaffected. On the basis of these data Boothroyd (1978) calculated the median frequency and bandwidth of the cues needed for the perception of the three features (Table 5.1). Voicing and manner are widely spread across frequencies, with much energy in the lower frequency regions; information about place, however, is of a much higher frequency and in a relatively restricted bandwidth.

Table 5.1   Median frequency and bandwidth for three subphonemic features (from Boothroyd 1978, p. 117)

Feature	Median frequency (Hz)	Bandwidth (octaves)
Voicing	500	3.0
Manner of articulation	750	2.6
Place of articulation	1900	1.6

We now know much more about the acoustic nature of consonant-feature information. Voicing information is conveyed via the presence or absence of the complex laryngeal tone, and through temporal relationships between onset of voice and the occurrence of aperiodic (random) consonant noise. Voicing information is thus available in most frequency regions, from the fundamental frequency of the voice (100–250 Hz) upwards through most of its harmonics and spectral peaks. Manner information is cued by a variety of signals, such as the presence of a long burst of noise or by a silent period followed by a short burst of noise, and is therefore not usually restricted to any one frequency region. Place information, however, seems to be carried largely by the second and third formants – particularly their transitions – which are found in consonant-vowel structures; this information is often confined to a narrow region between 1.5 and 2.5 kHz.

The significance of the shape of the speech spectrum is now evident:

The high-power, relatively low-frequency portion of the spectrum around 500 Hz contains first formant vowel energy, as well as information about consonant voicing and manner. The mid-frequency region between 500 and 2000 Hz contains second formant energy, which is important for both the identification of vowels and of the place of articulation of consonants. The high-frequency, low power end of the spectrum represents upper-formant energy and consonant noise associated with stop and fricative consonants. (Norlin and van Tasell 1980, p. 17.)

Phoneme-error analysis has been used with hearing-impaired listeners and inferences made about the speech-feature information available to them by examination of the error patterns. A number of studies with partially hearing listeners (slight, moderate or severe degrees of impairment) have demonstrated error patterns that are broadly predictable on the basis of considering the hearing loss as a simple filter, mainly low-pass (because most hearing losses are greater in the higher frequencies). Thus, fewer errors are made on vowels than consonants; front vowels are harder than central or back vowels; place of articulation is the predominant error type for consonants; manner errors occur less often, and voicing errors relatively rarely; voiceless fricative consonants (/f, Ө, s, ʃ/); are identified only with great difficulty (e.g. Owens and Schubert 1968, Pickett *et al*. 1972). Bilger and Wang (1976) were able to go a stage further and show that feature errors differed in a predictable fashion between flat and high-frequency hearing losses.

One might regard pure-tone hearing loss, therefore, as effectively acting as a simple filter on the incoming speech signal; and indeed speech passed through various types of linear filters (e.g. low-pass) and recorded onto magnetic tape have traditionally provided a popular if inaccurate demonstration of 'what a hearing loss is like'. However, it has been shown (Godfrey and Millay 1978, Wang *et al*. 1978) that normally hearing listeners handle filtered speech much more effectively than would be expected on the basis of observation of hearing-impaired people with given pure-tone audiograms. Additionally, it is now clear that perceptual processes other than detection thresholds are disordered in the hearing-impaired. It has long been evident to parents and teachers of hearing-impaired children that children with the same pure-tone audiogram may turn out to have quite different language skills; much of the unaccounted-for variability may be due to social, emotional and educational factors, but it is also plausible that at least part of the answer may be found in individual differences in aspects of peripheral auditory perception other than simple detection. This is a promising field for future work, and if established would lead to research and development of the next generation of hearing aids which might be intended not only to amplify specific areas of the frequency domain, but to compensate for other disordered perceptual processes on an individual basis (see Rosen and Fourcin 1986).

Predicting speech-hearing from detection thresholds

The quantification of the relationship between pure-tone sensitivity and receptive language performance goes back to Fletcher (1929), and Harris *et al*. (1956) have reviewed the earlier studies. The widespread introduction of calibrated electroacoustic systems for speech audiometry in the 1950s led to an upsurge of interest in the relationship between pure-tone sensitivity and speech-hearing, particularly with regard to the efficiency of predicting speech-hearing from different summary measures of the pure-tone audiogram (e.g. Mullins and Bangs 1957, Kryter *et al.* 1962, Young and Gibbons 1962, Seigenthaler and Strand 1964, Macrae and Brigden 1973, Erber 1974, Bamford *et al.* 1981). Details of the traditional approach to the assessment of speech-hearing in the clinic can be found elsewhere (Bench and Bamford 1979).

A variety of materials for 'speech audiometry' is available, the most common being lists of words or sentences which the listener has to repeat item by item. A complete test will consist of several lists of assumed equal difficulty, and often equalized for other dimensions such as grammar (for sentences) or phonemic content (for words). Sometimes the lists contain phonemes in the proportions in which they occur in the natural language (phonemically balanced lists). Age and linguistic ability have to be borne in mind when selecting a speech test for an individual, since it is of paramount importance to choose a test which will be within that person's linguistic competence. Speech-audiometry tests are designed to assess receptive linguistic performance uncontaminated by linguistic competence. Lists are presented via headphones or loudspeakers at a series of intensities (one intensity per list) which are chosen to span the area from (speech) detection to maximum score. The listener's task is to repeat back each item (word or sentence) immediately after presentation, and the item is scored according to the number of words or phonemes correctly repeated. Thus a percentage score can be derived for a list at a given presentation level. If several lists are presented at different levels, the complete 'speech audiogram' (performance/intensity function) can be plotted, with percentage correct on the ordinate and presentation level in dB on the abscissa (Fig. 5.3).

For normally hearing listeners the speech audiogram typically assumes a sigmoid (cumulative normal) function. The exact position of this function on the abscissa depends upon various aspects of calibration. The speech audiogram is assumed to reflect speech-hearing ability, although the degree to which it actually reflects speech-hearing in everyday situations is open to some debate. Nevertheless, as a crude measure of this ability it probably has reasonable validity. Some workers have argued that since much of everyday listening takes place against a background of noise, speech audiometry has increased validity if it is measured in noise. In this case presentation is usually via loudspeakers with white noise or speech-spectrum noise presented via the same loudspeaker as the signal or via a spatially separate loudspeaker. With speech-in-noise audiometry, the speech level is fixed at some appropriate level (e.g. 60 dB) and noise levels are varied between lists. The abscissa is then the signal-to-noise ratio, with 0 per cent correct at high noise levels and 100 per cent correct at low noise levels. Normally hearing listeners exhibit speech audiograms (in quiet or noise) which typically rise from 0 to 100 per cent within 30 dB or so, depending upon a variety of factors (Fig. 5.3). It should be noted that this brief description of speech audiometry has largely ignored the fact that

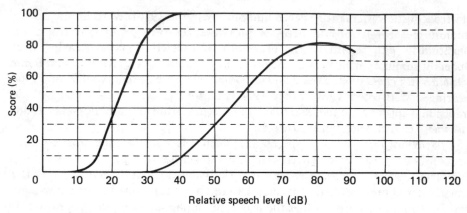

Figure 5.3   Speech audiograms: a typical normal audiogram (on the left) and an illustrative example of a speech audiogram from a sensorineural hearing loss.

workers often do not plot the complete speech audiogram, and may use specialized and different tests for the estimation of different parts of the curve; for the purposes of the present discussion, however, these details are not relevant.

The speech audiograms obtained from those with sensorineural hearing loss tend to show one or more of the following features (Fig. 5.3): *(i)* the audiogram curve is shifted to the right, reflecting the need for higher signal-presentation levels (or lower noise levels); *(ii)* the maximum score is less than 100 per cent; and *(iii)* the slope of the linear portion of the curve is flattened relative to the normally hearing case. The first two features are represented by two common measures in speech audiometry, namely speech-reception threshold (SRT) and maximum discrimination score (DS) respectively. The third feature, slope, is rarely measured except insofar as it affects SRT. The presentation level (or S:N ratio) at which the listener scores 50 per cent correct is the SRT, and DS is the maximum percentage correct at any level. Studies relating measures of pure-tone hearing loss to these measures of speech-hearing loss have been in good agreement, showing SRT well predicted by degree of pure-tone loss and DS less well predicted: Bamford *et al.* (1981) found from multiple-regression analysis of pure-tone and speech-hearing measures on 149 hearing-impaired children that the multiple correlations between pure-tone thresholds and SRT and DS were 0.88 and 0.53 respectively. Thus, SRT is well predicted by pure-tone sensitivity and the shift of the speech audiogram to the right in sensorineural hearing-impaired listeners largely reflects the elevation in detection thresholds (certain, uncommon, retrocochlear pathologies give an elevated SRT in the absence of elevated pure-tone thresholds, but this is a special case which need not concern us here).

If SRT were a completely exclusive and valid reflection of speech–hearing ability, then we could be satisfied that loss of detection fully accounts for impaired speech perception, and rehabilitation through amplification would be likely to be relatively successful. As we know, such is not the case, and speech perception as reflected by DS is not well predicted by elevated detection thresholds. Speech audiometry, therefore, provides a quantified if crude descriptive measure of the phenomenon that we have been discussing here, namely that speech perception depends only partially upon sensitivity levels. Language disability in the hearing-impaired is not to be understood solely in terms of the impairment in pure-tone hearing, and one has to look at other impaired perceptual processes which may be implicated.

Frequency discrimination and frequency resolution

We saw in Chapter 1 (p. 15) how recent studies have indicated that a substantial amount of filtering appears to take place at the peripheral end of the auditory system; thus, single-cell recordings from neurones in the eighth nerve of certain animals have shown physiological tuning curves which are tuned to particular characteristic frequencies (see Fig. 1.6). A number of studies have examined the effects of experimentally induced cochlear damage on the tuning curves (Evans 1972, 1975a, 1976, Evans and Harrison 1976, Dallos *et al.* 1977, Liberman and Kiang 1978). The damage is induced by the use of ototoxic drugs such as kanamycin, which if used in carefully controlled amounts can produce short or long-term effects on particular areas of the cochlea. It seems that the outer hair-cells are most commonly damaged, particularly in the basal and middle turns of the cochlear partition. The damage has marked effects on the tuning curves of the auditory nerve (Fig. 5.4).

A number of complex patterns of damage to the tuning curves have been identified (Pickles 1982) but in general the tips of the tuning curves are raised, indicating loss of sensitivity (i.e. elevated thresholds) and, more importantly, the narrow finely tuned tips become much broader, indicating a decrease in frequency resolving power. Thus, we have direct physiological evidence that damage to the cochlea produces elevated thresholds and broad, poorly tuned (essentially low-pass) tuning curves. As the frequency selectivity of the auditory system is predominantly determined by this cochlear filtering, then it might be expected that people with sensorineural hearing impairments (which most commonly involve pathological conditions of the cochlea) would exhibit psychophysical signs of deterioration in frequency selectivity. Such is indeed the case.

Frequency discrimination – the ability to discriminate on the basis of frequency sounds which arrive successively – has been studied in the hearing impaired (Butler and Albrite 1957, di Carlo 1962, Wightman 1981, Turner and Nelson 1982). The difference threshold for frequency has been found to be larger for hearing-impaired listeners than for normally hearing listeners, even for frequencies which exhibit normal sensitivity (Turner and Nelson 1982). This finding of reduced acuity in the hearing-impaired, not only in regions of reduced sensitivity (usually the high frequencies) but also in regions of normal sensitivity, is interesting. Turner and Nelson speculate either that the pathology responsible for the high-frequency hearing loss alters the mechanical properties of the basilar-membrane travelling wave such that discriminations from the lower-frequency regions of the cochlea are

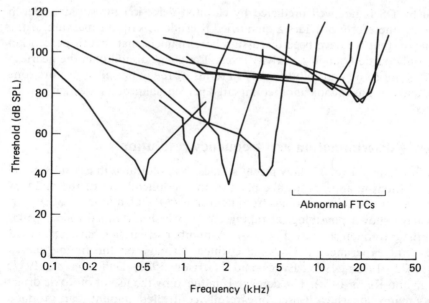

Figure 5.4   Physiological tuning curves in the guinea-pig: those in the higher frequencies are abnormal, showing loss of the sharply tuned tips. (From Evans and Harrison 1976, Fig. 1.)

also affected; or that normal neural firing patterns from the basal (high-frequency) turn of the cochlea contribute to acuity at lower frequencies. They also offer another possible explanation, that there are subtle sensory deficits in the lower-frequency regions, based upon pathological changes in these regions, which are simply not indicated by elevated thresholds at those frequencies.

We know, of course, that much of speech perception is based upon events that occur simultaneously, such as the peaks in spectral energy (formants) which are present at different frequencies and which are used as cues for phonemic discrimination. The ability of the ear to resolve the frequency bands of a complex signal which are temporally coincident is therefore more important than frequency discrimination.

The effect of sensorineural hearing loss on critical bandwidth has been investigated by a number of workers. While individual differences are large, and some studies do not show clear effects in hearing-impaired listeners (Bonding 1979), the more general picture is of abnormally widened critical bands (de Boer 1959, Scharf and Hellman 1966, Martin 1974, Florentine *et al*. 1980). Pick *et al*. (1977) used a psychophysical comb-filtered noise technique to estimate both the bandwidth of the auditory filter (critical band) at given frequencies and the shape of the filter skirts. Comb-filtered noise has a continuous spectrum, with regularly repeating peaks and valleys representing higher and lower areas of energy at particular frequencies. This was used to mask a tone signal at the frequency for which frequency resolution was to be determined. Interest centres on the difference between the tone thresholds masked by a spectral peak and by a spectral valley as a function of the fineness of peak spacing. The results of the studies showed that the hearing-impaired listeners showed elevation of the filter skirts with mild degrees of sensitivity loss, followed by a progressive widening of the auditory filter bandwidth as hearing loss increased. The reduction of frequency-resolving power evidenced by the change in shape of the effective critical band in sensorineural hearing loss would be expected to limit the ability of the ear to resolve the individual formants of the speech signal, to affect normal 'place' coding of the individual formants, and to cause an increased susceptibility to background noise. Broadbent and Ladefoged (1957) suggested that the fundamental voice pitch is used as the cue for grouping the high harmonics (and therefore individual formants) into a percept of one voice. As Darwin (1981) showed (see Chap. 1, p. 27), this may not be a very useful cue in multiple-speaker environments since, he argued, the individual harmonics from several voices to be resolved out would probably fall within the same critical bands. It might, however, be a useable cue with only one voice to be listened to. The abnormal bandwidths in the hearing-impaired may make the resolution of formants in even a single voice a difficult task for the auditory system.

Turek *et al*. (1980) studied the identification of synthetic /bdg/ stimuli by hearing-impaired listeners when the formants of the speech sound were presented either monotically, to one ear, or some to one ear and the remainder to the other ear (dichotically). One of the explanations for impaired speech perception in listeners with sensorineural hearing loss has traditionally been that such listeners exhibit an abnormal degree of upward spread of masking (see below), and the higher-frequency formants upon which phonemic identification depends are masked by the lower-frequency formants. If we assume, again, that peripheral (cochlear) filtering is the predominant source of auditory frequency selectivity, we might predict that upward spread of masking would be avoided by presenting different formants to different ears in an appropriate manner. Since such presentation did not markedly avoid the difficulties experienced by the sensorineural listeners in distinguishing the consonants, Turek *et al*. suggested that rather than any effects of masking, it is the poor frequency resolution *per se* which gives rise to poor performance through an inability to resolve the higher formants distinctly, resulting in a 'blurred' representation of the short-term spectrum. The question arises as to whether the blurring of the spectrum can be compensated for by any preprocessing using electronic devices.

Summerfield *et al*. (1981) attempted to compensate for poor frequency resolution by narrowing the formant bandwidths, thus enhancing the formant peaks acoustically if not aurally. The study involved varying the formant bandwidths associated with the synthesized words *bet, debt, get, bib,* and *big* from unnaturally wide to unnaturally narrow. In the event, the normal hearing subjects identified words at near-perfect levels with narrow and normal bandwidths, but performance deteriorated to near-chance as bandwidth increased; the hearing-impaired listeners, with poorer absolute performance levels, also scored worse as bandwidth increased but, contrary to expectations, did not improve as bandwidth was narrowed. The authors offer two possible explanations for the lack of improved scores with narrower bandwidths in the hearing-impaired group. Firstly, that the 'unnaturalness' of speech sounds with very narrow bandwidths outweighs any advantage to be gained from improved frequency resolution. This rather general proposal receives some circumstantial support from Remez et al. (1981), who substituted the formants of the vocalic portion of a syllable with sine waves which exactly matched the course of the formants they replaced. Listeners (normally hearing) initially perceived the sounds as nonspeech patterns of noise and tones, although after practice and the suggestion that they might be speech sounds, the listeners were able to perceive them as speech sounds which then exhibited the normal categorical phonemic identification and discrimination functions. Liberman (1981), from a 'speech is special' viewpoint, has argued that details of formant bandwidth are irrelevant for linguistic purposes (since they are beyond the control of the articulatory apparatus – here we see the influence of motor theories of speech perception), and the only effect of changed formant bandwidth will be to make the speech unnatural. The second possible explanation offered by Summerfield et al. (1981) is one which is derived, in contrast, from an acoustic perceptual view of speech analysis: they suggest that there may be little to be gained from making formant bandwidths narrower than the bandwidths of listeners' auditory filters. Admittedly it increases the separation between formants, and intuitively therefore would seem to make them more distinct; but perceptually this view has no substance, unless one takes into account the critical bandwidths of the listener.

A method for examining the frequency-resolving power of the auditory system other than critical band measures has been the use of psychoacoustic tuning curves (PTC) in which the intensity of tones at different frequencies needed just to mask a low-level probe tone of fixed frequency is measured (see Fig. 1.5, p. 13). The assumption is that the extent to which the masker tones just mask the probe tone gives a measure of the degree to which the two signals are resolved. A characteristic V-shaped tuning curve, with a steeper slope on the high-frequency side, is generally obtained in normally hearing subjects. Evans and Wilson (1973) found a strong similarity between physiological tuning curves in cats (single-nerve recordings) and psychophysical tuning curves in human subjects. In listeners with sensorineural hearing loss (but not, it seems, in those with conductive losses – see Zwicker and Schorn 1978), the sharply tuned tip of the PTC is reduced or abolished and the slopes become shallower, particularly on the low-frequency side (Leshowitz and Lindstrom 1977). Hoekstra and Ritsma (1977) found that with increased hearing loss the tip of the tuning curve gradually disappears until, at losses greater than 50 dB, it is completely absent. For some subjects a loss of 40 dB or more results in a dramatic alteration in the form of the PTC to a W-shape. Wightman (1981) and Gribben (1981) note that tuning curves are broader than normal, even when measured in areas of normal sensitivity in listeners with high-frequency hearing loss. Tyler (1986) gives a comprehensive review of the measurement of PTCs with hearing-impaired listeners.

Figure 1.5 (p. 13) shows two PTCs from a group of normal-hearing subjects, and Fig. 5.5 shows PTCs from two individual sensorineural hearing loss subjects. In normally hearing listeners the width of the tuning curve 10 dB above the minimum is approximately one-eighth of the probe frequency ($Q_{10} = 8$), although different studies have given average Q_{10} measures which vary from 6.7 (Florentine *et al*. 1980) to 11.1 (Tyler *et al*. 1982a). There is in fact considerable variability between normal-hearing subjects in this measure, even within studies, but this is negligible compared to the variability found between hearing-impaired listeners. For this reason, averaged Q_{10} values have little meaning for these groups, and often the data are more profitably examined individually. Gribben (1981) studied PTCs in eight subjects with sensorineural impairment, and found a large amount of individual variation. Nevertheless, subjects with more than 40 dB hearing loss exhibited PTCs that were markedly abnormal in shape and tuning, whereas subjects with slight hearing losses gave PTCs which overlapped with those from the normal group. The finding that the fineness of tuning deteriorates (possibly in complex ways) with increased sensitivity thresholds is a fairly general one. What may be of more interest, from the point of view of understanding not simply poorer speech perception with increased thresholds but individual differences in speech perception ability with similar pure-tone thresholds, is the possibility of accounting for such speech perception differences between people with similar thresholds on the basis of differences in PTCs (reflecting differences in frequency-resolution ability). However, a number of workers have pointed to various complicating factors in the measurement of PTCs, and it may be that individual variability in the susceptibility to these factors (rather than variability in frequency-resolution ability *per se*) is the source of PTC variability across hearing-impaired listeners.

The complicating factors include combination tones, lateral suppression and off-frequency listening. 'Combination tones' refers to the phenomenon that when two tones are presented to the ear, other tones which correspond to some combination of the original frequencies (e.g. $f_2 - f_1$) are generated because of non-linearities in the ear. These combination tones could be used to aid detection of the probe tone. 'Lateral suppression' refers to the fact that when two tones are presented simultaneously, the masker may not only just use the neural channels used by the signal but may in addition decrease (suppress) the signal's level of neural activity (Moore and Glasberg 1982); lower masking levels are thus required to mask the probe tone. Finally, Moore (1989) has suggested that in relation to lateral suppression the signal may be detected by the region of excitation where the pattern of excitation is suppressed the least – i.e. off-frequency listening. These complicating factors may be partially but not wholly circumvented by using non-simultaneous (usually forward) masking paradigms, in which for example a 200-ms masker is presented and followed immediately by the 20-ms probe tone. In nonsimultaneous masking, the masking effect of the masker is somewhat diminished, though still present. Since our interest is primarily in differences in frequency resolution between individuals, the reduction in the absolute amount of masking is not a problem.

We noted in Chapter 1 that the asymmetrical shape of normal PTCs is consistent

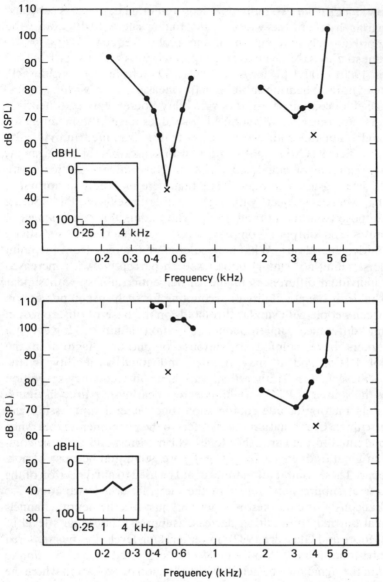

Figure 5.5 Psychoacoustic tuning curves from two individuals with sensorineural hearing loss. Pure-tone audiograms from the test ears are shown in the insets. (From Gribben 1981.)

with the 'upward spread of masking' phenomenon (see Fig. 1.4, p. 11). That is, maskers of lower frequency than the probe tone can, if intense enough, mask the probe, whereas the same is less true for maskers of higher frequency than the probe, as evidenced by the steep slopes of PTCs on the high-frequency side of the probe tone. The observation that the low-frequency slope in particular of PTCs is shallower in subjects with sensorineural hearing loss indicates that one might expect pathological spread of masking to the higher frequencies in such subjects, and this is indeed so (e.g. Rittmanic 1962, Danaher *et al*. 1973, de Boer and Bouwmeester 1974). Increased amounts of upward masking would be expected to reduce the ability of the auditory system to resolve out the higher formants in speech signals. Thus, Danaher and Pickett (1975) found that, while discrimination of higher formants presented in isolation was only mildly affected in hearing-impaired listeners, their ability to discriminate the formants was drastically reduced in the presence of the first formant. In cases of moderate or greater hearing loss, the high frequency slope of the PTC is often reduced, giving rise to some degree of pathological downward spread of masking (Gribben 1981, Tyler *et al*. 1982a); however, this is perhaps of less interest since *(i)* it is generally the higher formants which are of particular value for speech perception; and *(ii)* in any case, the upward spread is more marked than the downward spread of masking.

The implications for hearing aids of the pathological upward spread of masking is clear, and one would suppose that, for the purposes of speech perception, reduced amounts of low-frequency amplification would provide optimum benefit. Indeed, attempts have been made to design hearing-aid systems which incorporate automatic low-frequency noise suppression (Iwasaki 1981). De-emphasis of low frequencies has been a general feature of the design of hearing aids for some years. However, it is interesting to note that Punch *et al*. (1980) and Punch and Beck (1980) have shown that both normal-hearing and hearing-impaired listeners prefer speech which is reproduced through amplification systems which have extended low-frequency emphasis. There is therefore some contradiction between patient preference (represented by quality judgements) and speech-intelligibility performance. Indeed, despite evidence from the shape of the low-frequency side of PTCs in the hearing-impaired, it appears that the precise nature and amount of increased upward spread of masking in such patients remains uncertain. Thus, as we mentioned earlier, Turek *et al*. (1980) found that dichotic presentation of the frequency components of synthetic speech sounds (thus presumably avoiding peripherally-based upward spread of masking) did not substantially improve the discrimination of consonants articulated at different places of production. Earlier workers suggested that increased amounts of upward spread of masking simply reflected the production of more aural distortions in sensorineurally impaired ears (e.g. Lawrence and Yantis 1956), but this view has since been discredited. Gagné (1982) initiated a series of experiments which attempt to resolve the issue of the degree of upward spread of masking in impaired ears. Results from small numbers of normal and hearing-impaired listeners indicate that in certain experimental conditions some hearing-impaired listeners display excess upward spread of masking: thus, the masking functions (cf. Fig. 1.4, p. 11) of some impaired listeners were abnormal, showing higher masked thresholds than the masked thresholds obtained for the normally-hearing listeners, and masking-function slopes that were less steep than the slope of the masking functions of the normal-hearing listeners.

Wightman (1981) turned his attention to the issue of the extraction of the pitch of the speech fundamental. Having demonstrated the reduced ability of hearing-impaired listeners to discriminate two successive pure tones on the basis of frequency, he asked his subjects to listen for a change in the fundamental frequency of a complex tone. The listener was presented with a two-interval, forced-choice task in which each interval contained four upper harmonics of some fundamental. The fundamental for the interval was fixed, and that for the second was either higher or lower than the first. The listener's task was simply to judge whether the pitch of the second complex tone was higher or lower than the first. The specific harmonics for each stimulus were scrambled from interval to interval, in order to avoid the changes in frequency of the harmonics serving as a reliable cue for change in fundamental frequency. The data showed that the performance of the hearing-impaired listeners was markedly impaired relative to normally hearing listeners. At best, the pitch-discrimination threshold was twice that of the normal subjects.

Temporal integration and temporal resolution

Temporal integration (or temporal summation) refers to the integration of acoustic power over short durations: the sensitivity threshold in normally hearing listeners decreases as the duration of the stimulus increases, below a critical duration of 400 ms or so (e.g. Zwislocki 1969, Gengel and Watson 1971). Temporal integration may be assessed indirectly by obtaining thresholds as a function of stimulus duration; the slope of such functions gives a measure of auditory temporal integration. For normal adult ears, this slope is approximately –3 dB for a doubling of duration (Gengel and Watson 1971). A number of studies have reported impaired temporal integration in listeners with sensorineural hearing loss (e.g. Jesteadt et al. 1976) but the results are not unequivocal. Dempsey and Maxon (1982), for example, measured thresholds for tones at three frequencies (0.5, 2 and 4 kHz) as a function of duration (25, 100 and 200 ms) in 8–12-year-old children with sensorineural hearing loss. Although the threshold-duration functions were flatter than those previously obtained on normally hearing children, there was some overlap; and furthermore, the functions were steeper than those obtained from a group of hearing-impaired adults. Pedersen and Pulsen (1973) failed to find a marked deterioration in temporal integration in hearing-impaired ears. Stephens (1973), Tyler (1976) and Tyler et al. (1982b) have also assessed temporal integration in subjects with hearing loss. Again, some effects were noted, but large inter-subject variability and overlap between normal and hearing-impaired groups was common. No strong relationship was found between pure-tone thresholds and temporal integration. These equivocal results may reflect the fact that to date there is little evidence of time-processing effects from physiological studies of cochlear-nerve-fibre discharge patterns in pathologically altered cochleas (Evans 1975b, Kiang et al. 1970). It may be that disordered temporal processing is associated not with cochlear pathology so much as with lesions in the auditory nerve and cochlear nuclei, and this might explain why temporal integration is apparently worse in hearing-impaired adults than in hearing-impaired children, since it could be argued that degeneration of retrocochlear processes would be more likely in adults because of ageing and other factors. Ginzel *et al.* (1982) have shown a decreased ability to identify phonemes on the basis of initial consonant length and vowel length in older subjects.

Temporal resolution refers to the minimum time required to segregate or resolve acoustic events. It is most popularly measured by means of a gap-detection task, in which listeners have to detect the presence of a temporal gap in a burst of noise. On a simple physical realization of the auditory filter, the widened bandwidths in the hearing-impaired would predict shorter time constants and consequently *better* temporal resolution. This does not seem to be the case. Boothroyd (1973, reported in Giraudi-Perry *et al.* 1982) found larger gap-detection thresholds in his profoundly-impaired subjects compared with normal subjects, although there was some overlap in the results of the two groups. Similarly, Fitzgibbons and Wightman (1982a) have found elevated gap-detection thresholds in subjects with moderate flat sensorineural hearing loss, although again there was considerable intersubject variability, with some listeners showing normal performance. In a study of chinchillas with noise-induced hearing loss, Giraudi-Perry *et al.* (1982) demonstrated normal gap-detection with thresholds elevated by 15 dB, longer than normal gap-detection thresholds with a hearing loss of 30 dB if compared at the same sound-pressure level, but not if compared at the same sensation level, and longer gap-detection on either scale with hearing loss of 40 dB or more. The authors interpret their results in terms of an orderly breakdown of temporal resolution as the degree of (noise-induced) hearing loss increases.

The large variability and the performance overlap between normal and hearing-impaired listeners, which has made interpretation and modelling rather difficult, was not evident in the results of a further study by Fitzgibbons and Wightman (1982b), in which gap-detection was investigated in different frequency regions. They investigated the minimum detectable gap in five normal and five hearing-impaired subjects, using octave-band noise signals at three different frequency bands: 400–800 Hz, 800–1600 Hz, 2000–4000 Hz. Noisebands were embedded in broad-band notched noise to remove unwanted spectral cues. Gap thresholds decreased (i.e. performance improved) as the centre frequency of the octave-band noise increased, for all subjects. However, the hearing-impaired listeners exhibited significantly poorer gap thresholds at all frequencies, both at equal sound-pressure level and at equal sensation level. Temporal resolution, the authors conclude, is poorer than normal in hearing-impaired subjects. The results indicated that temporal resolution is affected by signal level, implying that with a signal of given SPL, temporal resolution will decrease as the degree of hearing loss increases. The authors also suggest that the higher frequencies may prove to be dominant for temporal resolution (cf. better gap-thresholds in higher frequencies) and that if this is so it would impart a further relative disadvantage on the hearing impaired, who generally show greater sensitivity loss at higher frequencies.

Zwicker and Schorn (1982) have devised a rather different task to tap temporal resolution, in which the threshold of a test tone-burst is measured as a function of its position in relation to a short burst of narrow-band noise. The masker is repeated periodically so that forward, backward and simultaneous masking of the test tone-burst is combined into a 'masking period pattern'. The tone-burst is triggered by the masker, and its threshold is measured as a function of its temporal position within the masker. The results for patients with conductive hearing loss showed normal temporal resolution; patients with noise-induced, age-induced and sudden hearing loss showed normal resolution at low and mid-frequencies, but reduced resolution at 4000 Hz; and patients with retrocochlear loss and Menière's disorder showed reduced resolution at all frequencies (though greater effects still at 4000 Hz).

As we have already seen, Wightman (1981) used nonsimultaneous masking to derive psychoacoustic tuning curves to assess frequency resolution. He implicated temporal processes in the performance of his subjects by comparing PTCs obtained with a gap of 30 ms between masker tone and probe tone with PTCs obtained with no gap between masker and probe. In the case of his normally hearing listeners, the effect of the masker-probe delay was to cause a general upward shift in the PTC, reflecting the expected decay of the masker's effectiveness. While one of his hearing-impaired subjects showed the same tendency, the other did not, and that subject's PTC shifted hardly at all from the condition of no interval between masker and probe. Wightman did not speculate as to the implications of this difference, noting that more data are required, except to comment that the difference between the hearing-impaired listeners is 'highly suggestive of a difference between the listeners in the rate of decay of masking and may indicate general differences in temporal resolution' (1981, p. 17).

In a comprehensive study of a variety of temporal processing tasks with normal and impaired listeners, Tyler, Summerfield, Wood and Fernandez (1982) found in general that most of the hearing-impaired subjects performed significantly worse. The authors measured temporal integration, gap detection, temporal-difference threshold (the increase in duration required to just detect a difference in duration of a noise-burst), and gap-difference threshold (the increase in duration required to just detect a difference in the duration of a silent interval between two noise-bursts). Also measured were speech identification in noise, and identification and discrimination of synthetic speech stimuli varying in voice-onset time (i.e. temporal cues). The results from the speech stimuli will be referred to later when we attempt to account for speech perception in terms of psychoacoustic performance. Finally, frequency resolution was assessed by means of a simplified five-point psychoacoustic tuning curve (PTC). Performance on all psychoacoustic tasks was measured at 500 Hz and 4000 Hz.

Although some individuals exhibited normal performance on some tasks, taken as a whole Tyler *et al.*'s results show that temporal processing is substantially impaired in cochlear hearing loss. Most of the hearing-impaired listeners displayed poorer temporal analysis than the normal listeners on all tasks, regardless of whether the comparisons were made at similar SPLs or similar sensation levels (the significance of this distinction in stimulus presentation level will become evident when intensity coding is discussed; briefly, because of abnormal loudness growth in the impaired ear once threshold is exceeded, the functioning of the impaired auditory system with inputs of 30 dB above threshold may be unlike the normal ear with inputs of 30 dB above its threshold, but perhaps similar to the normal ear when the latter receives higher levels of input). These results confirm others already cited, and show that, despite considerable individual variability, both frequency and temporal resolution are impaired in sensorineural hearing loss.

The results from studies on frequency resolution may provide some leverage on the variability in speech perception left unexplained by differences in threshold sensitivity, although there is much individual variability and as yet a lack of extensive normative data. We shall see later to what extent it may be possible to account for speech perception problems in this context. But, excluding one or two recent studies, the results from most studies on temporal discrimination and resolution are even more variable, equivocal and under-researched than those from frequency-resolution studies. In general, patients with sensorineural hearing losses exhibit poorer performance, but the gross nature of the data is unlikely yet to take us far along the path of accounting for the speech-perceptual skills of hearing-impaired individuals except in the most general terms.

Intensity coding

A diagnostic sign of cochlear hearing loss, as opposed to conductive or retro-cochlear hearing loss, is the phenomenon of recruitment, or abnormal loudness growth. In normal ears (see Fig. 1.2, p. 7) there is a certain 'dynamic range' of hearing which lies between the minimum-audibility threshold and the loudness-discomfort level (LDL). LDL is at approximately 100 dB SPL across frequencies in normal ears, though its exact level depends considerably upon the stimuli used and the task instructions given to the listener. In conductive hearing loss, where the various peripheral perceptual processes are little affected other than in terms of loss of sensitivity, both thresholds and LDL tend to be elevated. In cochlear hearing loss, on the other hand, detection thresholds are elevated but LDL may remain at normal or near-normal levels. This results in a much reduced dynamic range across the frequencies where the sensitivity thresholds are elevated. In other words, whereas a normal ear may go from minimum loudness ('just hear') to LDL in, say, 100 dB of signal intensity, the pathological cochlea might go through the same range of loudness for an intensity change from 60 dB HL (threshold) to 110 dB HL (LDL)–that is, a much smaller change in intensity produces the same (normal) range of subjective loudness.

Evans (1975a) has proposed a neural model to account for recruitment, and this is illustrated in Fig. 5.6. In the normal ear the physiological tuning curves, as indicated by single-cell recordings from the auditory nerves of animals, have a characteristic shape and tend to be highly tuned to a specific frequency. As stimulus intensity of a signal is raised from some level below threshold, at first

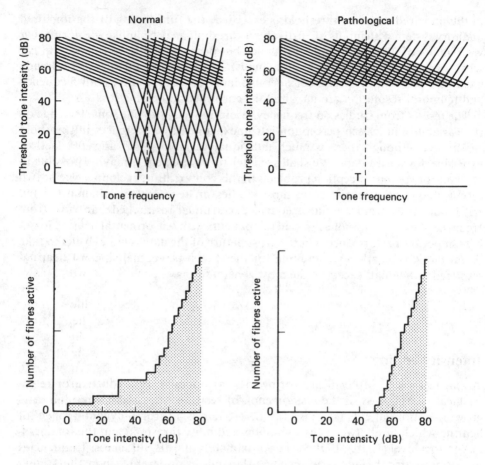

Figure 5.6   A neural explanation of loudness recruitment. Loudness in the abnormal ear grows abnormally quickly with intensity once threshold is reached, because the tips of the tuning curves are missing. (From Evans 1975a, Fig. 8.)

only the tips of the curves are activated, and the number of fibres involved will be small. With increased stimulus intensity there comes a point when the tails of other tuning curves are encountered, and the number of fibres activated thus rises abruptly. The term 'recruitment' refers to this activation of other fibres (i.e. other tuning curves) as the stimulus intensity increases. In the pathological ear, the effect seems to be to destroy the fine tuning of the curves, leaving only the broad shallow tails. Stimulus intensity has now to be increased considerably before any fibres at all are activated (i.e. before the threshold is recorded), but as soon as threshold is exceeded, the fibres are recruited rapidly, since the stimulus has already reached the area of the broad tails where the fibre tuning-curves overlap. Furthermore, because of the marked asymmetry of the tuning curves, most of these additional fibres are of higher characteristic frequency: thus, upward spread of masking is exhibited, with intense low frequency sounds recruiting a greater number of higher frequency fibres. Finally, it should be noted that apart from the recruitment or activation of new fibres, any one fibre has a dynamic range of activity (of about 40 dB) from threshold to saturated firing, and the functions relating cochlear-fibre discharge rate with stimulus level are steeper in pathological fibres than normal. Evans' model does not entirely account for recruitment, since Moore *et al.* (1985) have shown that recruitment is not abolished by the presence of flanking noise bands on either side of the signal tone. The noise was designed to mask the tone-evoked neural activity in other tuning curves, thus limiting the spread of excitation produced by the tone. It was concluded that the spread of excitation could not wholly account therefore, for the phenomenon of recruitment. Nevertheless, Evans' model gives at least a partial explanation, and it does account for the upward spread of masking and difficulties encountered by the hearing-impaired with speech perception in background noise.

It is difficult to know or predict the consequences of abnormal loudness growth upon speech perception. It is certainly one reason why cochlear hearing-loss patients may complain that they can 'hear' speech all right, but they cannot 'distinguish' it – in other words, provided the speech signal is above the listener's detection thresholds, loudness (or lack of it) is not the problem. Recruitment is, however, a problem for hearing-aid prescription, and the history of progress in this area has been dominated by the need to come to terms with reduced dynamic range in cochlear-loss patients. Put simply, the problem is that if you provide a hearing aid with sufficient gain (amplification) to raise sensitivity thresholds by a suitable amount (although not back to normal levels, even if this were possible: presumably because of abnormal loudness growth, experienced wearers choose to adjust the gain to be about half of their hearing loss (e.g. Martin 1973)), then there will be some speech sounds and some background noises which will exceed LDL. There is evidence that loudness discomfort is a major reason for the rejection of hearing aids (Beattie *et al.* 1979).

One solution to this is to provide a hearing aid with the appropriate amount of gain, but to limit its maximum output. The simple way to do this is to 'peak-clip' – i.e. to fix some maximum amplitude for the amplification and to 'clip' the tops of any waveform peaks which exceed that criterion. Such peak-clipping introduces distortions to the speech signal, however: in its simplest form, it will change a sine wave into a clipped sine wave, which will look something like a square wave, and which in turn will not contain just one frequency component but can be shown to contain a number of components. More sophisticated solutions to the problem of maximum output include the use of compression amplification systems, in which quiet signals are given maximum amplification but higher intensity signals are given progressively less amplification. This approach tends to give less distortion than peak-clipping, although some difficulties remain.

Central auditory processing

Theories of pitch perception and the extraction of the speech fundamental envisage a peripheral spectral analysis followed by a central pattern recognition process acting on the outcome of the peripheral analysis. Little is known about the neurological basis or the location of the central processes, and they could involve any structures in the brainstem and above, upwards of the locus of convergence of information from the two ears (Houtsma and Goldstein 1972). When people talk of hearing disability they are generally referring to the effects of impairments in peripheral function – sensitivity loss, reduced frequency selectivity and so on – which make up the overwhelming majority of the hearing-impaired population. Recent years have seen an increasing interest in the possibility of impairment in central auditory processes, and early attempts have been made to produce measures of these processes.

It is of course important for the therapist who is considering intervention because of cognitive or linguistic problems to rule out defects in the earlier stages of signal processing. That can be achieved reasonably routinely for the peripheral processes by standard audiometric tests (although this is not to deny the need for better tests of peripheral functions other than sensitivity), but tests for central auditory dysfunction are relatively new and untried, particularly in the UK where there are no established norms for the existing (largely American) tests. Disorders of central processing can occur in the absence of impaired peripheral mechanisms, and the current test batteries are designed primarily for use with those who have normal peripheral sensitivity. The prevailing view is to regard such patients as having a central auditory dysfunction which is within the domain of 'hearing' impairment, since hearing is seen to be represented by both peripheral and central processes. This group of patients might be seen as a subgroup of that population of children who exhibit receptive language disorders, often of a severe nature. However, we would argue that although the dividing line is diffuse, there is a useful remedial and possibly organic distinction to be made between those with lower-level central auditory disorders, who find difficulty in complex acoustic and auditory conditions, and those whose 'hearing' is adequate but whose comprehension begins to break down as *linguistic* complexity increases. Other writers (e.g. Eisenson 1968) have not found such a distinction useful and have included 'auditory dysfunction' in the description of developmental aphasia.

The deterioration of central processes of many kinds with ageing is well known; but of more interest in the present context is the phenomenon of central auditory dysfunction in children. Martin and Clark (1977), for instance, compared a group of normal children with a group of 'language learning-disabled' children on a binaural fusion task, and found significant differences in performance between the two groups. Peripheral and central auditory processes thus seem to be potentially susceptible to dysfunction independently, although of course peripheral processes are of most immediate impact and are reasonably easy to assess. There is therefore no reason to deny the possibility of children who exhibit peripheral dysfunction *also* exhibiting central auditory dysfunction – although if the likelihood of impairment in one is indeed independent of the likelihood of impairment in the other, then the number of cases with dysfunction in both would be rather small. There is another possibility, that the integrity of central processes can be compromised by impairment of peripheral processes, and there is some evidence from animal developmental studies that this occurs (Webster and Webster 1979, Ruben 1980). Thus it may be that early childhood peripheral impairment gives rise to central auditory dysfunction in addition; the possible dysfunction of central processes in the presence of peripheral hearing impairment will be difficult to isolate, however, and must await the emergence of new assessment procedures.

Furthermore, we are bound to point out the lack of a coherent theoretical framework for so-called central auditory dysfunction in those with normal peripheral sensitivity. As Keith (1981) has pointed out, there seems to be considerable confusion of terminology. At least three distinct levels of processing are confused: nonlinguistic 'central' auditory perception skills, such as localization and binaural release from masking; phonemic analysis and linguistic decoding; and such higher-level skills as speech discrimination and sequential short-term memory. In addition, there is little evidence that therapy in any of these skills has any effect on language ability; and Rees (1981) has furnished a convincing critique of the concept of central auditory dysfunction, in which she rightly emphasizes that, quite apart from the lack of theoretical underpinning in the area, the demonstration of correlations between 'central auditory processes' and language ability says nothing about causality. The subject of central auditory dysfunction will be dealt with in more depth in Chapter 10.

The relationship between peripheral processes and speech perception

We saw at the start of this chapter that, as we would expect, pure-tone sensitivity predicts what might be called 'sensitivity loss' for speech quite well; but, more importantly, it does not account for more than about a quarter of the variability of speech-discrimination scores (PTA $\propto 1/DS$, $r \simeq 0.5$, $r^2 = 0.25$). Whereas the 'attenuation' of speech because of sensitivity loss can be largely corrected by amplification (hearing aids), discrimination or the intelligibility of the speech is another matter. The question we must now ask is whether the deterioration in peripheral perceptual processes other than sensitivity loss can be correlated with deterioration in speech perception, and can help us therefore to account for the unexplained variability.

Plausible though the peripheral processes have been as determiners of speech intelligibility, the answer is that the relationships remain to be demonstrated unequivocally. Dreschler and Plomp (1980) studied 10 hearing-impaired children aged between 8 and 13 years, 8 of whom had sensorineural (or mixed) hearing loss of a moderate degree, and 2 of whom had mild conductive hearing loss. Their measures included frequency selectivity (critical bandwidth and critical ratio) and a measure of speech intelligibility for sentences in different levels of speech-spectrum background noise. The speech scores gave a correlation of 0.90 and 0.79 with critical ratio and critical bandwidth respectively; however, correlation between pure-tone hearing loss and speech intelligibility in noise was 0.90 for mean loss and 0.87 for the slope of the loss, so it is difficult to ascribe deterioration in speech intelligibility either to the separate effect of the audiogram (sensitivity loss) or to the separate effect of reduced frequency selectivity. The data of Tyler and Summerfield (1980) is similarly inconclusive: measures of the sharpness of psychoacoustic tuning curves and gap-detection performance correlated well with speech intelligibility (Four Alternative Auditory Feature (FAAF) test of Foster and Haggard, 1979), but 'these analyses do not allow for the effects of other variables (e.g. age, pure-tone threshold), which may mediate [the] correlations' (Tyler and Summerfield 1980, 465).

In a more detailed study Tyler, Wood and Fernandez (1982) examined the relationships between thresholds in the quiet, thresholds in noise, pure-tone masking, psychoacoustic tuning curves, temporal integration, the Fry Word Lists in noise, and FAAF in noise for groups of normal subjects and subjects with cochlear hearing loss. For the latter group, pure-tone thresholds correlated significantly with speech intelligibility (correlations of 0.55, 0.39, 0.48 and 0.64), indicating as always that sensitivity loss can act as a gross indicator of severity of disability, but can account for little over a quarter of the variability in speech scores. Tyler *et al.* assessed psychoacoustic performance at both 0.5 and 4 kHz, and several of the frequency-resolution measures, particularly those measured at 4 kHz, correlated significantly with speech intelligibility. Thus, for example, the low-frequency slope of the PTC at 4 kHz gave a correlation of 0.439 with score on the FAAF speech test. Again, however, much of the variability remains unaccounted for, and again it is not possible to separate the effects of poor frequency resolution from the effects of pure-tone sensitivity loss: score on FAAF correlated with threshold at 4 kHz by $r = 0.643$. When the effect of threshold at 4 kHz on speech intelligibility was partialled out, the correlation between FAAF and PTC low-frequency slope fell from 0.439 to a non-significant 0.184. As the authors note, this does not mean that frequency resolution is unrelated to speech intelligibility, merely that both are correlated highly with pure-tone threshold. Tyler *et al.* also took an estimate of temporal integration by measuring the difference between thresholds for signals of 10 and 1000 ms duration. As we noted previously, the temporal integration scores for the normal and hearing-impaired groups were not different at 500 Hz, but the hearing-impaired listeners were poorer at 4000 Hz. There was however some overlap between the two groups, and much intersubject variability. Nevertheless, a significant correlation between temporal integration at 4000 Hz and pure-tone threshold at 4000 Hz ($r = 0.563$) was found, whereas there was no significant correlation between speech scores on FAAF and temporal integration (there was a low but significant correlation of 0.324 between speech scores on Fry Word Lists and temporal integration).

The relationships between temporal and frequency psychoacoustical tasks and speech discrimination is further elucidated by Tyler, Summerfield, Wood and Fernandez (1982). Multiple regressions of psychoacoustic measures (irrespective of degree of hearing loss) on FAAF percentage correct scores for heterogeneous group of 16 hearing-impaired listeners gave the following multiple R^2 values for the psychoacoustic tasks when included stepwise and cumulatively into the regression: temporal difference threshold at 4 kHz, 0.552; temporal integration at 4 kHz, 0.682; gap-detection at 4 kHz, 0.789; high-frequency slope of PTC at 4 kHz, 0.825; temporal integration at 0.5 kHz, 0.838; and low-frequency slope of PTC at 4 kHz, 0.851. The authors comment that the preponderance of 4 kHz variables found in this best regression analysis 'can be attributed to the emphasis on high-frequency spectral contrasts evident in the consonants of the FAAF test' (Tyler *et al*. 1982, p. 747). In further analyses of their data, Tyler *et al*. examined the correlations between all their psychoacoustic and speech perception measures. As they point out, we know that higher absolute hearing thresholds are correlated with poor PTC tuning, poor temporal processing, and poor speech intelligibility in noise. In order to dissociate the 'attenuation' and the 'distortion' characteristics of hearing loss and their effect on speech perception, interest again centres on those correlations between speech intelligibility and performance on psychoacoustic tasks which remain statistically significant even when the effects of hearing loss are partialled out. In the event, of eight variables with significant correlations with speech in noise performance, only two remained signficant after the effect of hearing loss is removed. These were gap-detection and temporal difference thresholds, giving significant but not high correlations of −0.482 and −0.422 respectively (correlations were −0.732 and −0.743 respectively when pure-tone thresholds are not partialled out). Tyler *et al*. (p. 750) conclude that 'the discrimination of difference in stimulus duration and the detection of gaps of silence may represent two important underlying processes that contribute to the poor speech perception in the hearing impaired'.

Festen and Plomp (1983) examined by correlational technique the relations between a whole series of auditory functions for 22 adults with moderate sensorineural hearing loss. The implications of the results may be somewhat limited by their use of older subjects: average age was 58 years, with one subject aged 72 years. There were 20 auditory measures taken, including audiometric loss, several different measures of frequency resolution and temporal resolution, and speech intelligibility in quiet and noise. A principal components analysis was performed on the correlation matrix of test scores, and it transpired that the scores could be summarized by two significant principal components. Examination of the relationships between individual test scores and these two principal components indicated that tests of frequency resolution formed a cluster which was fairly independent of sensitivity loss. The other significant principal component was centred upon measures which reflected aspects of sensitivity loss. It would have been useful to predict speech intelligibility from the two principal components, but the authors did not attempt this. Instead, they included speech perception performance in the principal components analysis, and found that speech in noise was closely allied to the frequency resolution measures. However, it should be noted that together the two principal components accounted for 65 per cent of the total test variability (48 per cent for the sensitivity loss component and 17 per cent for the frequency resolution component), leaving 35 per cent unaccounted for. The influence of frequency resolution on speech perception has been extensively discussed by Rosen and Fourcin (1986), with the general conclusion that there are significant correlations between measures of frequency resolution and speech perception in noise, but not in quiet. Glasberg and Moore (1989) have confirmed that speech discrimination in quiet is related chiefly to absolute detection thresholds, while discrimination in noise is related more to a range of suprathreshold abilities, including frequency resolution.

At least two reasons may be offered for why we are not yet able to state with much confidence the effect of various perceptual impairments upon speech intelligibility. Firstly, most of the perceptual processes investigated to date correlate highly with pure-tone hearing loss, and few attempts have been made (e.g. with multiple and step-wise regression) to assess the effects separately from sensitivity loss. In view of our starting observation that the successful development of language in hearing-impaired children can vary dramatically between people with similar audiograms, it would be useful to adopt such an approach to try to tease out the independent effects of frequency selectivity, temporal resolution, and so on. If no effects were to be found, one would have to look further afield, to other perceptual and contextual possibilities and, in addition, to social, psychological and educational factors. Secondly, it may be that the use of gross speech-intelligibility scores is not the most appropriate method for investigating the effects of different perceptual processes on speech reception, since normal speech is so far removed in terms of the interactive complexity of its various components – phonetic, semantic, syntactic, contextual etc. – from these simple perceptual processes that direct relationships may be swamped by variability from a variety of other sources. The alternative approach is to simplify the speech perception task such that it becomes easier to relate it to the underlying perceptual process of interest. This approach has been adopted with some success, using speech sounds generated synthetically. Such sounds can have their acoustic properties precisely controlled, thus allowing experimental manipulation of acoustic cues which in natural speech would occur in combination.

Studies with synthetic speech sounds

We saw earlier that the detailed analysis of confusion errors for single phonemes has been used by some investigators. Franks and Daniloff (1973) reviewed studies on vowel confusions, and concluded that hearing-impaired subjects use the same features as normally-hearing subjects. Dreschler and Plomp (1980) studied the perception of eight Dutch vowels by means of triadic comparisons, in which the hearing-impaired subjects had to judge for each triad of vowels which pair was most similar and which pair was most dissimilar. Principal components analyses of the confusion matrices indicated two significant dimensions which could be interpreted as the first and second formant positions, with correlations between dimensions and formants of 0.89 and 0.95. The individual characteristics of vowel perception in this task could thus be summarized by two parameters represented by the amount of F_1 and F_2 information utilized. While some of the listeners relied equally upon F_1 and F_2, others showed distortion of vowel perception, resulting in a high F_1 weighting with a low F_2 weighting. The influence of the pure-tone audiogram is clear here, since all those who made little use of F_2 (i.e. low F_2 weighting) had sloping audiograms with greater degrees of loss in the higher frequencies. However, once again it is difficult to partial out the separate effects of pure-tone sensitivity loss and reduced frequency selectivity, which are significantly correlated with each other. Dreschler (1982) studied the confusion patterns for initial consonants, vowels and final consonants in the presence of background noise. The noise had the effect of impeding the use of low-frequency features such as voicing and F_1 position, and forced them to rely where possible upon higher-frequency cues such as sibilance and F_2 position.

Godfrey and Millay (1978) synthesized test stimuli along a continuum from /be/ to /we/. A sufficient cue for the distinction between the stop /b/ and the glide /w/ is the speed of the formant transitions – the stimuli can be synthesized with formants at the same frequencies and formant transitions at the same starting-point; the only difference between stimuli is then given by the speed with which the formant transition alters. A standard phoneme identification task was used, in which the listener is presented with one of the eight stimuli which make up the continuum from /be/ to /we/ and has to identify the stimulus as either /be/ or /we/. Results can be plotted in terms of the percentage of /be/ responses as a function of stimulus position. Not surprisingly, normally hearing listeners on such tasks typically show 100 per cent /be/ identification for stimuli at one end of the stimulus continuum and zero (i.e. 100 per cent /we/) at the other, with a very steep slope (the 'phoneme boundary') somewhere in the middle. From the theoretical point of view (see Chapter 1), it is of particular interest that, with such speech stimuli, listeners exhibit similar functions when, rather than being forced to identify stimuli as belonging to one or other category, they are asked simply to discriminate two stimuli on any trial – the well established phenomenon of categorical perception of some speech sounds. Godfrey and Millay used the identification task to examine the performance of 15 hearing-impaired listeners with mild to moderate sensitivity loss. Six of their subjects performed poorly and evidenced grossly abnormal identification functions, while the remainder performed normally. The authors concluded that the acoustic cue of formant transitions caused some subjects great difficulty.

They pursued this in a later study (Godfrey and Millay 1980) in which they constructed pairs of contrasts with a hypothesized hierarchy of difficulty with respect to formant transitions. They predicted that the identification of vowels differing only in steady-state formants (e.g. /u/ vs /o/) should represent an easier task for the impaired listener than /ba/ vs /wa/, where the distinction must be based upon the speed of formant transitions. They further predicted that a voiced/stop contrast differing only in place of articulation (/ba/ vs /da/) would present a more difficult task than the stop/glide contrast, since the stop contrast requires that subjects distinguish between very rapid formant transitions using only the direction and/or extent of the frequency change to make the distinction. Schematic spectrograms of the stimuli used are shown in Figure 5.7.

Listeners in the study were 15 moderately cochlear-impaired adults, and a group of normally hearing controls. The latter gave the clearcut identification functions generally expected with forced-choice labelling. The hearing-impaired subjects performed similarly to the normals on the vowel contrasts, somewhat poorer on the stop/glide contrasts, and very poorly on the /ba-da/ contrast. The grouped identification functions for hearing-impaired subjects are shown in Figure 5.8 and these show clearly the deterioration in performance for the hearing-impaired on the predicted more difficult stimuli. Bearing in mind the individual variability in their previous study, Godfrey and Millay also examine individual data. They were able to define the normally hearing identification functions in terms of the mean of the cumulative normal distribution of the identification function. This mean is the centre of the crossover point, or phoneme boundary, and its standard deviation is a measure of variance among the normal subjects. Applying a fairly relaxed criterion, it was found that all the hearing-impaired listeners gave means and standard deviations which were 'normal' for the /u-o/, the /o-a/, and the /ba-wa/ contrasts; 10 (out of 15) gave normal identification for /da-ya/, and only two gave normal identification for /ba-da/.

The authors conclude that sensorineural hearing loss causes difficulty in identifying sounds which are cued by formant transitions, and they imply that the hierarchy of difficulty found from vowels to glides to stops is a reflection of greater difficulty with short-duration stimuli. The impaired subjects could cope with spectral peaks in a steady-state vowel of 190 ms; some were unable to cope when the distinction depended upon the perception of more versus less rapidly changing formants at onset; and almost none were able to cope with identification based upon the perception of the direction and/or extent of rapidly changing formants (several hundred Hz in 40 ms). The question arises as to whether this poor performance is indeed a direct reflection of the inability of the impaired auditory processes effectively to handle formant transitions *per se*, or whether other impaired processes (e.g. masking) are to blame. The latter is a distinct possibility for the /ba-da/ contrast, since in order to identify the stimuli correctly the listeners would have to detect the direction of the frequency change in the second or third formant. The first formant provides no useful cue for distinction of /ba/ from /da/, whereas it could be used (as could F_2 and F_3) for the separation of /ba/ from /wa/ and /da/ from /ya/ (see Fig. 5.7). The F_2 and F_3 transitions are located at higher frequencies and have lower relative amplitudes than the F_1 transitions, and this of course could disadvantage the hearing-impaired listeners. Furthermore, Danaher and Pickett's study (1975) showed that sensorineurally impaired listeners' ability to resolve the higher formants was severely reduced in the presence of lower formants, because of abnormal upward spread of masking.

To decide whether the greater difficulties encountered by the hearing-impaired listeners with the place of articulation distinction in /ba-da/ is due to problems with rapid transitions *per se* or due to other effects such as upward spread of the F_1 masking, it may be that we have to revert to experiments requiring purely

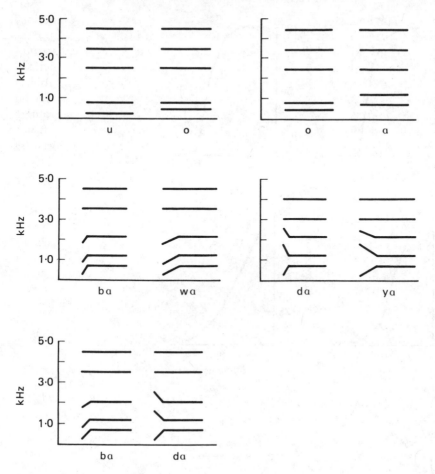

Figure 5.7   Schematic spectrograms of the endpoint stimuli used by Godfrey and Millay (1980, Fig. 1).

perceptual, rather than linguistic, discriminations. One possible approach would be to examine the ability of subjects to deal with unidirectional frequency-modulated sweeps (e.g. Gardner and Wilson 1979). The observer could be asked to discriminate a short (e.g. 40 ms) signal which changes in frequency (an upward or a downward sweep) from a similarly short signal which does not change in frequency. The ability of listeners to do this as a function of the duration of the signals and/or the rate of change of the sweep would throw light on their ability to handle rapid transitions in isolation. The importance of this ability is evidenced by the role transitions play in linguistic contrasts (e.g. /ba-da/), and also by the role which they may play in preventing the auditory streaming of Bregman and Campbell (1971). The tendency for the normal auditory system to stream a series of short tones of varying frequency into high and low-frequency streams, such that the temporal order of the tones is able to be preserved within but not between

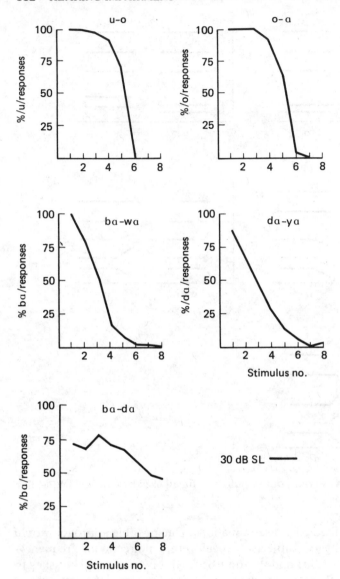

Figure 5.8 Identification functions for the five identification tasks by Godfrey and Millay's hearing-impaired listeners ($n = 12$ for /u-o/, $n = 15$ for all others) (from Godfrey and Millay 1980, Fig. 3).

streams, was discussed in Chapter 1. Bregman and Dannenbring (1973) showed that if short glides (transitions) were added to the tones such that the frequency transitions 'pointed' towards the next tone in the series, then order information between all tones (high or low) could be preserved – i.e. auditory streaming was much reduced.

There have in fact been few reported studies of the discrimination of short-duration tone glides with normally hearing subjects, and almost none with the hearing-impaired. Van Bergeijk (1964), Nabelek (1978), Collins and Cullen (1978) and Cullen and Collins (1982) have studied the perception of tone glides in the normally hearing. Cullen and Collins (1982) measured thresholds for rising and falling frequency sweeps presented at 60 dB SPL. The sweeps were centred around 2000 Hz, and changed frequency linearly at rates of 24, 48, 96 and 192 Hz/ms over durations of 5, 10, 20 and 40 ms. The design of the study aimed to minimize the confounding effects of signal duration and frequency change, and the results indicated that the rate of frequency change is the primary determinant of performance. They also found that rising glides were detected more easily than an explanation for this effect in terms of basilar-membrane mechanics; this may be incidental to the present discussion, although it could be a factor in the greater difficulty of the hearing-impaired listeners in Godfrey and Millay's (1980) study with the /da-ya/ distinction than the /ba-wa/ distinction, since in /ba-wa/ all three formant transitions are rising while in /da-ya/ two of the three transitions are falling (see Fig. 5.7, p. 111).

As far as hearing-impaired subjects are concerned, Thyer (1984) studied 10 adults with mild to moderate degrees of sensitivity loss on a same–different task in which listeners are required to discriminate isolated frequency glides. Performance was compared with a group of normally hearing listeners at both the same sensation level and the same sound-pressure level. The glides were chosen to be similar to the F_1 and F_2 formant transitions in Godfrey and Millay's (1980) study. Godfrey and Millay's explanation of their data – that hearing-impaired listeners exhibit perceptual difficulties in processing rapid frequency transitions – was not upheld, since the hearing-impaired listeners performed as well as the normally hearing controls; furthermore, they gave near-perfect performance on the condition in which they had to discriminate upward-going from downward-going very rapid transitions (as in the /ba-da/ discrimination). Tyler et al. (1983) found different thresholds for frequency glides of 2.7 Hz/ms for hearing-impaired listeners compared with 1.2 Hz/ms for normal hearing listeners. Thus, although hearing-impaired performance was worse, it was quite good enough to cope with the 5 and 10 Hz/ms slopes used in Thyer's study, and the similar slopes used by Godfrey and Millay (1980). Other explanations for Godfrey and Millay's results have therefore to be sought, and as we have noted upward spread of masking of F_2 by F_1 is one possibility, and there may be others. In any event, the interesting point is that here is a case where the isolated perceptual task is not impaired, yet when embedded in linguistic–perceptual context the task is impaired relative to normally hearing performance. If speech perception involves central pattern-recognition processes working on a complex peripheral input which in hearing-impaired ears is degraded, it is of considerable interest to know how well the hearing-impaired can process isolated features of the peripheral input pattern. If in isolation these can be processed effectively, it points a way forward to signal-processing hearing aids which could be designed to isolate aspects of the complex pattern in order to aid perception.

What aspects of the context of compound stimuli are responsible for poor discrimination performance are not yet clear; Gordon-Salant and Wightman (1983) studied different types of masking stimuli and suggested from their results that intelligibility differences in the presence of competing segments of speech are 'primarily attributable to phonetic interference rather than to spectral masking' (p. 1756). Let us return, therefore, to a consideration of studies which use the discrimination of linguistic, rather than purely perceptual, stimuli in an attempt to elucidate impaired speech perception in hearing-impaired listeners.

While it is to be hoped that explanations in terms of purely perceptual processes will be forthcoming, it has become necessary to use synthesized linguistic segments in certain circumstances. In so doing one trades the simplicity of isolated acoustic parameters for the realism of more complex stimuli (e.g. multiple formants) which involve phonemic decisions.

Apart from sheer complexity, one source of realism of linguistic stimuli is that the acoustic cues they contain are context-dependent. A similar argument can be applied against the use of distinctive-feature analyses. Distinctive features (such as place, manner, voicing) are linguistic properties which characterize a phonetic segment independent of context, and they thus have limited value in assessing the perception of context-dependent cues. The linguistic status of voiced versus unvoiced stops is the same, be they in syllable-initial or syllable-final position; but hearing-impaired listeners might be expected to handle the voiced/unvoiced distinction more easily in syllable-final position, where substantial differences in vowel duration are available, than in syllable-initial position, where the relevant cue is to be found in very small differences in voice-onset time (VOT). It is therefore the underlying acoustic cues and their processing rather than the linguistic features alone which are likely to lead to a fuller understanding of impaired speech perception. A recent notable example is a study by Revoile et al. (1982), in which a number of detailed acoustic cues to final-stop consonant voicing (vowel duration, occlusion duration, presence of voiced murmur, and the offset transitions of the vowel formants) were progressively neutralized; the results indicated that vowel transitions are an important cue to correct perception, but that the hearing-impaired subjects may rely relatively more on the vowel-duration cue – further evidence, incidentally, of the possible importance of processing of temporal cues compared with frequency cues.

Parady et al. (1981) studied the identification and discrimination of an initial stop-consonant voicing contrast (/da/ vs /ta/) in children with moderate, severe and profound hearing loss of sensorineural pathology, in order to see whether the pathology affects the perception of VOT for the voicing contrast in the same way as it clearly affects the perception of the acoustic cues for place contrasts. The cue for the identification of an initial consonant as voiceless is a lag in the time of onset of the first formant relative to the time of onset of the second and third formants. For normal listeners, an onset asynchrony of the formants of about 25 ms defines the phoneme boundary between /d/ and /t/. Parady et al. found that the perceptual boundary between /da/ and /ta/ did not differ between normal listeners and those with moderate sensitivity losses, whereas of 10 listeners with severe sensitivity losses, three showed longer than normal boundaries and two could not identify the stimuli at all. Of three listeners with profound hearing losses, one could identify normally and the other two could not identify at all. In a few cases the listeners who were unable to identify the stimuli *were* able to discriminate between them, and the authors argued that these subjects had the 'auditory capacity' to resolve differences in VOT but could not use this capacity to make phonetic identifications. It is of considerable interest that these difficulties with auditory temporal resolution were not directly related to sensitivity loss, and this may therefore be one cause of the variability in speech perception ability which is left unaccounted for by pure-tone hearing loss. Parady *et al.* examined their subjects post hoc, and speculated that factors such as early amplification or later onset of hearing loss (e.g. at age three rather than age one year) might be important for the formation of central representations of phonetic categories, and might lead to normal identification ability in the face of profound hearing loss.

The finding that for some impaired listeners discrimination was better than identification suggests that the two tasks may tap different auditory phonetic processes. This view is supported by the findings of Tyler and Summerfield (1980) who used VOT continua (rather than the fixed 30-ms differences in VOT used by Parady *et al.*) to study identification and discrimination of /ba/ vs /pa/ and /bi/ vs /pi/ in normal and moderately sensorineurally impaired listeners. Identification performance by subjects with moderate degrees of sensitivity loss was similar to that of the normally hearing listeners, but in a VOT difference threshold task (i.e. discrimination rather than identification) the performance of the two groups was different, with the hearing-impaired unable to match the fine discriminations of the normally hearing listeners.

In a study of 35 language-impaired and 38 normally developing children aged between 5 and 8 years, Tallal and Stark (1981) examined the discrimination of a variety of speech stimuli which involved the use of various spectral and temporal cues. Both groups of subjects had normal hearing sensitivity, and were matched by age, performance IQ and socioeconomic status. They differed only in terms of receptive and expressive language ages. The results showed that the language-impaired children made most errors discriminating syllables which were differentiated by consonants and fewest errors on those differentiated by vowels; they performed significantly worse than the normal children in discriminating syllables that incorporated brief temporal cues followed rapidly in succession by other acoustic cues. These findings accord with those from an earlier study on language-impaired children (Tallal and Piercy 1975), which showed them to be specifically impaired on tasks of discrimination, sequencing and serial memory when stimuli were presented rapidly. When stimuli were presented more slowly, performance improved. The authors argued that it was the brevity rather than the transitional nature of the formant spectra that accounted for discrimination difficulties, because when the duration of the formant transitions for stop consonants was extended, performance improved.

The results from these two studies and others on language-impaired children point to dysfunctions and deficits in central auditory processes unaccompanied by obvious peripheral sensitivity loss. Once again, therefore, we have evidence for the possibility that auditory processes other than simple sensitivity loss can be impaired, and that such other deficits may go some way towards accounting for the discrepancies between pure-tone hearing and speech perception. The term 'hearing loss' is widely interpreted in terms of peripheral sensitivity loss. Audiology in both its diagnostic and rehabilitative role is heavily committed to this view, perhaps understandably. It is clear, however, that a more proper view of hearing must take account not only of auditory sensitivity but for other more complex processes and of centrally mediated processes.

Concluding remarks

Although this chapter has examined some of the evidence for speech perception difficulties in the hearing-impaired by recourse to studies using linguistic stimuli, in particular the phonetic segments which lie near the surface of language, nevertheless much of our approach has been to try to account for speech-perception problems in terms of purely psychoacoustic deficits. This does seem to us to be particularly appropriate to the hearing-impaired whose deficit is, in the first instance at any rate, largely perceptual rather than linguistic. The interfacing of molecular-level auditory deficits with molecular-level phonetic/linguistic deficits is an unresearched area of great promise for the study of hearing impairment. The last decade or so has seen considerable advances in our knowledge of auditory perceptual processes. In particular, it is now clear that a considerable amount of quite sophisticated processing takes place at the periphery. Thus, for example, frequency resolution is fully coded by the level of the auditory nerve, and is largely realized at the level of hair-cell microsystems. With regard to people with cochlear hearing-impairments, the evidence clearly shows perceptual deficits not only in terms of sensitivity loss (elevated thresholds) and intensity coding, but deficits in both frequency analysis and temporal analysis. Frequency and temporal information is known to provide crucial cues for the perception of speech signals.

Despite these marked advances in our knowledge about normal and impaired audition, the goal of accounting for variability in speech-perception ability between hearing-impaired individuals remains elusive. Correlating speech-perception performance with performance on various perceptual tasks other than sensitivity loss in hearing-impaired listeners has not allowed us to account for speech-perception ability much better than by using sensitivity loss alone. Broadly speaking, measures of frequency discrimination and resolution tend to add little to prediction of speech-hearing from pure-tone loss.

We are unlikely to forget that the interfacing of auditory and phonemic deficits may not be so easy to discover as we might imagine. Liberman (1981) has argued strongly in favour of the 'speech is special' view, and that the processes underlying speech perception are not simply auditory in the sense of being the same processes which underlie the perception of the rustle of leaves in the wind (or unidirectional frequency sweeps for example). For Liberman and others, the processes underlying language perception are biologically specialized for the task. In support of this view, Liberman quotes a number of studies, one of which we will briefly describe (Mann *et al*. 1981). If one or other of nine possible third-formant transitions from the continuum which describes the contrast from /da/ to /ga/ is presented in isolation to one ear (normally hearing listeners) it will be heard as a time-varying 'chirp' – that is, 'like reasonably faithful auditory reflections of the time-varying acoustic signal' (Liberman 1981, 115). The 'bases' of the two phonemes /da/ and /ga/ – that is, the first two formants and all but the initial transition of the third formant – are identical, and if this base is presented to the other ear in isolation it will be heard as one or other of the stop-vowel syllables. If the two stimuli are now presented dichotically there is a double percept: first of |/da/ or /ga/, depending upon the identity of the isolated transition on one ear, secondly of a non-speech-like chirp. Furthermore, when these dichotically presented stimuli are presented as part of a typical discrimination paradigm, the listener will give a typical discrimination function which matches the phoneme-identification function, with a high peak reflecting the phoneme boundary. However, this occurs only if the listener's attention is drawn towards the speech-like nature of the 'stimulus'. If, however, attention is drawn towards the non-speech or 'chirp' aspect of the percept, the discrimination function becomes continuous: acoustic rather than phonetic. 'The integration of the formant transition into a phonetic percept is owing to a special process that makes available to perception a unitary phonetic object well suited to its role in language' (Liberman 1981, p. 117).

This view of perception suggests that when we see an object, we do not 'see' a range of visual cues and features which are somehow synthesized into the appropriate percept. Rather we have a range of experience of such objects which, at least in the adult, enables us to go straight to a categorical perception, ignoring many of the underlying cues. Likewise, normally hearing adults have implicit experience and knowledge of the vocal tract, and percepts of linguistic units such as phonemes may be determined and constrained by this knowledge (i.e. the phonetic mode) in such a way that underlying nonlinguistic cues may be partially or wholly irrelevant.

This compelling view, that speech is special, has tended to focus research interest and activity on linguistic rather than perceptual processes. While this is perhaps understandable from the point of view of the normally hearing, it has rather left alone the acoustic–preceptual side of things. For the hearing-impaired this is a pity, and we have seen in this chapter how the impetus of the needs of this group has begun to encourage interest in the perceptual end of the chain. Nevertheless, if in the end speech perception has to be accounted for by reference to processes which cannot be wholly or adequately described in acoustic terms, then we must be aware of this. And if this is the case, it will be of great importance to discover the biology of speech perception from developmental and crosscultural studies. We will need to know what has developed by evolution of the human species, and what therefore remains to develop in the history of the individual (see Chap. 2). The impaired perceptual processing of those with a hearing loss then comes to have a further significance – not only for its degradation of the acoustic input, but for its interference with the optimum development of the phonetic mode.

6

Language disability and sensorineural hearing loss

The heterogeneity of 'hearing impairment'

It is as well to open this chapter with a cautionary note regarding the heterogeneity of children with prelingual sensorineural hearing losses. Degree of peripheral sensitivity loss can vary from mild through to profound, and although the number of children with partial hearing losses is greater than the number with severe and profound hearing losses, the research emphasis has been directed more towards the severe end of the range. Configuration of the hearing loss, in terms of the sensitivity to different acoustic frequencies, can vary widely. Individual differences in other auditory perceptual skills (see Chapter 5) can be large. Onset of the hearing loss may be congenital, or it may be congenitally determined but progressive in its manifestation. We have restricted our terms of reference to children with prelingual impairments, but a precise definition of prelingual is elusive. In the USA census of 1910, 'deaf mutes' were defined as children losing their hearing at any time before the age of 8 years; and Reamer (1921) observed from her data that 'onset of deafness before age six makes no difference in later educational work' as compared with onset at birth.

As the significance of language acquisition in the early years and even in the early months of life has come to be realized, so our estimate of the length of the 'prelingual stage' of development has had to be shortened. It is, of course, futile to attempt to be specific about the dividing line, but we can now be sure that normal hearing for the first year of life will confer linguistic advantages compared with congenital onset. The delay between onset and diagnosis (or at least identification of a hearing loss) is another source of variability between individuals, since it is only at the latter point that amplification and other rehabilitative and educational procedures get underway. In addition social, emotional and educational factors are likely to be atypical and variable, and the psychological strategies which a hearing-impaired child develops in order to make sense of the world will be to some degree idiosyncratic. Always, therefore, the reader should beware of thinking of 'the deaf' or 'the hearing impaired' as a homogeneous group with similar patterns of behaviour and a common 'hearing-impaired language'.

Background and underlying issues

In view of the heated debate about the efficacy of oral, manual and 'total

118

communication' methods of education for the hearing-impaired, it is perhaps surprising that relatively little rigorous work has been published on the language of hearing-impaired children and its acquisition. In this chapter we will consider and review what we know of spoken-language comprehension and spoken-language expression in children who suffer from bilateral sensorineural hearing loss of congenital or prelingual onset.

Reference to language expression as evidenced by the written word has been a favoured approach of some workers, and we shall refer to it where necessary, although it is not the case that spoken and written language skills tap identical processes. However, while some reviewers (e.g. Kretschmer and Kretschmer 1978) do make a distinction between written and spoken language, the clarity of that distinction may not always be great. Thus, for example, a number of studies have used highly controlled written responses to examine the underlying knowledge of linguistic rules by the hearing-impaired (e.g. Cooper 1967 for morphological rules). Such studies merely use a very restricted written response as a convenient way of getting at rule knowledge: in the context of short-duration morphological items, spoken responses would be unreliable. Studies which make use of such controlled written responses will not be treated separately in this chapter from spoken-language studies. Research into the language of free written responses (e.g. as in picture description, or free composition) *is* clearly distinguishable, and there is ample evidence that the linguistic data from this source are qualitatively different from spoken language data in hearing-impaired children. Free written responses will therefore be given separate consideration, although not in the first part of the chapter where earlier studies (roughly pre-1970) are reviewed, since these studies are so few, the data generally so global, and the implications so limited as to render separate treatment worthless. Comprehension of the written word (reading) will be reserved for consideration in Chapter 8. Non-verbal sign languages used by a proportion of the hearing-impaired population are not part of the subject-matter of this book and will not therefore be discussed (see, however, Schlesinger and Namir 1978, Woll *et al.* 1981).

It would be attractive to the tidy mind to be able to organize this chapter on the same basis as Chapter 3, in which (despite its interactive nature) we are able to summarize normal language development under the successive headings: the earliest stages; phonological development, segmental and then non-segmental; vocabulary; grammar; and contextual aspects of language development. Work with hearing-impaired children is less advanced and is not so easily sectioned. The overwhelming emphasis remains (rather like the normal language studies of the 1960s) on grammar and vocabulary, with the primary aim, intended or not, of providing a comprehensive description of these aspects of the language of hearing-impaired children. This descriptive approach uses normal language development as a comparator and essentially attempts to answer the question '*What* are the stages of language development in hearing-impaired children?' Great interest has focused upon the issues of whether the language of the hearing-impaired is simply delayed or whether it is 'deviant' with regard to normal language acquisition, and much effort has been expended in collecting large amounts of descriptive normative data.

This chapter will review this work in some detail, but in so doing we do not intend the reader to be seduced into regarding this approach as necessarily the most useful or the most appropriate. It has its limitations. In particular it may tell you 'what' but it does not tell you 'how' or 'why'. The language of a hearing-impaired child may be 'delayed' by comparison with the normal sequence of development; but whether it really is appropriate to view his language skills as the same as those of a younger normally hearing child is very doubtful. There are other cognitive processes which may be quite different and more sophisticated, and what may be called the component processes underlying language development in the two children may be utterly dissimilar. In other words, the descriptive normative approach tells us little about *how* language develops in the hearing-impaired and the nature of the underlying processes. To ask the first, descriptive 'what' question is thoroughly justifiable, but is really a preliminary. Certainly, before we can find out how children learn language, we must first determine what it is they have learned (Braine 1963). But if we find that language is delayed, deviant or whatever, and by how much, the question about how and why this occurs automatically follows. The significance of this question is that the answers are likely to reveal something about the underlying processes which will have implications for rehabilitative and educational strategies. The descriptive approach, using normal language development as a model, tells us what is wrong – which is important. It tells us that hearing-impairment is associated with poor language performance, and it can describe in detail the nature of this performance deficit. However, it does not tell us *why* it is wrong (except in the broadest sense – i.e. because of hearing impairment), and therefore it will be unlikely to point to possible remedial pathways.

Ivimey (1982) has listed six questions to which research in this area must be directed, and the traditional descriptive approach provides us with information relevant to only two or three of these questions:

(i) What do hearing-impaired children actually produce in the way of language?

(ii) What changes, if any, can we perceive in their language productions as they grow older?

(iii) How are their linguistic productions related to the use and development of language by hearing children?

(iv) Are the differences to be seen between the communicative performance of deaf and hearing children due to delays in normal development, or do they represent a totally deviant system; indeed, do they represent any system whatsoever?

(v) How may any observed differences between the deaf and hearing most reasonably be explained?

(vi) What, if anything, can be done to improve the situation?

The descriptive approach to the study of hearing-impaired language has concentrated on questions *(i)*, *(ii)* and *(iii)*, and tended to ignore the remainder, which in the final analysis may be more important.

The descriptive approach continually emphasizes comparisons with normal language development. That may be appropriate, and it is something with which speech pathologists would feel familiar. It has, however, been called the 'normalization conspiracy' by some (Merrill 1979) which leads, they say, to an effort to focus the education of deaf children onto the development of hearing and speech skills, rather than on traditional educational goals (i.e. achievement in substantive fields such as literature, mathematics and science). On the other hand, one could argue that the cavalier dismissal of comparisons with normally hearing children as irrelevant may lead to lowered expectations on the part of teachers, resulting in lower levels of success by the hearing-impaired pupils. The wide implications of the approach one adopts are clear.

The chapter will examine the descriptive research which makes up the historical background to work in this area; in so doing we may appear to over-emphasize the usefulness of this approach. We so not wish to do so, and the relative emphasis here must be taken as simply reflecting the volume of published work. Only recently has the nature of the learning processes themselves been studied, and although we consider this a major advance the space devoted to it will be somewhat less, since published studies are yet few. The foregoing might be taken to imply that a large amount of work has been reported on the descriptive approach, not just relative to the more contemporary studies (which is true) but in absolute terms as well. This is not so. Bearing in mind the heterogeneity of the hearing impaired child population, in terms of age, hearing loss, background, and so on, there are insufficient data to allow us yet to give a comprehensive description of the development of language in the various groups. Furthermore, what studies there are of language skills in hearing-impaired children have tended to be static, one-off looks at a particular group: longitudinal developmental studies have been rare. Thus, as we shall see, we are nowhere near yet fulfilling even a developmental description of the language of hearing-impaired children.

Poor language performance associated with sensorineural hearing loss comes about not only because of depletion of sensory input – the 'primary' cause – but also because of associated secondary effects which may be just as important. These secondary effects are concerned with the contextual aspects of language acquisition. Contextual aspects can be divided into processes which are external to the individual – adult–child interactions, turn-taking, adult control of the communication process in the face of reduced communicative abilities in the child, and so on – and processes which are internal. Recent research has begun to be directed towards the external contextual aspects of language development in the hearing-impaired, in an attempt to go beyond the descriptive 'what' and to understand the 'how' of language disability, and we shall examine these research trends later in the chapter.

Internal contextual aspects of language development, that is, the cognitive processes and strategies brought to bear by the hearing-impaired child in the face of reduced sensory input, have a rather longer history, and it is possible to discern two distinct trends in the literature. One approach, examplified by Myklebust (1964), takes the view that the depleted auditory input of the child with sensorineural hearing impairment results in qualitatively different cognitive processes, which not only give poor verbal language performance but more significantly, perhaps, impose theoretical limitations on the further development of normal spoken-language skills. In order to make sense of the world in the face of severely depleted auditory input, it is argued that the child learns to rely on alternative sensory modalities, and in so doing fundamentally alters his developing linguistic and cognitive processes. Myklebust examined evidence from tasks of intellectual development, personality development and language behaviour. In the first category, for example, he looked at a variety of memory tasks such as digit span, picture span, memory for movement and so on. He found distinct differences between the deaf and hearing and argued that 'if the memory task, visual or tactual, does not lend itself to auditory associations, the deaf are superior . . . . This highlights the shift in psychological organization which results from the sensory deprivation of deafness.'

With regard to deafness and language behaviour, Myklebust demonstrated that the mean sentence length of spoken language of the deaf in response to pictures increased only slightly with age (7–15 years) and was markedly less than that of hearing controls; score on a syntax measure produced similar results; and scores on a scale reflecting the use of concrete rather than abstract ideation showed the deaf to be significantly more concrete (and less abstract) in their thought than hearing children of the same ages. Myklebust concluded (p. 385) that 'sensory deprivation alters the psychological response mechanisms of the individual . . . . There seem to be important implications for the "laws of learning" for those who have sensory impairments.' This tradition, with its pinpointing of possible theoretical limitations to aural language development, has been used by some to support the notion that the way forward to more adequate communicative skills must be via non-aural languages – that is, via sign language of some description.

The second and quite distinct approach to language and deafness adopts the view that prelingually hearing-impaired children possess normal cognitive processes but suffer from general restrictions in experience, interactions, and opportunities to learn (Furth 1964, 1966a). This view suggests that if adequate linguistic experience can be provided, language development will be essentially normal, although very likely delayed, and it is quoted by those who believe that an aural/oral approach to language teaching and general education in the hearing-impaired is appropriate. Furth (1964) reviewed a number of studies on deaf people's performance on cognitive tasks of various kinds; on the majority of tasks (25 out of 43) the deaf performance was not inferior, while on the remaining 17 tasks it was inferior. Furth argued that an explanation of experiential deficiency would seem to be a parsimonious one in understanding these results: the reduced performance on the minority of tasks reviewed could be attributed either to a lack of general experience or to specific task conditions which favour linguistic skills. Furth (1966a) examined the performance of the deaf on a number of Piagetian tasks, and argued that any observed deficits on such tasks are due to limited linguistic skills rather than to altered conceptual or cognitive structures. Thus, for example, the failure of deaf children to demonstrate an understanding of the concept of conservation of quantity until about 5 years later than normally hearing children is attributed to cultural deprivation and limited linguistic skills, rather than to a general cognitive deficit. It is also clear that performance on such tasks does often improve with age, without any obvious improvement in language, and this is argued to support the view that cognitive development is delayed rather than changed by deafness.

The issue of which of these two approaches is correct remains very open. Partly this is due to the lack of homogeneity of 'the deaf', who may have been deafened at different ages and by different degrees, who may have been exposed to different educational strategies, different social and psychological backgrounds and different amounts of amplification via hearing aids. But also it is due to a past reliance upon descriptive studies of hearing-impaired language. One of the reasons for recent disenchantment with the descriptive approach to the study of language development in hearing-impaired people is that descriptive studies merely extend our quantification of what is wrong, but, as we said before, do little to help us understand why this is so and do little therefore to resolve the issue of cognitive limitations versus reduced experience.

It is of course well known in the fields of deaf education that although the issue remains open, minds do not. The schisms between those who advocate oral/aural methods of education, those who hold that these must be supplemented by manual systems (total communication approaches) and, more recently, truly bilingual approaches, continue to divide the deaf education world, to the undoubted detriment of the hearing-impaired child. Educational research comparing different methods of intervention is notoriously difficult to control adequately in the normally hearing; in the hearing-impaired, the problems of adequate control and unwanted variability which are discussed by Kretschmer and Kretschmer (1978) are almost insurmountable. The failure of such studies to achieve a consensus is clear, and faced with the evident lack of success (compared with normally developed language skills) of a particular approach to teaching, a proponent of that approach is able to claim that its poor success is due not to any theoretical or underlying limitations but simply to poor educational practice. The occasional highly successful pupil is always there 'to show what can be achieved'.

Faced with this blind alley, researchers have begun to turn away therefore from purely educational research to studies which may throw light on the underlying processes themselves, and which may pinpoint unequivocal limitations to cognitive or even physiological processes. Thus, the recent interest in external contextual aspects of language in the hearing-impaired has shown that some of these aspects (e.g. adult–child interactions) are different for such children, and indeed there is some evidence that with suitable intervention these aspects *can* be altered in such a way as to have beneficial effects (Wood 1982). Studies on the internal contextual aspects of language performance (e.g. cognitive variables) in the hearing-impaired continue to be of importance for resolving the fundamental issues; many of these relate to reading ability (e.g. Conrad 1979) and will be covered in Chapter 8.

There have been a number of studies in which animals have been deprived of auditory inputs at or shortly after birth. Deprivation has sometimes been total, sometimes partial (e.g. induced conductive losses in the 30–40 dB range). Kyle (1978), Ruben (1980) and Webster (1982) have reviewed these studies, which in general terms provide convincing evidence for physiological (neuronal) degeneration in the auditory pathways, possibly irreversible although this is by no means certain, consequent upon the auditory deprivation. Some workers (e.g. Conrad 1980) quote the animal auditory deprivation studies as evidence of theoretical limitations imposed by deafness, and propose that the poor verbal language skills of deaf children are related to disturbance of neurological function.

The early animal studies were concerned with total sensory deprivation, and their relevance to hearing impairment in humans was open to question on the grounds that hearing loss is only very rarely total. Bench (1979a) for example, argued that, since most hearing-impaired humans are only partially deprived, the problem was one of linguistic rather than sensory deprivation (i.e. an 'extrinsic' rather than an 'intrinsic' problem). (This 'linguistic deprivation' view has also been proposed by Conrad (1980), but in addition to the sensory deprivation hypothesis, not instead of it.) Bench quoted the celebrated case of Genie (Fromkin *et al.* 1974), a severely environmentally deprived child who only began hearing language in early adolescence, and who less than two years after discovery showed considerable and ongoing advances in receptive and expressive language skills. Bench argued that this case points to the reversible nature of linguistic deprivation given adequate rehabilitation procedures, and he therefore pointed an accusing finger at the inadequacy of the rehabilitative procedures used with hearing-impaired children. In fact later reports of Genie (Curtiss 1977) indicate that the extent of language function *was* restricted, and that language acquisition was slower and more tediously learned than in normal acquisition. These later observations do incidentally support the notion of an optimum period for language acquisition: maximum language growth is apparently facilitated during a period characterized by rapid and flexible development of neurological maturity, the so-called period of resonance between 2 and 12 years (Lenneberg 1967).

Bench's arguments against the involvement of sensory deprivation have been superseded somewhat by the more recent evidence from animal studies, which shows that structural changes may occur as a result of *partial* hearing loss, and suggests that the defence that all will be well if hearing aids are fitted (e.g. Arnold 1982) may be a rather complacent view. Identification of congenital hearing impairment is unfortunately still often not made until after the first birthday at least, and there is therefore considerable time during which the congenitally hearing-impaired child is without hearing aids. Furthermore, since for a variety of reasons (including the reduced dynamic range typically associated with sensorineural hearing loss) it is not the aim to use hearing aids to restore normal detection levels (i.e. 0 dB HL or thereabouts), partial 'loss' will remain even when aids are worn. Although the precise relevance of the animal studies is still open to debate, it is now hard to resist the prudent view that central physiological and morphological changes may occur as a result of peripheral pathology.

Webster (1983) has argued that the two approaches – one that hearing impairment gives rise to qualitatively distinct cognitive processes which impose theoretical limitations, the other that hearing-impaired children have normal cognitive abilities but are the victims of reduced experience and reduced opportunities for learning – are extremes, and that a more 'serviceable' view is midway between the two:

> If . . . the nature of early interactions and early experience of the deaf child are atypical, then this will be reflected in the psychological strategies which the child develops in order to make sense of the world. At the same time, since there is also evidence that some parents and teachers are more gifted than others, and that some teaching strategies adopted by some schools are much more effective than others (Wood 1982), then we must be cautious about accepting an overly pessimistic view.

We saw in Chapter 3 that the current views of the relationships between language and cognition eschews both the extreme Whorfian notion that, put simply, language determines cognition and the more recently influential Piagetian theory that language development follows on and is significantly determined by cognitive development; rather, the relationship is seen as interdependent and interactive, with development on one front having implications for development on the other. The pragmatic view taken by Webster (1983) with regard to language development in hearing-impaired children can be seen as more analogous to current notions of language and thought in normal development than either of the two extreme views. Webster's reference to pessimism about language development reflects the accusation that the Myklebust (1964) tradition, emphasizing as it does cognitive deficiencies resultant upon prelingual deafness which impose absolute limitations to the potential success of verbal language development, is an essentially pessimistic theory, at least *in extremis*.

In fact, the accusation could be levelled at either approach: Arnold (1982), for example, in a defence of the oral approach to deaf education, argues that the language disability of deaf children is due to deafness *per se* and that 'deafness imposes a constellation of handicaps on a schoolchild, which developmentally interact together. Word meaning, morphology, syntax and semantics are all difficult to acquire . . . . We do not know in any detail why the majority of deaf children find speaking, reading, writing and arithmetic so difficult' (p. 284). It is tempting to regard *this* view as fundamentally pessimistic, with the implications of the alternative view – that recourse to non-verbal languages offers a way of circumventing or avoiding cognitive deficits which come about by an insistence on solely oral input in the face of profound deafness – as somehow optimistic, since they offer the potential of full communicative competence, albeit largely within a restricted (i.e. deaf) community. Further discussion of this deep-rooted pedagogic controversy is, however, beyond the remit of this book; interested readers are referred to, for example, Quigley and Kretschmer (1982). Suffice it to say that the charge of inherent pessimism can be levelled against proponents of either view, but such charges are rather unproductive. We need to extend our knowledge about the nature of language disabilities of hearing-impaired children and, perhaps more importantly, about the secondary or underlying processes involved in these deficits; only then are we likely to gain insight into those rehabilitative routes which offer a successful way forward. These are major issues, not simply pedagogic. What is meant by the foregoing phrase 'a successful way forward' will be influenced by individual moral and philosophical views; the results by which people achieve independence, growth, compassion, humour, opportunity and access to power are highly relevant, and it is this wider context that determines people's views on the efficacy of different approaches, including positive images of deafness and sign language as an appropriate way forward for some.

We will proceed in this chapter to study the 'what' of the language disability, and then discuss the 'how' and 'why' of the process. One thing to point out at this stage is that the majority of work has been done with severely or profoundly hearing-impaired children, and it is to this population that the issue of 'qualitatively different' or simply 'restricted' particularly applies. Partially hearing children (who make up a much larger group) are generally able with suitable amplification to manage quite well with an oral education and often with full integration in normal schools. Language-development research on this group has been somewhat limited, perhaps because their educational/communicative success is more assured, perhaps because they present as less 'pure' example of sensory deprivation than those who are profoundly impaired, and may therefore be of less interest to the theoretical cognitive researchers. This research neglect is unfortunate, and what studies there have been cannot, as we shall see, lead to a complacent view of the effects of partial hearing loss on language.

Definitions of profoundly deaf and partially hearing vary from study to study and many published reports contain data from subject samples representing a whole range of hearing losses from mild or moderate to profound in degree. To organize into neat categories of 'deaf: written vocabulary' or 'partially hearing: spoken grammer' would therefore be difficult; but more than that it would in the end give a somewhat sterile compartmentalized view, consisting of many rather separate little pieces. For these reasons the literature will be discussed under broad headings, but it is hoped that the framework of normal language development discussed in Chapter 3, and the introductory comments to the present chapter which have outlined some of the important issues, will allow the reader to organize the material in a coherent manner.

Early studies

It is customary to acknowledge the contribution of the pioneers in a given field of study, but it always poses the problem of deciding where historical interest ends and current theories begin. Certainly it is a trifle harsh to regard all the studies prior to 1970 as being of mainly historical interest; much of the published work in earlier days laid down important (if only descriptive) data for later theorists. Nevertheless, since we wish to give particular emphasis to current views, say in the last decade or so, we have chosen to deal less comprehensively with the work prior to 1970.

Early and extensive studies of deaf school children by Pintner (e.g. 1928) and his associates (Reamer 1921) represent the first attempts to quantify their educational retardation; the results indicated severe delays compared with hearing children, and started the line of thought which culminated much later in the 'simply restricted' (albeit severely) view of deaf language skills. Reamer concluded that not only were the deaf retarded educationally by five years on average, but that deaf children exhibit mental retardation of about two years. Pintner found that the average deaf child of age 12–15 years achieved levels on educational tests equivalent to 8- to 9-year-old hearing children. Heider and Heider (1940) used written compositions about a short film to evaluate the linguistic skills of over 1000 deaf and hearing children enrolled in shools in the USA. The hearing children were aged between 8 and 14; the deaf between 11 and 17. Analysis of the compositions showed amongst other things that the sentences of the deaf children were shorter both in number of words and in number of clauses; they used more simple sentences and avoided subordination and coordination; and in most respects the performance of the deaf resembled that of the younger hearing children.

Reay (1947) presented further analyses of these data with respect to the use of verbs and nouns. The analyses showed that the number of different verbs used was less for deaf children than for hearing children of the same age, and the deaf tended to use a greater percentage of verbs and nouns from high-frequency classes. Reay noted that these differences increased with age, and argued therefore that the vocabularies of the deaf and hearing children were developing along different lines. This suggested something more than simple retardation, and the author was thus prompted to observe that *(i)* the deaf children's compositions contained more of the most frequently used words. This made the style appear clumsy; the deaf child had words which enabled him to describe only the basic facts, and 'everything that is seen, regardless of its importance in an event, receives equal attention. . . .'; and *(ii)* the deaf children's descriptions were written in more concrete terms than those of the hearing children. Reay's conclusions concerning the concrete nature of the language of deaf children, and their relative inability to deal either with abstract concepts or with things removed from the here-and-now, has provided a familiar and perhaps over-used set of labels by which their language is very often characterized. Some have regarded these aspects as representing the 'egocentricity' of the language of the deaf, by analogy with Piaget's early stages of intellectual growth in normally hearing children. This view therefore emphasizes similiarities between deaf children and their younger hearing peers; but Kretschmer and Kretschmer (1978, 105) point to the likelihood that the older deaf children will be cognitively more sophisticated than their younger hearing peers and that direct comparisons, therefore, may be highly questionable.

Hardy *et al.* (1958) studied some aspects of language skills in partially hearing children. Their subjects consisted of two groups (*n* = 20 each) of hearing and hearing-impaired children aged between 6 and 15 years, matched for age and socioeconomic status. The hearing-impaired children had average pure-tone hearing loss in the better ear of 42 dB, sloping into the higher frequencies. Subjects were asked, amongst other tasks, to describe a set of action pictures, to tell a story, and to name and talk about some animal pictures. Performance differences between the two groups were not numerous. For example, the authors found no basic difference between their two groups in the ratios of four syntactic categories (actor, action, connective and modifier) to the total number of different words (types) and to the total number of words (tokens), which they found surprising. As Bench (1979b) points out in his critical review of the literature, however, the two groups were of high IQ, the hearing losses were in many cases slight in degree, and the syntactic categories were rather global. Hardy *et al*. did however find differences in the vocabulary quotients for their two groups, and comment that the language production of the hearing group was 'smoother, fuller, contained a broader variety of connectives and modifiers (more complex sentences). . . .'

Owrid (1960) devised three tests for the assessment of the spoken-language skills of over 300 hearing-impaired children aged from 5 to 8 years. Hearing losses ranged from mild (c. 30 dB) to severe. The three tests were a toy vocabulary test in which the child had to name objects; a comprehension test, which required the child to follow instructions which were graded from simple (e.g. 'show me the horse') to complex (e.g. 'show me the narrow one'); and a test of use of speech, in which the child described the contents of a set of pictures. Owrid analysed the effect of residual hearing on all three tests, and found a pronounced tendency towards better scores to accompany better hearing in children with hearing losses in the range 30–75 dB. For the more severe losses there were differences in the predicted direction, but somewhat less marked. The effect of age was also significant, test scores improving with age. However, the effects associated with age, and with variables such as sex, type of school and the amount of home training, were small or nonexistent compared with the effects associated with sensitivity loss.

A number of early studies indicated that deaf children use a larger proportion of nouns in their written or spoken language than their hearing counterparts. Indeed, Myklebust (1960) found a substantial number of deaf children who used only nouns. Thus, sentences were said to be short, simple, 'telegraphic' – i.e. with many words omitted (Heider and Heider 1940, Myklebust 1960). The words most likely to be omitted were the so-called 'function words' (Fries 1952) such as conjunctions, prepositions and auxiliaries (Myklebust, 1960).

Simmons (1962) examined the type-token ratio[1] within both spoken and written compositions (picture-elicited) from 112 hearing and 54 deaf children aged 8 to 15 years, and found that ratios were invariably higher in the hearing children's

---

[1]The type-token ratio is the ratio of number of different words used (types) to the total number of words used (tokens). The maximum possible ratio is of course unity, and high ratios are assumed to reflect richer, more diverse (i.e. more developed) language.

compositions. Analyses of ratios were examined for different word classes, namely nouns, verbs, adjectives and adverbs (lexical items), and determiners, auxiliaries, conjunctions and prepositions (function words). For all classes except adjectives, the hearing children had larger ratios. The deaf children used more nouns and verbs than the hearing children, but in both cases they used fewer different words and exhibited, therefore, smaller type-token ratios. The lower TTR in the deaf group was a reflection of the extensive use of four verbs – *have*, *be*, *go* and *feel*. Similarly, the use of auxiliaries by the deaf children was quite restricted, mainly to *was*, *did*, *were* and *had*, while the hearing children used in addition those denoting present tense, subjunctive mood etc. Conjunctions, whether subordinating or coordinating, were used much less by the deaf children, and prepositions – particularly those with 'vague meaning' – were often omitted or used incorrectly. Determiners, especially *a* and *the*, were used much more by the hearing-impaired group, partly a reflection of the large number of nouns in their compositions, partly also a reflection of inflexible overuse of determiners in inappropriate positions.

MacGinitie (1964) argued that the fact that deaf children tend not to use function words is not a demonstration that they *cannot* use them. He examined the ability of 30 deaf children (average age 12;7) and 30 hearing children (average 9;5 years, but matched for reading and nonverbal reasoning scores) to restore single words omitted from sentences, the omitted words being from four different lexical classes and six different functional classes. Although the hearing children were generally more successful in restoring the omitted words, the pattern of difficulty of the different form classes was similar for the two groups. MacGinitie pointed out that 'word classes based on a formal analysis of language patterns may not be suitable categories for a differentiation of the language behaviour of deaf and hearing children', and suggested for example that the dimensions of abstractness or concreteness for nouns might be more suitable.

Goda (1964) compared aspects of the spoken language of normal, deaf and mentally retarded adolescents. Subject groups comprised 28 normal subjects, 42 retarded subjects and 56 deaf subjects; all were aged between 12 and 18 years. The hearing-impaired children had pure-tone hearing losses of 75 dB or greater in all octave frequencies from 500 Hz upwards. Spoken language samples were elicited in response to a series of pictures. The total number of words spoken by each group of subjects was divided into successive 100 different word samples, which were then analysed using Fries's (1952) classification into Classes I, II, III, IV (broadly speaking, nouns, verbs, adjectives and adverbs respectively) and function words. Approximately the same number of different words (types) were collected from each group, although many more responses were collected from the deaf than from either of the other groups. All three groups used a similar proportion of Class I words, which were used more than any other class of words; but the deaf group used significantly more Class II words and significantly fewer function words than the other groups. Three-quarters of the output of the deaf consisted of Class I and Class II words. Goda speculated that these results reflected the stereotyped and concrete nature of deaf spoken language, and attributed this in part to the teaching the children had received, which 'needs to be highly concrete and specific' (Goda 1964, 403).

Tests of both vocabulary knowledge and vocabulary use were administered by Templin (1966) to 24 hearing and 24 deaf children who were aged 6, 9 and 12 years at the first test session and 8, 11 and 14 years at a follow-up test session. The study is a rare example of longitudinal design, albeit somewhat limited. Analyses indicated that deaf children at age 11, 12 and 14 obtained mean scores below those of hearing subjects at the same age level on all tests. The inferiority of the 14-year-old deaf children varied from 2 or 3 years to more than 8 years on some tests. Templin noted that the findings from one test

> suggest that the language experience of the deaf and hearing in relation to . . . common words differs significantly. The hearing seem to have had similar experiences, to have learned thoroughly a number of different meanings of common words, and to increase consistently with age in the number of meanings known. The extent of such similar language experience among the deaf would seem not only considerably less than that of the hearing, but also less universal among the deaf subjects, since they know many fewer meanings of the words, and they do not 'know' the several meanings as thoroughly or as consistently. (p. 351)

In one of the tests used, one, two or three words were presented to be used in the construction of sentences. Both hearing and deaf subjects were able to construct a larger number of adequate sentences when only one word was to be used than when two words were to be used, and when two words rather than when three words were to be used. The hearing, but not the deaf children, constructed significantly more adequate sentences with increasing age. The performance of the 14-year-old deaf children fell between that of the hearing at 6–8 years in construction of sentences using one given word; at about 8 years in the construction of sentences using two given words, and between 8 and 9 years in the construction of sentences using three given words. Hearing children increased the number of 'abstract' sentences with age, while the deaf children did not.

Brannon and Murry (1966) obtained picture-elicited spoken-language samples from 30 normally hearing and 30 hearing-impaired children. The normally hearing children were aged 12–13 years, while the hearing-impaired ranged from 8 to 18 years. The latter were divided into a group with partial hearing loss (pure-tone average from 27 to 66 dB (ASA)) and a 'deaf' group (average loss greater than 75 dB in the better ear). As in all these studies, onset of the impairment was said to be prelingual. Fifty sentences were obtained from each child in response to 14 coloured pictures, and these responses were analysed with regard to total number of words, sentence length, sentence complexity and syntactic accuracy. The partially-hearing subgroup resembled the control group in its total output of words, but the output of the deaf subgroup was significantly depressed. Mean sentence length for the normals was 7.7 words, for the partially hearing 6.9 words, and for the deaf 6.0 words. The differences were statistically significant. These sentence-length figures made allowance for structural omissions, and when this was ignored the differences were even more striking: 7.8, 6.4 words respectively. A syntax score was also derived for each subject, one point being subtracted for each word error (addition, omission, substitution or word order) and a percentage score reflecting the relationship between the number of correct words and the total number of words was calculated. The syntax score was 98.2 per cent for the hearing children, 82.2 per cent for the hearing-impaired. This latter figure broke down to 90.2 per cent for the partially hearing subgroup and 74.2 per cent for the deaf subgroup. These differences were all statistically significant, but the authors noted that the size of the difference between normal and partially hearing children was not great; on the other hand, the performance levels exhibited by the deaf children were widely separated from the scores of the other children. Brannon and Murry also noted that most sentences spoken by the hearing-impaired children were of the simple declarative SVO (subject-verb-object) type, with errors tending to occur in the middle. Words used to expand utterances from the centre, such as auxiliaries, were therefore thought to be under poor control.

The data which formed the basis of the report by Brannon and Murry (1966) were analysed by means of a word-classification system into one of 14 word classes; the results were reported by Brannon (1968). The number of both tokens and types was reduced in the partially hearing and deaf subgroups compared with the normally hearing children. The moderately impaired children used proportionately less adverbs, pronouns and auxiliaries than the normal children; while the deaf subgroup used less word tokens in *all* classes, especially adverbs, pronouns and auxiliaries. Hearing impairment was associated with a relative overuse of nouns and articles, and Brannon supposes that this is 'due to the limitations imposed by deafness upon the hearing of abstract concepts, particularly those related to time' (p. 286). Again, the results seem to show that the deaf use proportionally more content words than function words, relative to the normally hearing, and that this related to the concrete nature of many content words as opposed to the abstract nature of function words. Among the content words adverbs are an exception; and among the function words, articles are an exception 'because they (the children) overgeneralize from what they are taught, that nouns are preceded by articles' (p. 286).

In many respects the conclusions from these early studies add little to the ground already covered by the two major pieces of work in this section: Heider and Heider (1940) and Myklebust (1964). Taken together, the early studies provide us with the following pieces of information about the language of prelingually hearing-impaired children compared with that of the normally hearing children.

(i) Language output is depressed, and this can be demonstrated with reference to a number of measures: number of words (tokens), number of different words (types), number of sentences and length of sentences.

(ii) Sentence construction is generally simpler, complex sentences involving e.g. subordination being rare.

(iii) The style of the language is inflexible and stereotyped.

(iv) Content words, particularly nouns and verbs, are over used, while function words, particularly auxiliaries, conjunctions and prepositions, are underused or misused.

(v) Errors of omission, substitution, addition and word-order are frequent.

Ivimey (1982) dismissively concludes (and with some justification) that this information, although perfectly valid, is trivial in nature, and is gained by and known to the average teacher of the deaf through everyday observation. The standard defence to this common accusation is that it is one thing to observe in broad everyday situations, but quite another (and preferable) to confirm commonsense notions with controlled quantified studies. This may be so up to a point, but when all the research over a 30-year period has been confined to this purpose, some disenchantment is to be expected.

The problems with this early research are discussed by Cooper and Rosenstein (1966) and by Ivimey (1982) in similar terms. In essence, the use of broad descriptive global measures (type-token ratio, sentence length etc.) which are compared with these measures in 'normal language' is of very limited value because it tells us very little about the origins of the problems. The early studies measure aspects of linguistic performance, and yet the crucial issue for child language acquisition is linguistic competence. The rules which underlie spoken English are known to each speaker of the language. The speaker may not be able to list this finite set of rules, but he or she knows them in the sense of being able to apply them in a regular fashion in such a way as to produce or understand an infinite number of sentences which need not have been encountered previously. It is the speaker's or listener's implicit knowledge of these underlying rules which constitutes his or her linguistic competence (Chomsky 1965). For various reasons the underlying rules will be violated in the actual performance of speaking, writing or comprehending, and linguistic performance is concerned with this aspect of behaviour. Unfortunately, poor linguistic performance can, but does not necessarily, reflect impaired linguistic competence. As Cooper and Rosenstein (1966) point out, for example, 'the irrelevancy of quantitative indices of performance such as sentence length and type-token ratio to an assessment of linguistic competence can be seen from the fact that these indices continue to rise long after the child has mastered the complex system of rules represented by his language' (p. 55).

It is of great interest to examine the underlying competence of the hearing-impaired in order to determine the extent to which their rules conform to those underlying the language of the normally hearing English speaker, and to do this different research strategies are required. Such research began to emerge in the late 1960s, and we will examine it in the following section. These arguments should not be taken to imply that we think that research in this area should concentrate solely on the essentially linguistic question of competence; linguistic performance *is* of interest, and in particular the psycholinguistic question concerning the factors which determine language performances given a particular language competence are likely to be of considerable value in understanding the acquisition of language in the hearing-impaired, and in pointing to ways in which that acquisition can be facilitated. The early studies of hearing-impaired language tell us a little about the overall performance of some (generally older) deaf or partially hearing children. They are largely irrelevant to linguistic competence, they are too global to be of more than passing general interest with regard to performance, and none of them was directed towards the psycholinguistic processes which translate competence (possibly impaired) into impaired performance.

The studies to be examined in the remainder of the chapter are improvements on the early work, in that either they look at underlying competence; or they examine performance in realistic detail rather than in global summaries; or they are developmental in design; or they specifically examine processes which might plausibly reflect the interface of performance and competence.

Contemporary studies: older children and the grammatical emphasis

As before, the studies which will be described in this section are not easily categorized into neat areas of work. They will therefore be treated as a whole, with the exception of studies which aim to examine free writing (e.g. free composition). These will be dealt with separately. Amongst the studies of receptive and spoken expressive language will be found studies which *do* use written responses, but written responses of a highly controlled nature. These merely use a controlled written response of some kind as a useful procedure for identifying knowledge of underlying linguistic rules, and as such they are not appropriately included with studies of free written English.

Such an approach was adopted by Cooper (1967), who used a controlled written test to investigate the implicit knowledge of morphological rules in 140 prelingually severely deaf children (aged 7 to 19) and 176 hearing children (aged 7 to 18). The morphological rules of interest to Cooper were those controlling the use of derivational suffixes (e.g. -*er* as in *singer*) and inflectional suffixes (e.g. -*s* as in *singers*), and he used a test based on Berko's (1958) methods with nonsense words to investigate these rules. Thus, receptive knowledge of inflectional rules was tapped by a task in which the subject has to select the picture appropriate to, e.g. 'put an X on the picture of the *moggs*'. A picture of one imaginary animal is labelled as a *mogg*, and other pictures are presented, one of which shows two *moggs*, another of which shows one *mogg* with another animal, and so on. If the correct picture corresponding to two *moggs* is identified, this is taken as evidence that the subject has responded to the inflexional suffix -*s* and therefore has receptive knowledge of that morphological form. Productive knowledge of inflexional rules was assessed by sentence completion of the type, 'This is a man who knows how to *hibb*. He did it yesterday. What did he do yesterday? Yesterday he . . . .'. *Hibbed* as a response was taken as evidence of knowledge of the inflectional suffix -*ed*. Comprehension of derivational rules was tapped with a similar sentence completion task (e.g. 'Mary knows how to *zugg*. She *zuggs* every day. She knows a lot about . . . .'), although in this case the subject had to select the correct answer from four alternative given words. Productive knowledge of derivational rules was similarly assessed by sentence completion (e.g 'John's dog has *wabbs* on it. *Wabbs* are all over the dog. What kind of dog is it? It is a . . . dog.').

The results from this study showed marked superiority on the part of the hearing subjects. Mean test scores across ages were 18.3 for male deaf, 25.3 for female deaf, 32.9 for male hearing and 37.2 for female hearing children; standard deviations were of the order of 7.0–9.0. There was little evidence of any increase in test scores for the hearing-impaired children after about age 13 years, and the mean score of the deaf 19 year olds was less than the mean score of the hearing 9 to 10 year olds. Interestingly, the patterns of item difficulty between the deaf and hearing groups were similar, and the rank correlation coefficients of item difficulties were 0.68 for receptive items and 0.78 for productive items. Table 6.1 (from Cooper 1967, 84) shows the percentage of deaf and hearing subjects passing each test item. The items are arranged in order of difficulty for the deaf children. For both groups items testing inflectional rules were in general easier than those testing derivational rules, and the difference in performance between deaf and hearing children was more marked for the derivational rules than for the inflectional.

Table 6.1   Percentages of deaf and hearing subjects who passed the morphology test items (from Cooper 1967, Table 3).

Item	Percentage Deaf	Hearing
	Receptive test*	
Past, reg. or irreg. as in *bet*	94	92
Plural, reg. or irreg. as in *knife*	91	98
Plural irreg. as in *knife*	89	93
Superlative	89	97
Past, reg. or irreg. as in *sing*	88	95
Plural, reg. (*-es*)	87	90
Plural, reg. (*-s*)	69	82
Progressive[†]	67	69
Past, reg.	64	68
Deriv. adj. (*-y*) with noun stem	64	81
Third person singular (*-s*)	55	89
Past, irreg. as in *sing*	51	60
Deriv. noun (*-er*) with noun stem	48	86
Third person singular (*-es*)	45	84
Comparative	40	93
Past part., reg. or irreg. as in *sing*	35	63
Deriv. adv. (*-ly*) with deriv. adj. stem	35	66
Deriv. adv. (*-ly*) with adj. stem	25	50
Deriv. adj. (*-able*) with verb stem	20	66
Deriv. verb (*-ate*) with noun stem	17	70
Deriv. adv. (*-ward*) with noun stem	07	65

Item	Percentage Deaf	Hearing
Past, irreg. as in *Bet*	03	44
Deriv. adv. (*-wise*) with noun stem	−07	53
Deriv. noun (*-ness*) with adj. stem	−12	65
Deriv. noun (*-ing*) with verb stem	−14	90
	Productive test	
Plural, reg. or irreg. as in *knife*	86	89
Plural, reg. (*-s*)	85	92
Plural, reg. (*-es*)	85	89
Past, reg. or irreg. as in *sing*	85	89
Past, reg.	81	83
Progressive	69	89
Past, reg. or irreg. as in *bet*	63	80
Past part., reg. or irreg. as in *sing*	57	76
Third person singular (*-es*)	42	85
Third person singular (*-s*)	35	86
Deriv. verb with noun stem	34	68
Deriv. adv. with adj. stem	34	39
Deriv. noun with noun stem	30	75
Deriv. adj. with noun stem	28	63
Deriv. noun with verb stem	24	81
Superlative	22	66
Deriv. verb with deriv. noun stem	22	68
Comparative	16	67
Deriv. adv. with deriv. adj. stem	16	49
Deriv. adj. with verb stem	13	35
Deriv. adv. with noun stem	05	46
Deriv. noun with adj. stem	03	32

* Receptive items corrected for guessing.
† Average difficulty of two items testing progressive.

The hearing-impaired children who took part in Cooper's study all came from the same school, and the author therefore added a cautionary word regarding the generality of the conclusions. A later study on children from two residential schools by Bunch and Clarke (1978), using the same technique as that used by Cooper, produced somewhat poorer results with regard to the children's morphological rule knowledge. For example, only about a third of the children, who had peripheral sensitivity losses of at least 80 dB HL and who were aged from 9 to 17 years, could produce the plural *-s* with any consistency, and only about one in six of the children could produce the regular plural *-es*. The younger children showed little evidence of consistent use of the past tense form *-ed*, nor of the irregular past tense. The data from Cooper's study (Table 6.1) by comparison indicate a much more favourable picture, but it is not clear why this should be so.

Rather than the controlled technique for examining competence with morphological rules used in the preceding studies, Bamford and Mentz (1979) used a picture-description task to study the spoken language performance of 263 hearing-impaired children aged 8 to 16 years. Pure-tone hearing loss in the better ear ranged from 40 dB HL through to profound (defined by the authors as 95 dB or more). The spoken-language samples were analysed for grammatical content using the Language Assessment Remediation and Screening Procedure (LARSP) of Crystal *et al.* (1976). LARSP provides a checklist of syntactic and morphological items arranged into normal stages and normal order of emergence respectively (see Ch.3). We will refer later to the syntactic data, but in the present context the analysis at the word level – morphological items – is of interest.

These items were grouped and averaged across all hearing-impaired subjects onto 'mean' LARSP profile and compared with a mean profile obtained from analysis of the spoken language samples of a small group ($n = 11$) of normally hearing children aged 10–15 years. Marked differences in the use of some morphological items were found: past tense *-ed* was used considerably more by the hearing-impaired than by the normals (12.63 vs 5.45), whereas for the past participle form *-en* the ratio was 12.09 to 2.10 in the other direction, that is with much greater use by the normally hearing children. These data agree with those of Pressnell (1973), who similarly found that hearing-impaired children have less difficulty with the simple past tense than with the past participle form. This tendency to over use the past tense form at the expense of the past participle form applied to all the sub groups of the Bamford and Mentz (1979) study, irrespective of age, degree of hearing loss, or non-verbal IQ. On the other hand, it was found that all other word-level (morphological) entries on the mean LARSP profile were used less by the hearing-impaired children than by the normally hearing control group. Of those items which were used relatively frequently, plurals, contracted auxiliaries, third person singular inflections and, as already noted, past participles were particularly infrequent. One point of caution here is that this was a study of spoken language, and the poor output-phonology skills of some of the children may have given rise, despite the use of tape recordings, to transcription errors – particularly, of course, at the morphological level, where items are generally very shortlived.

Picture description was used by Elliott *et al.* (1967) in an important study which sought to determine indices of language development which would be applicable to young hearing-impaired children. Fifty-five children aged from 4 to 10 years, and with hearing losses ranging from moderate to profound, were studied, along with a group of normally hearing children ($n = 19$). Spoken-language samples, elicited by picture description, were recorded and then transcribed for later analysis. Elliott *et al.* evaluated the language samples by a number of objective measures and a number of subjective ratings. The objective measures were based upon either the features of the spoken output or aspects of the written transcription. In the former category come total length of utterance in response to a picture; total pause time; and total time of unintelligible speech. Measures based on the transcription consisted of number of words (types and tokens), frequency of usage, and classification by Fries' system (1952). Subjective ratings of the written transcriptions were made by college students and by teachers of the deaf along four dimensions: structural sophistication, grammatical accuracy, content and creativity.

The subjective ratings were highly intercorrelated, and this led the authors to suggest that all ratings were measuring one global dimension of language goodness. This is an interesting finding which emphasizes the interactive nature of language development, and suggests that advances on one front (e.g. grammar) go together with advances on other apparently quite separate fronts (e.g. creativity). Mean ratings (on a seven-point scale) for children classified as profoundly deaf (average hearing loss greater than 90 dB HL) were approximately 1.5, compared with 2.5 for the partially hearing and 3.5 for the normally hearing groups. Multiple stepwise regression techniques showed that the overall subjective measure of language goodness (derived from the ratings) could be predicted from four of the objective measures, namely total speaking time, a measure of total word output, a measure of word frequency, and a measure of word classification. The multiple correlation (R) was 0.84, which means that 74 per cent (R^2) of the total variability in the subjective ratings could be accounted for by the four objective measures.

One interesting finding in this study was that as the total number of different words used increases, the partially hearing children showed a more rapid increase in use of high-frequency words than the deaf children, while the latter more rapidly increased their use of words of lesser frequency. The authors note that 'the deaf may have acted as if maximizing information transmitted per unit time. Although this strategy may succeed in communicating discrete concepts . . . it becomes woefully inadequate in transmitting meanings which depend upon well-related word sequences' (Elliott et al. 1967, 151).

Elliott et al. administered their tests on several different occasions to a number of their subjects, and Table 6.2 shows the development of one (severely hearing impaired) child's responses on four sessions spread over 4 years. The children in Elliott et al.'s study were apparently provided with good amplification, and the authors comment that such children accomplish at least the early stages of language development in a manner which resembles normal patterns. However, they also note that it is rather unexpected to find a unitary dimension of language goodness which is well predicted by mere objective counts. Fully fledged language behaviour has always been thought to encompass rather more than a combination of word counts. Examination of some subjects who were high scorers and some who were low scorers on the dimension of language goodness did reveal that the intercorrelations between ratings for the high scorers was less than that for the low scorers. This suggested that, as language develops, so global language ability diversifies into mulitple dimensions; and there is evidence for this from normally hearing children, in whom such diversification begins at quite an early age. Elliott et al. comment that, although it is possible that normal but delayed development

Table 6.2 Responses to the same picture on four separate occasions by a hearing-impaired child. In the top panel are the transcriptions of the responses. The bottom panel shows the counts for the judges' ratings and for the variables in the predictive equation. The child had an average pure-tone sensitivity loss of approximately 90 dB HL (from Elliot *et al.* 1967, 154–5, Tables 6 and 7).

FIRST TEST
Age: 5.6   Date: 10/61
– dog – the bath tub then – boy – water – nose – mouth

SECOND TEST
Age: 8.1   Date: 5/64
all the children is washing the dog and the rug is all wet the dog got all dirty – I think that's all

THIRD TEST
Age: 8.6   Date: 10/64
yes the children are washing the dog in the bath tub and the water fall on the rug and the rug is getting all wet and her mother will come and say hey – oh you are naughty you must not wash the dog you will take a nap that's all ok

FOURTH TEST
Age: 9.0   Date: 4/65
the girl and the boy are putting bubbles in the bath tub and turn the water on and they are washing the dog in the bath tub and all the water got on the rug and the floor and every got all over then his mother's going to come out and spank them because they got the water on the rug and floor and up on the wall

---

COUNTS

Administration	Age	Total time (sec.)	Σ Types	Σ 1a1 tokens*	Σ Function types
1	5.6	28	9	3	1
2	8.1	30	14	17	3
3	8.6	30	31	28	9
4	9.0	33	33	43	10

MEAN RATINGS

Administration	Age	Structure	Grammar	Creativity	Content
1	5.6	1.19	1.06	1.59	1.06
2	8.1	2.47	2.87	3.09	2.06
3	8.6	4.66	5.32	4.55	4.94
4	9.0	5.29	5.03	5.24	5.19

---

* 1a1 is a word-frequency category indicating the 100 most-frequent words.

and diversification of language takes place with the hearing-impaired, one cannot rule out the possibility that diversification or multidimensionality fails to occur in many hearing-impaired children, and that this may be a direct result of instructional methods used by parents and teachers, leading to 'more homogeneous behaviour and language patterns than would normally occur' (p. 158).

Pressnell (1973) also suggested that classroom instruction techniques might underlie some of the differences which she found in the comprehension and production of syntax by hearing-impaired children. The Northwestern Syntax Screening Test (NSST) was administered to 47 severely or profoundly-impaired children aged from 5 to 13 years; in addition, a spontaneous language sample elicited by toys and pictures was taperecorded for later analysis using the procedure of Lee and Canter (1971). In the latter, points are awarded for the correct use of a number of grammatical constructions, viz. indefinite pronouns, personal pronouns, main verbs, secondary verbs, negatives, conjunctions, yes/no questions, *wh*-questions and overall correct sentences. An overall index – Developmental Sentence Score (DSS) – is derived from these subscores. The mean receptive-language score on NSST for Pressnell's subjects was 24, significantly less than the score of 30 reported by Lee (1969) for young normally hearing children. Furthermore, Lee's data show a sharp increase in score with age from 3 to 8 years, whereas Pressnell's hearing-impaired children showed only a low and very variable correlation between age and receptive NSST score.

The results for the expressive portion of NSST showed a similar picture for Pressnell's children: slower improvement with age, lower mean score, and greater variability than the norm. The DSS was based on an analysis of 50 spontaneous spoken sentences, and this showed much variability (0.98–9.42), low mean score (4.05), and no correlation with age. Lee and Canter's (1971) normal children, on the other hand, showed increase in score with age from 3 to 7 years, and a mean score of about eight. Of the grammatical constructions under scrutiny in DSS, Pressnell's hearing-impaired children were least successful in their use of main verbs, and it was clear from the data that those verb-forms upon which they performed poorly were not necessarily those which normally hearing children would find most difficult. Thus, for example, of 385 attempts to use the *is* + verb + *ing* form, only 39 per cent were judged correct, yet this is thought to be one of the easiest forms.

The three overall scores (the receptive and expressive NSST and the DSS) were correlated with a number of possible background variables which intuitively might account for the data. These were: chronological age, severity of hearing impairment, age at onset of impairment, age at identification of impairment, age at which hearing aids were fitted, age at which training was commenced, and years of training. Surprisingly, age and hearing loss gave the only significant correlation with linguistic performance ($r = 0.721$). As we shall see later, Bamford and Mentz (1979) similarly failed to show any involvement of background variables other than age, hearing loss and, in their case, nonverbal IQ.

There is a tendency in these studies to use the sometimes rather limited data to come down in favour of one or other of the deviant versus delayed descriptions of hearing-impaired language. Pressnell, for example, took the evidence of relative differences in percentage correct for different verb-types as compared with normally-hearing norms as evidence of something more than mere delay. However, the difficulties her subjects had in producing correct forms of *is* + verb + *-ing* were not replicated by Wilcox and Tobin (1974). They used a sentence-repetition task to investigate the use of verb construction by 11 partially hearing children (mean pure-tone hearing was 61 dB HL) and 11 normally hearing children; ages ranged from 8 to 12 years. Subjects had to repeat sentences (e.g. *Mary is baking a cake*; *the plate was washed by Mary*) immediately after aural presentation at 39 dB sensation level (i.e. above each individual's speech awareness threshold). Separate analyses indicated that speech discrimination was not a significant factor in the results, which overall were that the hearing-impaired children gave poorer linguistic performance than the normals. However, the hearing-impaired children in this study performed relatively well on the *is* + verb + -*ing* form. Of the six verb forms under consideration the normally hearing children had little difficulty with any, while the proportion of correct responses for the hearing-impaired was 0.572 for present, 0.810 for *is* + verb + -*ing*, 0.351 for *have* + verb + -*en*, 0.589 for auxiliary *will*, 0.637 for passive, and 0.083 for negative passive.

Some workers have used agrammatical sentences or phrases to elucidate further the syntactic ability of their hearing-impaired subjects. Odom and Blanton (1967), for example, had their subjects recall phrase-type strings of (four) words; the word-strings were either grammatical (e.g. *paid the tall lady*), nonphrases with acceptable English word order (e.g. *lady paid the tall*), or nonphrases with unacceptable word order (e.g. *lady tall the paid*). The impaired subjects were aged about 17 years and were described as 'deaf'. The recall scores of these subjects was unaffected by the scrambled word-orders, whereas normally hearing controls performed better on the phrasally defined material. The authors argue that the hearing children possess memory mechanisms which integrate segments according to their phrasal structure, and that this is evidenced by the facilitation effects found when the material was phrasally defined and the interference effects when it was not. Since the deaf subjects showed no differential performance as a function of linguistic structure, Odom and Blanton conclude that the same mechanism is not present in the deaf. A not dissimilar approach was used by Bunch (1979) when he asked a group of hearing-impaired (deaf) children to write down on a sheet of paper a sentence they had just been shown. The sentences were agrammatical in varying respects (e.g. *they sleeping in their beds* – omitted auxiliary), and interest focuses on the spontaneous correction of the grammatical errors. Unlike the findings with hearing children, no evidence was found to indicate that such spontaneous correction occurred. Even when instructed to correct the sentences, at least half the hearing-impaired children failed to do so.

A series of studies using controlled written responses were initiated by Quigley and Power (1972). The major objective of these studies were to 'determine the underlying rules that generate the language produced by deaf persons at particular developmental levels and to trace the development of certain syntactic structures in the language of such persons' (p. 16). They criticized earlier work on the grounds that it often used a corpus of written or spoken language which was either spontaneous or picture-elicited. In both cases it is clearly possible for some grammatical structures not to appear, and one is not able to distinguish between lack of ability to produce the structures and lack of opportunity. Furthermore, some structures appear so rarely, with such ambiguity or with such poor phonology (if the response is spoken) as to make analysis virtually impossible. For these reasons Quigley and Power devised a number of controlled written tests that allowed them to investigate the underlying knowledge of hearing-impaired subjects for particular isolated grammatical rules. The tasks they made most use of were sentence completion and sentence correction. In the former a 'gap' in a given sentence is to be completed by inserting the appropriate word or words drawn from the subject's own lexicon or from given 'multiple choice' answers. Sentence correction is similar to the tasks used by Odom and Blanton (1967) and Bunch (1979), except that usually the child is presented with two strings of words, one of which is grammatically correct and the other incorrect. The subject has to choose the 'right' sentence. Alternatively, the child is presented with a sentence and is asked to judge if it is 'right' or 'wrong' – if the latter, the child is asked to correct it. Other minor variants of these tasks were also used from time to time. Since the tasks are not simple, Quigley's series of studies tended to concentrate on older deaf children in the range 10 to 18 years of age.

It has been known for some time that the passive voice is a relatively difficult structure for normally hearing children, and may not be fully mastered until 8 or 9 years of age (Turner and Rommetveit 1967). In one of the earlier studies of the series, Power and Quigley (1973) investigated the use of the passive voice in both comprehension (picture selection or object manipulation) and production (sentence completion) in severely hearing-impaired children. The children had pure-tone hearing losses of at least 85 dB HL across 0.5–2 kHz, and were divided into five subgroups, 10 children per group, by age: 9–10, 11–12, 13–14, 15–16 and 17–18 years. Their results are summarized and compared with the Turner and Rommetveit data for hearing children in Fig. 6.1. Although significant improvement took place with age, only about half the children by age 17–18 could successfully comprehend or produce correct passive sentences. Data from Tervoort (1970) using deaf Dutch children gave substantially the same picture, and the authors of both studies argued that the passive voice tends to be interpreted in terms of surface structure, guided in particular by word-order. The simple active sentence which is mastered early and used extensively identifies the actor with the subject and the acted-upon with the object, and the usual order is S-V-O. In such active sentences there is a simple relationship between subject and verb, whereas in passive sentences not only is the word-order, in terms of actor and acted-upon, reversed but there is a surface-structure relation between subject and the auxiliary verb and a deep-structure relation between the actor in the prepositional phrase and the main verb, of which this actor is the subject.

Similar arguments were used by Quigley et al. (1974a) to account for the poor performance of hearing-impaired children on relativization. In a large study, they examined the ability of 450 severely hearing-impaired children (50 at each age from 10 to 18) and 60 hearing children (20 at each age from 8 to 10) to comprehend sentences containing relative (i.e. subordinate) clauses. A variety of tasks was used,

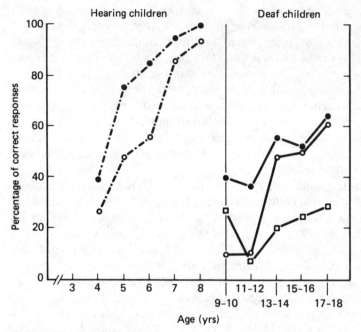

- Non-reversible sentences (e.g. *the car was washed by the boy*)
- Reversible sentences (e.g. *the girl was pushed by the boy*)
- Agent-deleted sentences (e.g. *the girl was pushed*)

–·–·– Turner and Rommetveit (1967)
——— Power and Quigley 1973

Figure 6.1 Comparison of deaf and hearing children on the acquisition of aspects of the passive voice. Data of Power and Quigley 1973, compared with that of Turner and Rommetveit, 1967 (from Power and Quigley 1973, Fig. 1).

including sentence correction and responding with yes/no answers to a set of simple sentences which referred to what might have happened in a complex (relativized) sentence.

Like the results from the study of passive sentences, the performance of the hearing-impaired children improved with age, but at age 18 years this was still significantly poorer than the performance of the much younger hearing subjects. The maximum number of different elements which a single clause can contain is four (e.g. S-V-O-A) and the development of mature, flexible and imaginative language is dependent upon the mastery of the processes whereby clauses can be combined within sentences, by coordination or subordination. The difficulties evidenced by the hearing-impaired on this task are therefore of some significance for the development of language in its later, more sophisticated stages. Although on all tasks the hearing-impaired at 18 years of age failed to match the performance of the 10-year-old hearing children, nonetheless the latter did not always reach perfect performance. Both groups had most difficulty with medially embedded clauses (e.g. *the girl who hit the boy went home; the man who bought a dog chased the woman*). Subjects often failed to connect the initial noun-phrase to its verb-phrase, from which it is separated by the embedded clause, and instead connected the closest noun-phrase to the verb-phrase and thus produced positive responses to *the boy went home* and *a dog chased the woman*. Again, surface structure dominated by proximity, word-order and simple S-V-O clauses seemed to be the source of the subjects' difficulties.

Finally, it should be noted that, although the hearing children were consistently better than the older deaf children, the order of difficulty of the various tasks was similar across the two groups; this, and the fact that all of the deviant (incorrect) structures used in the sentence correction tasks were accepted as correct by at least a few hearing children, tends to lend credence to the view that the development of the mastery of relativized clauses in deaf children is retarded rather than completely deviant, and that it tends to follow the normal pattern, albeit slowly. Nevertheless, and as Quigley *et al.* point out (1974a, 339), the fact remains that a high proportion of 'deviances' persist in the deaf subjects' language repertoires at age 18. The data in this form are not particularly definitive with regard to the deviant/retarded distinction.

Quigley *et al.* (1974b) reported on a further study, using largely the same subjects as before, on the mastery of questions. The children in the study responded to and judged the 'correctness' (i.e. grammaticality) of yes/no questions, *wh*-questions and tag questions. The results were again of the same form, showing in general a steady improvement of performance with age for the deaf groups, but with levels at age 18 still generally less than the levels achieved by the 10-year-old hearing children. Only for yes/no questions did the deaf groups approach the level of comprehension of the younger hearing children. Comprehension of yes/no questions was indeed easiest, and improved faster with age, followed by *wh*-questions and finally tag questions. Judgement of the grammaticality of yes/no questions was better than for *wh*-questions. Of the *wh*-questions, deaf children were able to judge grammaticality significantly better when the *who* was the subject than when it was the object. The perceived order of difficulty of yes/no questions, followed by *wh*-questions and then tag questions has been recorded as the order of emergence in young hearing children, and it appears that deaf children may therefore follow this same pattern.

Examination of the data from an essentially descriptive study by Sarachan-Deily and Love (1974) suggests a similar conclusion. Their subjects were asked for the immediate written recall of sentences presented visually which contained grammatical structures of varying complexity. Subjects were 42 deaf children aged 15-19 years and 21 hearing children of the same age range. Errors of recall were subdivided into agrammatical errors, which caused 'a gross violation of English sentence structure' (p. 696), and grammatical errors which resulted in a sentence that 'might be heard in spoken English or would be judged as grammatical by a native speaker of English' (p. 693). Less than 20 per cent of the errors of the hearing children were agrammatical, whereas almost 50 per cent of the deaf children's errors were of this category. These agrammatical errors consisted mostly of deletion of major sentence constituents, incorrect derivational or inflectional noun and verb-endings, agrammatical sequential word-orders, or inappropriate verb substitutions. The authors argued that under pressure (of the recall task in this case) one would expect only the best learned linguistic rules to remain inviolate; they conclude that the results show that the deaf subjects have an unstable or limited competence for these rules of English grammar.

This unsurprising result is elucidated further by examination of the order of difficulty of the various sub categories of grammatical and agrammatical errors, as evidenced by the error proportions: it is clear that, despite the difference in absolute error values, in many cases the error categories which were largest for the hearing children were also among the largest for the deaf children. Thus inflectional or derivational errors (agrammatical) were common for both groups; so was adjective deletion (grammatical), and synonym replacement (grammatical). On the other hand, a few categories gave relatively large proportions of deaf errors but were almost absent from the hearing children's errors: word-order, replacement of *was* and *has*, and deletion of *the* (all agrammatical-error sub-categories), for example. Studies such as this provide more detail about the language skills of deaf children than did the global studies discussed in the early part of this chapter, but they are nonetheless essentially descriptive, and allow no firm conclusions either about developmental trends or about the deviant/retarded distinction.

Wilbur *et al.* (1975) reported further data from the study of the 450 deaf children (aged 10 to 18 years) and the 60 hearing children (aged 8 to 10 years). In this case the authors were concerned with the ability of their subjects to use the process of conjunction which (along with relativization and complementation) is one of the three recursive processes for constructing complex (multiclause) sentences. Conjunction may be achieved at its simplest level by interposing *and* (*or, but* etc.) between two clauses; if, however, the two clauses contain identical subjects, verbs objects and so on, repetition of those elements can be avoided by a rather more sophisticated form of conjoining, which involves the use of the conjunction and the pronominalizing or deletion of one of the elements (*John went to school and he worked hard*; *John went to school and worked hard*). Wilbur *et al.* used their standard tasks of sentence correction and sentence construction (making one conjoined sentence from two given sentences) to examine subjects' ability to deal with conjoining. The results were similar in pattern to those reported in their previous studies, in that the deaf children exhibit an increase in their ability to master the process of conjoining with age, but in all tasks the grouped performance of the deaf 18 year olds still failed to come up to the performance levels of the 10-year-old hearing children. There was evidence that the rate of improvement with age of the deaf children was more rapid than that found for the process of relativization, but similar to the rate of improvement found for question processes. Again, some examples were found of deviances (e.g. object/subject deletion) which occur rarely in the language of hearing children and which were still present in the 18-year-old deaf children, but again it is not really possible to say that this represents conclusive evidence for the existence of deviant rules in the language of the deaf as opposed to examples of retardation which have yet to be 'learned out'.

The third process for achieving recursiveness – complementation – was also studied by Quigley and his colleagues and was reported in Quigley *et al.* (1976a). They used the task in which subjects judged the grammatical correctness of a sentence and were then asked to rewrite it correctly if they had judged it incorrect. The same subjects were used as in the previous studies. Again, the results indicated improvement with increasing age for the deaf children, with maximum performance at 18 years being less than the performance levels found for the 10-year-old hearing children.

Finally, in two further studies Quigley and his co-workers reported on the use of pronouns and the use of verbs by their 400 or so deaf and their 60 hearing children. Wilbur *et al.* (1976) reported on the results from tests in which subjects had to complete a sentence by the selection of an appropriate pronoun from a list provided. The deaf children's ability to select the correct pronoun increased steadily with age to levels of 65 to 90 per cent correct (depending upon pronoun case); performance levels of the younger hearing children were generally above 80 per cent and often nearly 100 per cent correct. When the pronouns were grouped according to case there were significant differences: for the deaf children, subject and object pronouns were approximately of equal difficulty and were less difficult than possessive adjectives; these in turn were less difficult than reflexives and possessive pronouns, the latter causing the most difficulty. Wilbur *et al.* point out that this order 'roughly parallels the theoretical order of difficulty', although little comment is made about the fact that the young hearing children performed better with possessive pronouns and possessive adjectives than with other cases. In general, singular pronouns were easier than plural, first-person pronouns were easier than third, which were in turn easier than second. It was also clear, however, that there was a large number of significant interactions, which made it difficult to generalize about orders of development. It appeared that both hearing and deaf subjects mastered the pronoun system pronoun by pronoun, rather than in terms of general categories of case, person etc.

Quigley *et al.* (1976b) reported on the development of aspects of the verb system in the same subjects. The task was to judge the correctness of presented sentences containing auxiliary verbs, or in which the verb had been deleted, or in which the verb tense was not marked. As before, subjects were asked to supply the correct written sentence if they. had judged the given sentence to be incorrect (i.e. ungrammatical). The results indicated that the deaf subjects had considerable difficulty with handling the verb system, particularly in three areas: auxiliary verbs, tense sequencing, and *be vs have*. Both hearing and deaf subjects showed poorer performance with passives than with perfectives, which in turn were poorer than present progressives. Overall performance on these auxiliaries was however poorer for the deaf than the hearing children. The formation of the correct tense and voice for auxiliaries was an area of particular difficulty. Tense-sequencing judgements revealed performance little better than chance for the recognition of sentences which were incorrect (in having only one verb marked for tense). The data from auxiliaries and tense sequencing were used by Quigley *et al.* to propose a tentative order of difficulty of acquisition for verb types, which incidentally reflects the cognitive complexity of the types: *(i)* simple past; *(ii)* future; *(iii)* present progressive; *(iv)* perfective; and *(v)* passive. Finally, the confusion of *be* and *have*, while found with the hearing children, was much evident in the results from the deaf subjects. If either *be* or *have* were deleted from a sentence, the deaf subjects generally recognized that it was missing. However, they were not good at restoring the correct form (although they tended to correctly restore *be* more often than *have*). If sentences were presented with an incorrect substitution of *be* for *have* or vice versa, the deaf subjects were poor at recognizing it as incorrect.

Mention has been made already of the detailed study of the picture-elicited spoken language of a sample of 263 hearing-impaired children (aged 8 to 15 years) by Bamford and Mentz (1979). This is a study which did not concern itself with the use of highly controlled tasks to examine the linguistic competence of subjects; instead it used one of the traditional, rather free methods of language sampling to examine linguistic skills at the surface level of performance. What perhaps makes this study of more interest than the early descriptive studies of linguistic performance is the size of the sample and the use of Crystal *et al.*'s (1976) LARSP profile, which allows a very detailed examination of the data. Each sample of spoken language elicited by description of a set of pictures was analysed onto a LARSP profile (see Chap. 3). Since the structures are arranged on the profile in such a way as to reflect normal grammatical development (the structures becoming more advanced with age as one moves down the profile), the patterns of the entries on the profile can be used as an indication of the degree to which the analysed language sample approaches that expected from a sample of normal language.

At the first and most general level of analysis, Bamford and Mentz compared the mean profile for the entries from all 263 hearing-impaired children, grouped and averaged, with a mean profile derived from a small group of normally-hearing children. In contrast to this 'normal' LARSP profile, the hearing-impaired profile showed a marked lack of entries at the word (morphological) level (the details of which were discussed previously); a lack of entries at the phrase level, the shortfall becoming larger the more advanced the structures; and a shortfall in the more advanced clause-level entries, balanced by an increase in the least advanced clause-level entries. Thus, the total number of mean word-level entries (i.e. the sums of the means at word level) was 74.1 for the hearing-impaired compared with 134.4 for the hearing group. The total number of mean phrase-level entries was 139.89 for the hearing-impaired compared with 211.63 for the normally hearing, divided by stages as shown in Table 6.3.

The lack of development at phrase level could be partly traced to a lack of recursiveness (coordination and subordination) at clause level or to a lack of clause expansion (i.e expansion of noun or verb elements into noun-phrases or verb-phrases). The totalled mean clause-level entries for each stage are shown in Table 6.4. These effects all combined to give a much shorter average sentence length for the hearing-impaired children (7.2 words) than for the normally hearing (15.92

Table 6.3 Total number of mean LARSP phrase-level entries at each Stage for hearing-impaired (*n* = 263) and normally hearing children (*n* = 11) (adapted from Bamford and Mentz 1979).

	Hearing-impaired	*Normally hearing*
Stage 2 phrases	66.14	83.56
Stage 3 phrases	63.99	105.91
Stage 4 phrases	8.73	14.08
Stage 5 phrases	1.03	8.08

words). Bamford and Mentz argued rather tentatively that the pattern of entries on the mean hearing-impaired profile was deviant rather than simply a delayed (retarded) version of normal profiles. To what extent such deviant patterning reflects underlying deviant linguistic competence is quite another matter, which is not best answered by reference to simple surface structures, as in the LARSP profile.

Table 6.4 Total number of mean LARSP clause-level entries at each Stage for hearing-impaired (*n* = 263) and normally hearing (*n* = 11) children (from Bamford and Mentz 1979, 387, Table 1).

	Hearing-impaired	*Normally hearing*
Stage 1 'clauses'	14.50	0.36
Stage 2 clauses	16.65	16.73
Stage 3 clauses	33.71	39.54
Stage 4 clauses	8.12	16.00
Stage 5 clauses	20.83	31.27
Connecting devices	17.89	35.08

Bamford and Mentz also examined the effects of age (three levels), degree of hearing loss (three levels), and non-verbal IQ (three levels) on various combined measures (e.g. Stage 2 clauses, Stage 4 clauses) from the profile. A factorial analysis of variance showed significant main effects of age, hearing loss and non-verbal IQ on each of the 13 profile measures; all effects were in the expected directions. That is, the more advanced grammatical structures were used less often as hearing loss increased, more often as age increased, and more often as non-verbal IQ increased. Although the other interactions were not significant, that between age and hearing loss was highly significant for nearly all the combined profile measures. Thus, the children with hearing loss greater than 80 dB HL showed significant improvement in grammatical performance with increasing age; the children with hearing losses of between 60 and 80 dB HL showed improvement with age between the youngest and middle age groups, but not between the middle and the oldest age groups; and the group with pure-tone hearing losses in the range

40–60 dB HL showed no improvement with age. By way of example, these relationships are summarized for a particular profile measure (total number of phrases across Stages 2–5) in Fig. 6.2. Notice that the level of performance of the 40–60 dB hearing-loss group is below that of a normally hearing comparison group who were aged 14 to 15 years and had below-average IQ scores. Thus, although extrapolation of the function for the severely hearing-impaired group suggests that, given a year or two more, these children would attain normally hearing performance levels, the functions for the less hearing-impaired groups suggest that this is not the case. It seems that the performance levels of the less impaired group may represent some upper limit to grammatical advancement. One can only speculate as to the social, auditory/perceptual and linguistic reasons why this might be so.

Bamford and Mentz completed their analyses of the LARSP profiles by a

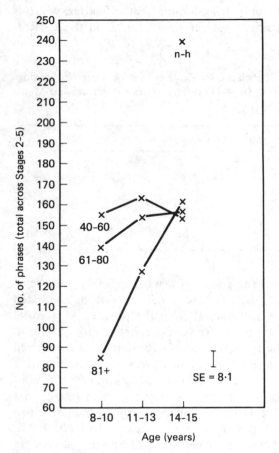

Figure 6.2   Total number of LARSP phrase level entries against age for groups of children with different degrees of hearing loss. n-h = normally hearing datum. (From Bamford and Mentz 1979.)

multivariate approach, in which a factor analysis of the 56 more important profile structures revealed the existence of one major factor which they called a measure of 'grammatical advancement'. This factor accounted for over half the total variability of the LARSP data. Having established such a measure, Bamford and Mentz were able to examine in further detail the effects of age, hearing loss, and nonverbal IQ, this time treating the variables as continua rather than dividing them into somewhat arbitrary subgroups. Correlation techniques showed that the three variables were related to grammatical advancement in the expected directions; furthermore, in combination (multiple regression) age, degree of hearing loss and nonverbal IQ accounted for some 45 per cent of the total variability of grammatical advancement scores. Surprisingly, and disappointingly, other variables which might be thought to influence grammatical advancement in important ways (onset age, diagnostic delay and social class) were shown to do so only weakly, and when included in the multiple regression accounted for only a further 3 per cent of the variability. This failure to find an effect of other plausible background variables was also reported, as we saw earlier, by Pressnell (1973). It should not be taken yet as an indication that these variables have no effects; much more likely is that the data are unreliable because of, for example, poor records.

Although the studies we have discussed so far in this section are an improvement on and tell us more than the early somewhat global approaches, there are nonetheless a number of problems associated with them. First, many of the studies (though not all) have been concerned with the linguistic skills of the deaf, and have ignored partially hearing children. Second, perhaps because some of the tasks involved are quite difficult, these approaches have tended to use older hearing-impaired children, and the early years – no doubt of vital explanatory importance for the understanding of performance in later years – have been under-researched. Third, very few of the studies discussed have been truly developmental in the sense of being longitudinal in design. Thus, the studies by Quigley and colleagues and by Bamford and Mentz (1979) compared groups of children of different ages. While the differences between such groups may be developmental, they may also be due to differences in a variety of uncontrolled variables, ranging from home background to patterns of educational intervention. Fourth, the studies which have taken place during the preceding decade have been very largely concerned with grammar, which is only one aspect of language skills. And fifth, we have to admit that, partly because of the foregoing, the studies of this era have remained, like the earlier work, largely descriptive in their approach. They have remained attached to the deviant/retarded argument, which in the face of descriptive studies is sterile and unlikely to be very productive.

The descriptive approach, albeit much more detailed than previously, and designed now to tackle the problem of competence rather than performance, still leaves us a long way from being able to link perceptual/auditory processes with linguistic processes. For this we turn to the most recent approaches which have appeared within the last few years. However, before we do this we will digress briefly to consider the data on written language which have been derived from free written sources.

Studies of free written language

Studies of free written language have been popular since the early studies of the Heiders (1940), presumably because written samples are relatively easy to obtain and do not involve complex experimental strategies, and also because, unlike many examples of spoken language, they provide a relatively unambiguous body of data. Although the underlying linguistic competence may be the same, the processes which are involved in written language performance may be quite dissimilar to the processes which are involved in spoken language performance. For one thing, there is no nonverbal support in written language, and 'all the problems of making meaning explicit in speech are magnified in writing because non-verbal support for communicating meaning is completely absent' (Cazden 1972, 198). It is therefore unreasonable to expect free written language to give exactly the same picture as the studies of spoken language. Bamford and Mentz (1979), for example, found few instances of deviant utterances in their spoken language samples ('deviant' in the sense of 'only those sentences which would be both structurally inadmissible in the adult grammar and not part of the expected grammatical development of normal children' (Crystal *et al.* 1976, 28)). On the other hand, studies of written samples from the hearing-impaired have often (although not always) shown apparently deviant language, as these two examples (from Davison 1977) shows:

I told the police that how the House of Parliament was exploses.

The purple men put their hands out and pointed to the dog turned purple and go with the purple men. The people looked out of the window and saw what had happened that the people had to watch out. The group of men went to the hall quickly without the purple men see.

Many of the classic early studies discussed previously were concerned with written language, and the lines of thought and controversies which pervaded these early studies are still to be found in the more recent free-written studies. The situation is perhaps slightly more confusing now, however, since there are at least three main approaches to the description of the written language of the hearing-impaired. On the one hand Heider and Heider (1940) argued that 'deaf children resemble younger or less mature hearing children' (p. 73). The differences in language skills which they do observe between deaf and hearing children were attributed to the different ways in which deaf children learn the language. These differences included shorter and simpler sentences, and 'a simpler style, involving relatively rigid, unrelated language units which follow each other with little overlapping of structure or meaning' (p. 98). At the other extreme there are those who have argued that the deaf have no linguistic system and they therefore lack any rules for the generation of language. Fusfeld (1955) observed that the written language of the deaf is 'a tangled web type of expression in which words occur in profusion but do not align themselves in an orderly array' (p. 70).

A third approach was suggested by Ivimey (1976), who found the notion of the deaf as a 'language-less' group decidely unhelpful. He examined the written language of a 10-year-old deaf child in great detail, using Chomsky's model of syntactic structures. The verb system in English is complex, and it is a common finding that hearing-impaired children exhibit greatest difficulties in this area. Ivimey's child was no exception. The studies of Quigley and his colleagues pinpointed the particular difficulty that deaf children seem to face with the verbs *be* and *have*. Most verbs have obvious reference and their 'meaning' can be demonstrated fairly easily. *Be* and *have* either indicate attributes or possession, or they act as carriers of semantic features such as tense and aspect. In either case, they are conceptually more difficult to handle than other more concrete verbs. Ivimey's subject showed great difficulty with *be* and *have*, to the extent of distress in tasks involving the copula. Dawson (1981, p. 48) quotes an example of a free composition written by a 9-year-old deaf child in which it is clear that the child confuses the attribute and possession functions of these verbs:

All about me. I am 9 year old. I am boy. I have live in Farm. Live Mummy, Daddy with Elaine. I am baby calf. I am have house. I am sheep . . .

Within the rest of the verb system, Ivimey found that forms were being used randomly, with past forms used for present and so on, and that within this confusion 'the verbs were used as generally unchanging units, significant markers occurring externally to the system' (p. 110). Thus, time would not be marked by an internal verb change but by an external marker (e.g. *now*) tagged on to an often inappropriate and fairly inflexible verb form: *the boy climbed up a tree now*, for example. The noun system was similar. Thus in the case of plurals the noun-form used, as regards marking for number, was random, and plurality was denoted by an external marker: *the two girl*. Although Ivimey does not acknowledge this, it is possible that some such errors are due to teaching strategies: the term *now* to indicate present tense is often used as a teaching prop, for example. Ivimey noticed significant differences between the noun-phrase in subject position and the noun-phrase in object position, in particular the overuse of determiners + noun in the subject position, but omission of determiners in object position. The same observation applied to the use of prepositions. Davison's (1977) study of 26 hearing-impaired 12-year-olds (see below) provided some support for these differences between subject and object noun-phrases: *she have friend* (absence of determiner), *the atom bombs . . .* (unnecessary determiner). The omission of function words such as determiners and prepositions from both spoken and written language samples from the hearing-impaired has been a common finding; and it has generally been argued that the reason for this is that, because such words are unstressed in spoken language, they are short in duration and difficult to lipread. They are therefore easily missed and tend not to enter the deaf child's repertoire.

Ivimey's results indicate that such speculation must be qualified with reference to the position in the sentence of the function words; those at the beginning (i.e. subject position) may be easier to perceive. On the more general front, Ivimey argued that the language of this child was rule-based, that the syntax was unlike normal English, and that 'the differences are so great that it seems more appropriate to categorize this corpus of data as a system of language *sui generis*' (1976, 112). If this is so for one deaf child it may be so for others, and if so it makes the application to deaf children of language tests which are standardized for hearing children of doubtful validity.

Studies by Charrow (1975) and Dawson (1981) provide a partial test of the notion that the language of the deaf is a separate rule-based language *sui generis*. They argued that if this is so, deaf English (DE) sentences should be easier for such children to process than standard English (SE) sentences. In their studies, hearing-impaired children were presented with a sentence (SE or DE) for immediate recall (by writing). Dawson's study looked in addition at the children's ability to recognize the sentences and also to recall and recognize sentences presented in sign-language format. Although recognition was better than recall, as one would expect, the interesting findings concerned the written recall of sentences. First, errors were numerous: in Dawson's study, 126 out of the 192 SE sentences were incorrectly recalled. The errors followed the usual pattern, being most numerous (55 out of 126) for verb tense (present or infinitive most often substituted); preposition omission (24) and substitution (14) accounted for the next largest error groups; then determiner ommission; and then incorrect use of plural and singular nouns. Secondly, both Charrow and Dawson found that the DE sentences were processed no more efficiently than the SE sentences, thus casting some doubt on the usefulness of the concept of deaf English other than at a purely descriptive level. As Dawson points out (1981, p. 60), it would be interesting to pursue studies such as these using individualized data – that is, there is no good reason to suppose that deaf English is unitary and homogeneous across what is a very heterogeneous population of deaf children. Deaf English may differ from child to child, and the DE sentences used should perhaps be based upon the DE structures generated by the particular child.

The heterogeneous nature of the hearing-impaired population was stressed by Davison (1977). She studied 26 hearing-impaired children of above average non-verbal IQ, and with pure-tone hearing losses ranging from moderate to profound in degree. The children were aged 12 years and all attended the same school, which selects for high verbal abilities and uses oral teaching methods. One might argue, as with many studies of hearing-impaired language, that this restricted sampling of a single school limits the implications of the findings, since particular linguistic skills (and errors) in hearing-impaired children are heavily influenced by the quality, style and method of teaching. Davison argues, however, that she is essentially sampling the 'best case' – i.e. high IQ children selected on verbal abilities to attend a well-resourced school – and she makes the explicit assumption that 'if some deaf children can write an English so perfect that it is indistinguishable from that of any competent hearing writer, then deafness in itself need not be an insuperable barrier in the acquisition of English' (p. 5). If this assumption were correct, the reasons for lack of language skills of some deaf children would have to be sought in areas other than the deafness itself – in educational, social, or psychological factors, for example. Of course these must be involved; but Davison's assumption is not convincing, because it in turn assumes that 'deafness' is somehow unitary. As we know, deafness is not just degree of loss of end-organ sensitivity; hearing involves other auditory perceptual processes, both peripheral and central, which may be impaired at least partly independently of sensitivity loss. Some children may do well because these other processes are relatively intact, some may do poorly (at least with verbal language) because the bases for auditory coding are completely scrambled.

The children in Davison's study were asked to write a story beginning with the phrase *You'll never guess what happened to* . . . . The stories were analysed for grammatical errors, punctuation, lexical choice and spelling errors. Of the grammatical errors, problems with the verb-forms were paramount (particularly tense sequencing and incorrect formation of finite verbs, participles and infinitives); there were a large number of mistakes in the choice of preposition, and in the use (and omission) of determiners; pronouns and subordinating conjunctions also gave problems. These error patterns were typical of deaf children's written language. Davison examined the errors and concluded that there was evidence of both delay and deviance. In the verb system, for example, it is of course true that normal children in their development use uninflected verbs, and make mistakes with tense formation and verb sequence. Nevertheless, there does appear to be a regular progression of acquisition so that the child is learning one aspect at a time. The deaf children, on the other hand, had often not mastered even the most basic inflections, and in a sense were 'acquiring' many aspects all at the same time.

Both Charrow (1975) and Davison (1977) conclude that deaf children exhibit an 'approximate system' of grammar, approximate to standard English, in which systematic errors are produced. Such a system can be transient or can become stable when learners reach a plateau of language development which is adequate for their communicative purposes. Such plateaux in hearing-impaired language have been widely reported. Davison also noted that

> A continuum of language development was seen, from systems which approximate more or less nearly to standard English through to complete acquisition . . . .The existence of a continuum is seen as evidence that deaf children are developing the English language rather than an idiosyncratic 'Deaf Language', although the pattern of development is not identical with that of hearing children.

We can see that even if authors deny the existence of deaf English as an underlying rule system, the finding of examples of deviant 'Deafisms' is commonplace. What then is the origin of these deviant structures? Some workers have suggested the interfering effects of sign language. Another possibility is simply lack of experience of the correct form, i.e. lack of input. The children in Dawson's (1981) study recalled sentences presented in sign language much better than they recalled DE or SE sentences. Although other variables such as sentence length may have been confounded, Dawson tentatively proposed that both the interfering effects of sign language and the lack of exposure to the correct form may intrude, and extrapolates this to a discussion of educational practices. Broadly, she argues that we might usefully regard the learning of English by the deaf as akin to second-language learning. This is a view supported by Tumim (1982) for some though not all deaf children. Tumim closely observed two hearing-impaired children of the same family, with similar degrees of sensitivity loss, and concluded that one of them learnt English relatively easily and quickly and as if it were a first language, while the other acquired it slowly with a great deal of effort, and similarly to the acquisition of a second language. Tumim made the suggestion that the essential early difference between the two infants was in terms of their ability to perceive the intonational and other suprasegmental patterns of speech.

This interesting idea may seem to give us a possible causal link between auditory perception and linguistic development – but the link may not be causal, simply correlational, and it does beg the question as to why one child was good at perceiving intonation and the other was not. Whatever the reasons, if acquiring English is to some children akin to second-language learning, then there is a strong case to be made for looking closely and critically at current educational practices, which may teach a 'second language' without any reference to a possible 'first language'.

These are speculative notions. By way of concluding this section it would be well to add a cautionary note. Many of these speculations are made on the basis of limited numbers of subjects, or on groups of subjects drawn from only one school. Furthermore, the writing task is not the same as the speaking task. When hearing-impaired children are faced with a perceived 'formal' and 'educational' task, it is unclear what strategies they bring to bear on what may be a fairly unnatural situation. Wilbur (1977) argues for example that many of the errors in deaf children's written English may be related to the deaf writer's approach to writing as a clause-by-clause task, rather than as a discourse task. Appropriate use of articles, correct tense sequencing, and pronominalization, all common sources of error in deaf children's writing, are principally concerned with discourse continuity.

A study by Webster (1983) provides a possible explanation for some of these effects in the writing task. He took two groups of deaf (average pure-tone hearing loss 70 dB HL or greater) and hearing children matched for (11–11;10 years), sex and nonverbal IQ and instructed them to write about a picture placed in front of them. Completed scripts were analysed using the LARSP profile of Crystal *et al.* (1976). The writing of the hearing-impaired children exhibited the expected features: little was attempted beyond Stage III (the S-V-O stage), there was little recursiveness, poor discourse and fluency, sentences were shorter, auxiliaries were omitted, tense sequencing was poor, determiners were overused or misused, and they were generally less advanced at clause, phrase and word-level than the hearing children. Although errors were more numerous for the hearing-impaired children, they nevertheless showed considerable awareness of their own syntactic abilities, and tended not to attempt to use grammatical structures which they were likely to get wrong – this, incidentally, is further evidence for rejecting Fusfeld's (1955) contention that the deaf simply do not develop a grammar of any kind.

All this, then, is to be expected. However, Webster employed an experimental condition in which his subjects wrote about a (different) picture using a stylus without ink. What the children wrote was recorded via carbon copy paper onto a sheet stapled below the top sheet, but in this 'invisible' condition none of what was written was visible to the writer. It has been argued that rehearsal of what is about to be written and inspection of what has been written are important aspects of the writing task which are performed concurrently with it. There is evidence, however, that deaf children lack access to internal speech (Conrad 1979) and to the articulatory loop systems of short-term memory (Baddeley 1979), and Webster therefore argued that the invisible condition for the deaf children would make little difference, since rehearsal and inspection are already severely compromised for these children. For the hearing children, however, whose internal coding and short-term memory processes are not already compromised, he predicted that the invisible condition would be disruptive.

The predictions were upheld. The overall mean error rates for the deaf children were 55 per cent (visible writing) and 52 per cent (invisible); but for the hearing children error rate increased significantly from 21 to 45 per cent in the invisible condition. There was little difference in the error rate for any LARSP stage for the hearing-impaired, but for the normally hearing per cent error rates for the visible and invisible conditions respectively were 8 and 25 (Stage II); 23 and 52 (Stage V); and 33 and 71 per cent (Stage VII). The effect of the invisible condition on the writing of the hearing children was remarkable. Lack of recursion, lack of sentence-linking devices, poor discourse and connectivity, were all noted. Fluency and coherence were lost, auxiliaries were misused, and pronouns were underused. Thus removal of written feedback in the invisible condition, preventing inspection and possibly disrupting rehearsal as well, produced what Webster labelled 'pseudodeafisms' in the hearing children.

These results, therefore, implicate secondary cognitive processes in the poor linguistic skills of the deaf, rather than poor language *per se*. The importance of looking for secondary effects of deafness is further emphasized by recent studies of the external context of language development, to which we now turn.

Contemporary studies: early development and contextual considerations

The overwhelming emphasis of the contemporary studies discussed so far has been on older hearing-impaired children. This has clearly demonstrated, in the descriptive tradition, the differences between the language skills of these children compared with the language of normally hearing children. One school of thought has it that such differences, albeit deviant in many respects, arise principally because the input to the child is restricted. Development of language, it is argued, takes place along much the same lines as language development in the normally hearing; delays caused by inadequate input may result in idiosyncratic and deviant examples of language. The other view, as we have seen, is that hearing-impaired verbal language is essentially deviant, since the impairment imposes cognitive limitations and changes which fundamentally alter the process of language development. The problem is that the descriptive studies of older hearing-impaired children do not provide us with the data with which to resolve this issue conclusively. It is partly because of this that recent studies have begun to turn to new approaches which are directed to determining not just what the differences are, but how and why they exist.

There is however another influence which has encouraged researchers to adopt new tactics. Faced with older hearing-impaired children whose language skills are markedly different from hearing children, one naturally wishes to devise remediation programmes which will be of value to those individuals. But taking a more general view – i.e. of future generations of hearing-impaired children as well as these particular individuals – the question arises as to how differences in language ability between hearing-impaired and normally hearing children came about. Some, convinced that it is essentially a manifestation of delay due to impoverished input, will argue that the path to normal linguistic competence must be the same (though longer) as that for normal children. This *may* be so; but equally it may not. Faced with an adolescent hearing-impaired child with reduced language skills, an obvious question to ask oneself is, how did this child arrive at this position? The answer to the question may help to throw light on the how and why of the process, and may therefore offer paths of remediation which hold some promise that future hearing-impaired adolescents will be less disadvantaged than those we have just studied. Thus, one would like to know how this hearing-impaired adolescent compared with hearing children when he or she was, say 6 years old; or 4 years old; or 2 years old. . .

Of course, what this leads us to search for is that age at which language skills in the hearing-impaired begin to differ from those in normally hearing children, for it is here that intervention will perhaps be most profitably applied in terms of later linguistic development. We saw in Chapter 3 that modern language-acquisition theory has turned more and more to the study of early verbal and preverbal behaviour in order to understand later processes; the same trend is becoming apparent in the study of hearing-impaired language.

The significance of the growing interdependence of perception and production for the hearing-impaired child in the very early stages may be illustrated by Smith's (1982) data on premeaningful vocalizations. It appears that the vocalizations of hearing-impaired children are similar to those of normally hearing children until about 12–15 months, in that velars and then alveolar consonants predominate, possibly for structural (i.e. anatomical) reasons. Thereafter, however, premeaningful vocalizations of the hearing-impaired differ, in that labial consonants come to dominate. Smith suggests that this is because labials are more *visible* than velars and alveolars, and that since the impaired child can attend to such cues more easily than to auditory cues, the velars become predominant.

Gregory and Mogford (1981) studied eight prelingually deaf children of hearing parents from when they were 15–18 months of age until their fourth birthdays. As well as video recording a free-play situation in the child's own home twice every three months, they interviewed the mother on aspects of the child's communication once every three months, and kept diaries on the children's progress. Degree of hearing loss ranged from moderate to profound. The authors were particularly interested in the children's acquisition of the first hundred words ('a consistent sound, spontaneously used by the child, with a particular recognizable meaning').

They found that on average the first word appeared at 16 months, and that the age at which the children reached 10, 50 and 100 words correlated highly with degree of hearing loss. Gregory and Mogford compared the rate of acquisition of words for their children with data on normally hearing children from Thatcher (1976), and the comparison is shown in Fig. 6.3.

The two children in Gregory and Mogford's sample who had the severest hearing losses (110 dB + in the speech frequencies) failed to reach the 10 word milestone by their fourth birthdays, and are not included in these data. It can be seen from Fig. 6.3 that the hearing children acquire their first words some 5 months earlier than the hearing-impaired children; that they move from 1 to 10 words in about one month, in contrast to some 7 months for the impaired children; and that both groups acquire new words at a similar rate of 6 to 7 a month from 10 to 50 words. Although the rate of acquisition of new words by the hearing-impaired children after the 50 word milestone increases to some 10 words per month, this compares poorly with the massive increase in new words acquired by the hearing children in this phase, when they move from 50 to 100 words in about a month. As we noted in Chapter 3, this very rapid increase in vocabulary from about 18 months coincides with the emergence of two-word utterances. Gregory and Mogford's children also moved into two word utterances at this stage, but at average age 30 months, and unaccompanied by a similarly rapid expansion of the vocabulary.

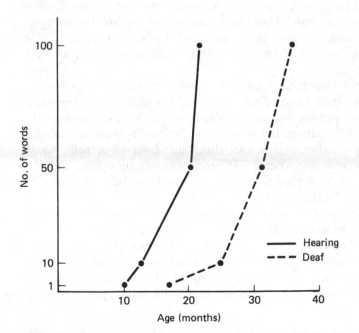

Figure 6.3 *The* rate of acquisition of words by a group of hearing-impaired children. (From Gregory and Mogford 1981, Fig. 14.1.)

On a qualitative note, the authors observed that whereas for hearing children first words are difficult to define because they exist on 'a continuum between making sounds in a conversational way and using words in a totally adult form', the same problem did not appear to exist for the hearing-impaired children:

> Sounds approximating to words do not exist in the interaction of deaf children with their mothers for several months before the true word is formed. Although they do vocalize, and these vocalizations have functions within the interaction, there is no impression that the vocalization may be words. The first words of the deaf child are deliberately elicited and trained . . . It seemed to us . . . that the deaf child 'performs' words, and that the saying of a word, in these early stages, is an end in itself, rather than part of a transaction within an interaction. (Gregory and Mogford 1981, p. 225.)

The implicit suggestion here is that while the language of a hearing child arises out of interactive dialogue, that of a hearing-impaired child tends to be taught (this is not to argue that it *should* be taught, merely that this often happens).

Gregory and Mogford proceeded to analyse the vocabulary content of the 50 and 100-word samples according to six categories: general nominals (e.g. *ball*), specific nominals (e.g. *mummy*), action words (e.g. *down*), modifiers (e.g. *wet*), personal-social words (e.g. *thank you*), and function words (e.g. *for*). Comparing the (rather limited) data from their hearing-impaired children with that from Thatcher's normally hearing children, they argued that although both groups used more general nominals and fewer function words than any other categories, there were significant differences; in particular, the hearing-impaired children used relatively fewer nominals (49 compared with 61 per cent) and relatively more personal-social words (8 compared with 3 per cent). Thus *thank you, no* and *bye bye*, for example, were much more common in the hearing-impaired children's vocabularies than in those of the normally hearing children, where words such as *car* and *shoes* were more likely to be found.

Gregory and Mogford suggest three possible reasons for this difference in the proportions of personal-social words. First, there might be differences in developmental cognitive levels, since the hearing-impaired children were chronologically older by the time they had produced 100-word vocabularies. Secondly, though this not really an explanation, they suggest that the higher level of personal-social words reflects a greater tendency to name features of social relationships. Thirdly, they suggest that many of the personal-social words are those that will be used to the child, with emphasis, by the mother.

These explanations are not mutually exclusive, and it may be that all play a part. It is interesting to note, however, that in the face of evident difficulty with joint reference (i.e. where adult and child are attending to the same thing) of objects, many adults (friends and relatives as well as mothers) will choose to fall back on the easier task of getting the child to label features of social relationships, presumably because joint reference of social situations is easier to achieve than joint reference to objects:

> The language that arises through interaction for hearing children seems to be a language of predominantly joint reference to objects, the language that is elicited

from deaf children seems to be one concerned with labelling features of social relationships and activity as much as with labelling objects. (Gregory and Mogford 1981, p. 230.)

This is a rather sweeping conclusion to draw on the basis of significant but relatively small raw-score differences between two separate studies, and it should not be overlooked that almost half the vocabulary of the hearing-impaired children in Gregory and Mogford's study was made up of general nominals. Nevertheless, it does point to the possible importance of contextual considerations, such as adult–child shared attention, in the development of linguistic skills. One should be guarded about the universal nature of results such as these: they may simply be a reflection of current nonoptimal intervention, or lack of intervention. A recent study by Stokes (1990) on a small group of early identified hearing-impaired children enrolled on an auditory–verbal early intervention programme did suggest a rate of vocabulary acquisition more like the normal hearing children in Fig. 6.3, and showed no strong evidence for the predominance of personal-social words.

Shafer and Lynch (1981) report on a similar longitudinal study of a small group of prelingually hearing-impaired children who were followed between the ages of 14 and 34 months. These children were severely or profoundly impaired, in terms of pure-tone hearing loss, and had hearing parents. Shafer and Lynch were interested to determine how the language acquisition of deaf children compares with that of the normal child 'in terms of emergence of specific semantic forms and functions' (p. 95). Their database was obtained from a number of videotaped sessions of mother and child supplemented by parental diaries of utterances, teacher's notes, and classroom-language samples taken by the investigators.

The study was divided into two parts, Part I being concerned with the acquisition of single words ('any sequence of sound . . . which was consistently used to refer to a specific object or event', p. 97), Part II with the emergence of two-word utterances. By the age of 18 months, of the four children studied in Part I, one had yet to acquire his first word, another had three spoken words, another five, and the final child had acquired 12 spoken words. By the conclusion of Part I all four children were aged between 20 and 24 months and were using words; the number of different spoken words in their vocabularies (estimated by mother) was eight, 13, 18 and 31. These totals are very different, of course, but they do confirm the delay in single-word acquisition relative to normally hearing children. The picture is slightly confounded because two of the children (those with 28 and 32 spoken words) also used signed words, and if these are included the size of their vocabularies increases to 62 and 58 words respectively. Some of the signed words were, for example, social words such as *thank you*, which Gregory and Mogford (1981) had found to be heavily used by their hearing-impaired children.

Shafer and Lynch found marked delay in the acquisition of first words and two-word utterances; this apart, they found both similarities and differences between the pattern of acquisition of the deaf children compared with hearing children. Like normally hearing children, their subjects exhibited both over extension and under extension of concepts; similarly, two of their subjects used person names first to point out a person, then to call a person, and finally to name objects associated with a person. On the other hand, the proportion of object names (general nominals) to person names (specific nominals) to action words for the two children with sufficient words to make such an analysis useful was 42 per cent to 11 per cent to 24 per cent, which is much more like the proportions found by Gregory and Mogford (1981) for hearing-impaired children than the proportions found by Nelson (1973) or Thatcher (1976) for hearing children at the 50 word stage.

In Part II of the study, Shafer and Lynch turned their attention to the transition from single words to multi-word utterances. They continued to monitor the vocabulary growth in four subjects (only two of whom had taken part in Part I), and concluded from perhaps rather limited individual data that while two of the children expanded their vocabularies over test sessions, the others appeared to reach a plateau. Three of the four children achieved between 50 and 100 words and all three began to move into two-word utterances; the child who used only about 20-25 different words in the later videotaped sessions of Part II did not move on to multi-word utterances by 34 months of age. Even those three subjects who did progress past single words gave mean length of utterance no greater than 1.37 words, which is considerably less than the 1.75 proposed by Brown (1973) for his Stage 1 grammar in which two-word utterances dominate. As with normally hearing children, the most frequent combinations of words were action + object (e.g. *climb stairs*) and attribute + entity (e.g. *nice doggie*). Development at the morphological level was very poor.

Shafer and Lynch were somewhat cautious in their interpretation of the results, and suggested that it is premature to draw conclusions about deaf children in general until more longitudinal early language studies are conducted. Gregory and Mogford (1981) are less constrained, and argue that their findings indicate 'fundamental differences' in the language development of deaf children even at this early age. In a field which has been beset for many years by important linguistic and educational inferences being made on the basis of insufficient data, it is perhaps unfortunate that these and other authors, who have posed new and interesting questions for research to answer, should so readily continue the practice. Nonetheless, this issue aside, Gregory and Mogford speculate interestingly on three contextual aspects of infant development which they feel may be difficult for the hearing-impaired child, and which may therefore be implicated by these early language differences: turn-taking, joint reference and anticipation games.

Turntaking between mother and child can be observed as early as the first few months of life. The mother's voice comes to have special significance quite early on, and the infant's behaviour will reflect this. Similarly, when the child takes the initiative the mother will moderate her behaviour. This results in a turn-taking sequence in which one is active while the other is responsive, and vice versa, and overlapping responses are largely avoided. Gregory and Mogford (1981) argue that, although other aspects of behaviour such as eye contact, gesture and facial expression can serve as cues for turn-taking, auditory information must be a major component, and the hearing-impaired child will therefore find it that much more difficult to turntake efficiently and smoothly. Gregory *et al.* (1979) have shown that deaf child–mother pairs exhibit more 'vocal clashes' (i.e. a breakdown of smooth turn-taking) than do hearing child–mother pairs. Joint reference refers to activity where both mother and baby are attending to the same thing. At first mothers will follow the child's gaze and will often then initiate 'conversation' about the object of that gaze. Thus objects and events become the focus of joint attention and form the subject matter of early speech input to the child. At a later stage the joint reference is not simply determined by the child's gaze or wandering attention, but by the mother using vocalization and especially intonational markers to direct the child's attention to some joint reference.

Gregory and Mogford (1981) suggest that joint reference may be more difficult to establish with the hearing-impaired child; furthermore, this may account for the significantly fewer general nominals found in the language of their hearing-impaired subjects. Anticipation games are those mother–baby games 'which are characterized by a build-up of tension, and then release, often accompanied by laughter' (Gregory and Mogford 1981, 232). Examples are 'peek-a-boo' and 'round and round the garden'. Although, unlike the other joint activities, there is no obvious reason why anticipation games should be more difficult for deaf children, nevertheless Gregory and Mogford claim that mothers of deaf children tend not to play them. Turn-taking, joint reference and anticipation games may help to foster a knowledge of language and help to develop dialogue and communication skills. The suggestion is that there are therefore aspects of hearing impairment which are secondary to the primary deficit of reduced or distorted auditory input, but which may be nevertheless devastating in their effects.

Evidence which implicates these secondary, contextual aspects in the difficulties with language which are faced by the hearing-impaired child has come from a number of recent sources. Gross (1970) examined the communicative interactions of mothers with normally hearing children and of mothers with hearing-impaired children. The mothers of normally hearing children used more questions and asked for more opinions and suggestions (rather than giving them) than did the mothers of the impaired children. Collins (1969), reported by Kretschmer and Kretschmer (1978), found that mothers of deaf children communicated mainly to direct the activities of their children, and that the mother–child communication was limited to events and ideas related to the immediate environment. Hughes (1983) examined the verbal interactions of 30 mothers and their hearing-impaired children in comparison with 26 mothers and their hearing children. Taperecordings were made of mother and child in free play at the child's home, and the mother's speech was analysed for 20 features. The features were in four categories: structural (e.g. MLU, sentence complexity, TTR); functional (e.g. percentage questions, declaratives, deictics); interactive (e.g. per cent maternal expansions, and self-repetitions); and conversational style features (e.g. ratio of mother to child speech). Mean scores on each feature were computed for the mothers of the normally hearing children and for the mothers of the hearing-impaired children, and *t*-tests were used to determine if the differences were statistically significant. Sixteen of the features showed no significant differences, and Hughes interprets this as supporting the view that 'the verbal interaction between mothers and hearing-impaired children is usually very much like that between mothers and normally hearing children'.

Three points need to be made. First, Hughes's hearing-impaired children were by no means all severely impaired: degree of hearing loss (pure-tone, averaged across the four frequencies 0.25, 0.5, 1 and 4 kHz) was only 'greater than 55 dB'. It is likely that here, as in other aspects of language and hearing-impairment, deficits become more marked with increasing hearing loss, and Hughes's moderately impaired children may have diluted the overall picture somewhat. Secondly, four of the measured features *did* show significant differences in the expected direction. Mothers of hearing-impaired children showed more maternal self-repetitions, more naming, more declaratives and less questions than did the mothers of hearing children. And finally Hughes presents evidence, in the form of a relatively weak correlation between features of the mothers' and features of the hearing-impaired children's language, that mothers of hearing-impaired children find it more difficult to gauge accurately their child's level of comprehension. In other words they find it more difficult to 'tune' their own output to the appropriate linguistic level.

Further evidence for the different language context provided by mothers of hearing-impaired children is provided by Cheskin (1981). She studied three severely hearing-impaired children of hearing mothers; the children were aged between 1 and 3 years. Each mother–child pair was studied for about an hour in the child's own home, and recordings were made of the language interactions. Analysis of the language environment provided by the mother's speech revealed that each mother spoke in short sentences (MLU of 3.2 to 3.7 words) and used repetitions and restricted vocabulary (type-token ratios of 0.42 to 0.47). Not unexpectedly, they repeated sentences far more frequently than do mothers of hearing children – perhaps 40 per cent compared with the 15 per cent reported for hearing children. Cheskin did not herself present any data on hearing children, so the significance of some of her quantitative data is not absolutely clear. On the more qualitative aspects, many of the questions asked by the mothers could be answered with a simple yes/no response and opportunities were therefore missed to involve the child in a more active role in the verbal interaction. Furthermore, when questions which required more than a yes/no answer were asked, the mothers tended to provide the answers rapidly rather than wait unduly for the child to reply; in so doing they were using the questions for the primary purpose of controlling and directing the child's attention, rather than to involve the child in genuine verbal interaction. Similarly, on those occasions when the child initiated 'conversation' with a verbalization, the mother tended to interpret the verbalization not as a conversation initiator but simply as a label for an object or event in the immediate environment. Cheskin suggested therefore that these mothers 'automatically interpreted their children's verbalizations as attempts at labelling rather than conversation starters' (1981, 495). It is well known, however, that early utterances can and do carry a variety of communicative intents other than simply labelling.

It is becoming clear that the development of language has to be viewed within a framework of communication. The emergence of speech in the normally hearing child is not evidence that language acquisition is beginning, but is the culmination of a stage in language-acquisition in which there is a shift from largely non-verbal to verbal communication. If, as it seems, the processes of early non-verbal communication are disrupted in the hearing-impaired, then language acquisition is being disrupted. Why are the early interactive processes such as joint reference disrupted? Wood (1982) provides a plausible explanation in terms of the cognitive load on a deaf child who is required to divide his attention in a serial fashion between objects and communicative interaction. The mother of a hearing child can fairly easily time her language and communication to fit the child's immediate experiences and perceptions, such that her language and communication is contingent upon his activities. For a deaf baby, however, joint reference and language input about the referent cannot occur in parallel. By taking up joint reference of an object or event, the child will have to avert his gaze from the mother and in so doing the channel of communication (i.e. speech-reading) is closed or much reduced, since little or no auditory input is available at the same time as he is making the object or event the focus of visual attention. The deaf child therefore has to handle a more difficult task in which he must learn that what his mother says refers to an object or event just experienced or about to be experienced.

The integration of language and reality thus becomes cognitively more difficult for the young infant, the amount of 'comprehensible input' available to the child decreases, and the whole communicative process slows down. It seems that in the face of such problems parents often respond by exerting greater control over the communication process. Instead of taking the lead from the child's behaviour, actions and communicative initiations, and providing language input concurrent with these activities, the parent begins to take a more active and deliberate role. This will often take the form of frequent interruptions of the child's ongoing activity in order to direct his attention, and a tendency to 'teach' early language skills. This in turn further distorts the already 'unnatural' communicative inter-actions, and further helps to disrupt language acquisition.

The tendency to take control of the conversation when reciprocal communica-tion breaks down may be a 'normal' response. Schlesinger and Meadow (1972) studied the interaction patterns of deaf children and their mothers, and found the mothers to be more inflexible and controlling than mothers of hearing children. Brinich (1980) found that 'mothers of deaf children used attention-related behav-iours much more often than did mothers of hearing children . . . [and] questions and instructions much more often than did mothers of hearing children' (p. 79). Similar findings have emerged for the mother–child interactions of mentally retarded children (Kogan et al. 1969), which suggests that the response of greater control may be widespread whenever it is difficult to establish interactive commu-nication – because of deafness, ageing or whatever.

Wood (1981) has identified similar disruptions of the communicative process in deaf children of school age in their interactions with teachers. Severely hearing-impaired children of, say, eight years of age are likely to be grammatically delayed such that their utterances are restricted to two or three words with simple Stage II structures (LARSP). When normally developing 2 year olds pass through this stage of grammatical advancement, the linguistic structures, although simple, are sufficent to carry the child's communicative needs, which are largely concerned with simple ideas based in the here and now of his environment. Any ambiguities can usually be solved by the parent by reference to the situation, gestures and other nonverbal cues. The severely hearing-impaired 8 year old, however, can plan, reason, remember, imagine, predict and generally perform a whole range of much more sophisticated cognitive functions. As Ivimey and Lachterman (1980) have argued, the child's developmentally primitive language is inadequate to cope with the pressure of his communicative needs. Severe problems and ambiguities in the surface structure and conversational patterns thus emerge which are not amenable to being resolved by reference to the here-and-now context of the conversation.

For some teachers and parents the response to this ambiguity is to exert more control over the conversation: halts, repeats, repetitions, and closed questions requiring single-word answers are all used extensively in order both to resolve the ambiguities and presumably to 'teach' him simultaneously a whole range of speech and language skills which will perhaps help him learn to avoid these ambiguities in the future. The danger of this response by teachers and parents is that there is so much being 'taught', or at least practised simultaneously, that the child is merely further confused and fails to learn anything very much; and that the resulting 'conversation' is so distorted as to become bereft of interest for the child.

Wood (1981) examined the verbal interactions of deaf children with their teachers. He identified seven major types of conversational 'moves' which a teacher can make in response to a child's utterance (there are other more complex moves, but these are little used in the present context). The first three moves, enforced repetition (e.g. *say bye bye for me*), closed question (e.g. *was it mummy or daddy?*) and open question (e.g. *when did you go?*), exert a greater degree of control over the conversation than do the remaining four moves. These are contribution (e.g *I don't like tea*), phatic (e.g. *oh lovely!*), tag contribution (e.g. *I'm always happy, aren't I?*) and tag phatic (e.g. *that's lovely, isn't it?*). Wood noted that hearing preschoolers and deaf primary school children responded similarly and consistently to the teacher's moves. Children generally answered questions and then stopped talking. On the other hand, contributions and phatics from the teacher usually evoked a contribution or question from the child, and helped therefore to continue the dialogue. More importantly, it was found that 'different types of moves were correlated with loquacity of the child being addressed' (Wood 1981, p. 34). Thus, teachers who exerted more control over the conversation by using more repetitions and questions elicited shorter utterances, fewer multiple turns and fewer spontaneous contributions from the children. In other words, it appears that, like some parents of very young deaf children, the teachers of school-age deaf children may, in response to the many ambiguities present in the child's contribution to the conversation, produce a conversational framework which actually inhibits the expressive language behaviours of the child. The suggestion is, of course, that this may in turn inhibit the linguistic development of the child.

Wood (1981) also analysed the function of the teacher's contributions to the dialogue. He and his colleagues found that the incidence of repair – in which the teacher goes back over what the child has just said in order to correct the phonology and/or syntax, or clarify the meaning – was far greater in teachers' conversations with deaf children than in teachers' conversations with younger hearing children. In addition; there was a significant positive correlation between degree of hearing loss and amount of conversational repair. Wood argues that repair makes the conversational task much more difficult for the child than it would otherwise be, since he now has to work out whether the teacher's utterance is concerned with advancing the conversation onto new territory or whether it refers back to what has already been said. It may be that a high degree of control and much repair results in a less ambiguous conversation, although Wood cites an example of a piece of dialogue in which this approach actually serves to increase ambiguity: one problem with control, repair, and questions is that they tend to elicit short utterances that lead nowhere. If the next utterance is 'correct' in terms of the conversation, the teacher can at least initiate a new conversational direction leaving behind some degree of resolution. Often, however, the next utterance will be 'incorrect' or inappropriate, and since it leads nowhere, and tends to be accompanied by the child ceasing to talk, the only way forward is to initiate conversation on a new tack, but leaving the uncertainty unresolved. This type of conversational failure is unlikely to reinforce verbal behaviour. The alternative strategy for the teacher, to exert less control, to let the conversation flow more freely, to encourage by appropriate moves contributions from the child, may seem to carry the danger of deeper and deeper degrees of ambiguity. This does not, however, tend to happen; instead, the increased conversational flow and longer utterances from the child brings increased clues to meaning, so that with a degree of perseverance the ambiguity may resolve itself. The other possible danger of this less controlled approach is that its opportunities for 'teaching' or improving the verbalizations of the child are passed up.

Two important questions, therefore, follow on the work of Wood and his colleagues. First, can teachers' and parents' conversational styles be changed by intervention, and if so does this give rise to greater conversational contributions from the hearing-impaired children? Secondly, does this in turn promote improved language ability in the child, or is the reduction in repair by the teacher necessary for this approach detrimental to language development?

Results from studies by Wood (1981), Wood et al. (1982) and Wood and Wood (1984) suggest that intervention can alter the teacher's style, and that the children become more or less conversationally active in the expected direction. Thus, when the teacher changes style to make more contributions and exert less control, the child's conversational behaviour changes such that he says more, uses longer utterances, and plays a more equal role in the dialogue. As to the second question, whether this style of teaching gives rise to improved language performance, there is simply too little evidence to be able to give an answer. It is worth noting, however, that this question appears to refer back to an old dispute in language teaching for the hearing-impaired, namely the choice between highly structured and naturalistic approaches. Linguists have argued that the dichotomy between the highly structured early support programmes for families and teachers of deaf children and the naturalistic approach, in which the child is immersed in bathfuls of 'natural language' in a fairly unstructured manner, is a false dichotomy. They argue this, convincingly, on the grounds that natural language is in fact highly structured in any case. To a large extent the argument has not been concerned with communication and the dual roles of initiator and responder (McKirdy and Blank 1982) that communication demands. The studies from Wood and colleagues, however, begin to take communication as well as language into account. The early results suggest that although the structured language approach may be unsound, any approach which leaves the parents to their own 'natural' devices may well end up with a very controlled and stifling language environment, since recourse to repair, repetition, questions and other controlling devices is a natural response to the ambiguity in hearing-impaired children's utterances.

These studies also raise the interesting possibility that the process of communication may be as important as the medium of the language (manual vs oral). It is too early to be sure, but these recent studies of language and deaf children appear to have opened up new pathways with considerable promise which research in the next decade will be likely to follow. Progress over the next ten years in this field may be faster and more productive than the rather ponderous descriptive research of previous decades. It also appears likely that the emphasis will change from the 'deficit' model of hearing impairment, in which one examines what hearing-impaired children cannot do, to a more positive approach in which one examines what these children *can* do, both in terms of performance and cognitive processes.

Closing remarks: rehabilitative issues

This chapter and the previous one have attempted to review the current state of knowledge about auditory perception and language skills in sensorineurally hearing-impaired children. We have presented a broad descriptive analysis of these skills, with some attempt to understand the underlying processes. It is this understanding, it is argued, that will eventually lead to theoretically underpinned rehabilitative procedures which offer some hope of success. Current rehabilitative procedures are based upon incomplete, surface (i.e. descriptive) knowledge; and while they may be notably successful in a large number of cases, we know neither precisely why they are so, nor why some hearing-impaired children fail to achieve reasonable linguistic competence. These chapters deal of necessity largely in grouped data, and in statistically significant trends. The reader who has never worked with hearing-impaired children may now have a more thorough knowledge of the trends, yet may lack a feeling for individual cases and for the wide differences to be found between individuals. Many partially hearing children are fully integrated into normal classes, and their progress linguistically and educationally is apparently normal. Some severely impaired children develop good linguistic skills, and may be educationally well above average. Nevertheless, many severely impaired children do not progress 'satisfactorily' – if one takes normal language development as the yardstick. Anyone with first-hand experience of the more severely impaired population will know that – again, in terms of normal development – the educational and linguistic achievement of these children is often still very poor.

Quigley and Kretschmer (1982) define the primary goal of education for typical prelingually deaf children as literacy – the ability to read and write the general language of society. They point out that reading is an indispensable tool for mastering academic subjects, but that it may depend upon a pre-established language system that is a product of, amongst other things, a stimulating early environment and good communication with parents. Some of the data in this chapter have suggested that at least some hearing-impaired children fail to develop reasonable linguistic skills, even by the age of 18 years or so. Data on reading ability (see Ch. 8) for severely impaired children are depressing: Conrad (1979), for example, found a median reading age of 15- to 16-year-old deaf children of about 9 years. Other related skills – auditory memory span, lip-reading ability, intelligibility of uttered speech – were also 'poor'. Again, the pejorative judgement is in relation to these skills in normally hearing children, and this deficit model may be a harsh or negative way to examine deaf children's progress. It is not entirely inappropriate, however.

Most educators would not disagree that there is a large number of hearing-impaired children who fail to develop adequate literacy skills. The pedagogic argument rages, and has done for over a century, as to the reasons for this. We have suggested that the descriptive approach to research into hearing-impaired language has provided little theoretical underpinning and little rigorous basis for choosing between alternatives. The arguments are pervaded by poor data, examples of individual cases rather than overall trends, and religiously held beliefs. We are not going to go over this pedagogic discussion here; it is well-documented elsewhere (e.g. Conrad 1979, Quigley and Kretschmer 1982). But in response to Ivimey's last question – 'what if anything can be done to improve the situation?' – let us consider those rehabilitative issues upon which we *can* comment, if only briefly.

The thrust of research into language acquisition in the last decade has shown clearly the importance of the early months of life. As a consequence, it throws doubt upon the view that fitting hearing aids to congenitally hearing-impaired children by 9 months, or a year, is early enough. The importance of early processes in language acquisition suggest that fitting hearing aids to such children at, say, 3 months of age would not be too early. This view is becoming more widespread, although it does beg certain further questions:

(i) Can we identify hearing impairments this early in life?

(ii) Can we fit appropriate hearing aids this early?

(ii) What can we do, rehabilitatively, this early which is effective?

(iv) Are we sure that, in terms of early parent–child relationship, we do no harm in identifying the child as impaired so early in life?

The early identification of congenital hearing loss remains a problem throughout the world. In the UK all babies are screened for hearing by trained Health Visitors at the age of 8 months or so; such screening utilizes noise-makers and distraction techniques, and is performed in the home or at the local clinic. There are two problems with this infant screening procedure, however. First, it is, not surprisingly, known to be somewhat unreliable (e.g. National Deaf Children's Society, 1983) with relatively large false positive and false negative rates. This is probably not a reflection on the testers so much as on the nature of the test itself, the small numbers being searched for, and the acoustic test conditions under which it has to be carried out.

Various strategies have been tried recently to improve the screening: formal questionnaires, for example, or even the simple question posed by the Health Visitor to the parent: 'Do you think your child is hearing normally?' (Hitchings and Haggard 1983). These approaches make explicit the value of parental observations and parental suspicion, which are known to contain a high degree of validity. In conjunction, improved communication and publicity with primary health care teams, family doctors and so on can help encourage such people to refer on if in doubt, rather than take the 'don't worry' or 'he/she will grow out of it' attitude.

The second problem with the health visitor screen is that it takes place too late. By the time a child has failed twice (there is always a retest before referral), been referred either direct to a hospital audiology or ENT department or via an intermediate Community Health clinic, the child may be nearly a year old. Why, then, is the original screening not performed earlier? The chief reason is that clearly observable behavioural responses (e.g. localization) to auditory stimuli are not present much earlier than 7 months of age, at least to the relatively naive observer. Even in the best case, then, the health-visitor screening is unlikely to result in hearing-aid issues prior to 9 months or so. Nevertheless, a properly organized, properly trained health-visitor screening programme, with quick and unambiguous referral routes and a well-resourced paediatric audiology department, backed up by good communication and ample publicity and information can achieve much. Age of first identification of hearing loss has in the past been poor, often as late as two to three years of age, when it is observed that speech and language is failing to develop adequately, and there is therefore considerable slack to be taken up by a good health visitor programme, as McCormick et al. (1984b) have shown.

This aside, there are approaches to early screening which offer ways forward and which are not constrained by the need for easily observable behavioural responses. Thus, screening neonates (while still a captive population in the maternity units) using brainstem electric response audiometry (e.g. Galambos et al. 1982) or otoacoustic emissions (Stevens et al. 1989) is under trial at present. Since the uptake of rubella immunization is increasing, and since neonatal paediatrics are now so advanced, it may be that these machines are most cost-effectively used in neonatal care units, where the numbers of hearing-impaired children may be 10 times the numbers in the normal neonatal population (McCormick et al. 1984a, Davis 1990).

It is quite possible to fit hearing aids to infants as young as 3 months. In order to select the aids with the appropriate power for the degree of loss, full-scale audiological assessment is required, and at this age this would probably have to include electric response audiometry. Assuming that this assessment gave a reasonable idea of auditory thresholds (not always a foregone conclusion) then appropriate aids could be fitted. The basis upon which aids are selected is in any case controversial and so details of fine tuning can wait until the child is older, provided that the degree of amplification in the various frequency bands is sufficient yet not too much to cause discomfort or even damage. With very young children, the provision of well-fitting earmoulds for the aids is not a simple matter, and new moulds are required often, as the child grows. This is not an insurmountable problem, however, for an adequately resourced service.

Suitable amplification may be the cornerstone of auditory rehabilitation, but it is also only the beginning. Parental guidance and counselling, and the early involvement of the preschool peripatetic educational services will be vital. Aids in addition to the traditional hearing aids may be useful; in particular FM or radio hearing aids, where the speaker (e.g. mother) wears a microphone from which the voice signal is transmitted by radio frequencies to a small receiver and amplifier worn by the child, can improve signal-to-noise ratios at the child's ears considerably, and there is much to be said for the early home provision of such aids. Although appropriate amplification systems are crucial, they are not sufficient. As we know from Chapter 5, sensorineural hearing loss gives rise to dysfunction in various auditory perceptual processes, and while hearing aids can compensate for loss in threshold sensitivity in various frequency bands, they can do nothing about the other perceptual problems. They have to be regarded as communication improvers rather than as prosthetic devices. For this reason, various professionals will need to be involved in the rehabilitative effort quite early on. In the UK this has traditionally been the teachers of the hearing-impaired for children with sensorineural hearing loss; but recently the contribution to be made by educational psychologists and by speech pathologists who have specialized in childhood hearing impairment has increasingly been recognized. The nature of early intervention, the assessment procedures available and the contingent decisions about detailed intervention made on the basis of these assessments remains a pressing area for research. A discussion of some aspects of one such early intervention programme is given by Stokes and Bamford (1990).

Early identification, early issue of appropriate amplification devices, good counselling and support services, early involvement of teachers, psychologists and speech pathologists as appropriate will do much to reduce the communication handicaps faced by congenitally severely hearing-impaired children; more open-mindedness on pedagogic issues in the face of our limited knowledge and sometimes limited educational success will be helpful; but in addition we do need to know more about the underlying processes of language acquisition in hearing-impaired children, and the reasons therefore why some individuals make progress and others do not.

7

Fluctuating conductive hearing loss

Hearing loss, secretory otitis media and screening

The presence of fluid in the middle ear due to secretory otitis media (SOM) generally results in a hearing loss. As the air volume in the middle ear decreases, the stiffness of the eardrum increases and the sensitivity to low-frequency sound decreases. This threshold then further deteriorates across all frequencies, as the air in the middle-ear cavity is replaced by fluid. Estimates of the degree of the average hearing loss caused by SOM vary widely for two main reasons. First, the test population is frequently preschool and thus determination of hearing threshold can be imprecise. Secondly, there are inconsistencies between the presentation of the results in the different studies, that is, in the distinction between *hearing level* and *hearing loss*. The hearing loss affects predominantly the conductive pathways, so that measures of bone-conduction thresholds are normal, or near normal, depending to some extent on the vibrator placement in the test procedure. For the true extent of the hearing loss to be appreciated, it is most meaningful to present this type of loss in terms of the difference between the air- and bone-conduction thresholds; but more often the air-conduction thresholds are presented only in relation to bone-conduction population norms.

There have been attempts to predict the hearing loss which might be expected at different points of the disease process from data obtained in animal studies. For example, Goodhill (1958) made electrophysiological measures of cochlear sensitivity in cats, where the bulla of the middle ear was filled with fluids of various viscosities. His results indicated that as the viscosity of the fluid was increased and became more glue-like, so the hearing loss increased. It is now understood, however, that hearing loss is dependent on the volume of the effusion, rather than its viscosity (Wiederhold *et al.* 1980).

There are two commonly used methods of estimating the average hearing loss caused by SOM reported in the literature. In the first, thresholds in children before and after surgical treatment have been compared, yielding predicted mean hearing losses of 18–29 dB, with standard deviations of about 10 dB (Kersley and Wickam 1966, Harbert *et al.* 1970, Richards *et al.* 1971, Eagles 1972). In the second, authors have obtained thresholds from a large number of children know to have SOM. A range of results from 0 to 55 dB HL have been reported (Harbert *et al.* 1970, Cohen and Sade 1972). Apart from subject

170

selection and other methodological differences, the large range of results probably reflects the differing middle-ear conditions at the time of assessment. Cohen and Sade, in agreement with other studies (e.g. Bluestone *et al.* 1973, Kaplan *et al.* 1973, Kokko 1975, Paradise 1981), found the most common hearing level in the speech frequencies to be 25–28 dB HL with about 20% of cases being unilateral.

A hearing loss of so mild a degree is not always easy to detect behaviourally, particularly in the young child. The level denoted as the pass criteria in screening, and often in clinic assessments, is usually 20 or 25 dB HL (under headphones) or 30 dB SPL or dBA (in the soundfield); as previously indicated, the presence of SOM does not always result in a hearing level of that order. It has become a matter of great concern that some children with SOM will pass the pure-tone screen and be declared as normal hearing, and yet be experiencing difficulties in normal speech perception as a result of the disorder. The significance of a mild, fluctuating hearing deficit to the developing child will be discussed in this chapter, and may be regarded as a controversial topic, but it is noted here, in the context of hearing screening, that Downs (1976) has argued that hearing losses of 15 dB should be regarded as having a potentially negative effect on optimal language development. It is clear that the efficacy of pure-tone audiometry as a means of detecting the presence of otitis media of sufficient severity to cause developmental difficulties, is very questionable.

Studies have been carried out to investigate the sensitivity of pure-tone audiometry as a means of identifying SOM, where the presence of the disorder has been confirmed by other means. The results vary but suggest that as many as 60 per cent of children who have SOM may not be detected by pure-tone audiometry (Eagles 1972, Brooks 1973, Renvall *et al.* 1975, Fiellau-Nikolajsen 1983). This is a disturbing underestimate, and is probably explained by:

(i) The wide intersubject range and intrasubject fluctuations of hearing loss which result from SOM.

(ii) Limitations of behavioural testing techniques, particularly with young children.

(iii) Unacceptable background noise levels in the test environment, often varying from 40 up to 70 dB SPL.

(iv) Variation in the standard of equipment calibration has been shown to be very common, resulting in misleading data.

(v) The skill of the test personnel varies. Bennett and Mowat (1981) reported that the Regional-screening failure rate varied from 5.6 to 20.4 per cent across U.K. Regions in 1971 – a difference which is unlikely to be explained epidemiologically. A second experiment showed that in one District, three different nurses testing the same children found failure rates of 3.4, 7.4 and 10 per cent respectively, demonstrating the variability introduced by different degrees of skill.

Pure-tone audiometry does not then appear to be an approach sensitive to this disorder. Identification by this means alone leads to an underestimate of provision and mismanagement of individual cases. In order to obtain a more sensitive screening procedure, the validity and sensitivity of other methods have been investigated and compared with pure-tone audiometry.

One such method is pneumatic otoscopy, used routinely in ENT clinics, in which the appearance and mobility of the eardrum is examined under high magnification and illumination. It is quick,and requires no active participation from the child, but it is an inexact method of determining the presence or absence of SOM, because of the large interobserver error that has been shown to exist, even between trained observers who know that they are being assessed. As an example, Paradise *et al.* (1977) report a study in which 15–20 per cent of effusions which were confirmed at myringotomy were missed by otoscopy, and other studies support this finding (e.g. Rose *et al.* 1977).

A method which objectively detects changes in the compliance of the tympanic membrane and changes in middle-ear pressure is called tympanometry. This technique has the advantage of eliminating the need for a behavioural response from the child, and does not require such a degree of training as otoscopy. Like otoscopy, tympanometry identifies middle-ear disorder, not hearing loss, and as such middle-ear disease which has not caused a hearing loss will be detected. Also, changes in the disease status may be monitored. Measurements are carried out by hermetically sealing a probe tip into the ear canal. The tip carries three tubes, connected respectively to an oscillator receiver that delivers a tone of fixed frequency and intensity, usually of 220 Hz and 90 dB SPL, a microphone to monitor the sound-pressure level in the sealed cavity created between the tip and the eardrum, and a pump manometer that varies and measures air-pressure. The input sound is fixed in intensity, so that the sound-pressure level recorded in the cavity formed between the probe and the eardrum will depend on how much sound is reflected back from the tympanic membrane. This will in turn depend on the flexibility of the middle-ear system. Accordingly, measurements of sound-pressure level in the cavity may be translated into changes in the compliance of the tympanic membrane, demonstrating the flexibility of the middle-ear system. By using the pressure pump to vary the pressure in the cavity, changes in the compliance that occur in response to these pressure changes may be plotted. The resulting graph is known as a tympanogram. As maximum compliance will occur when the pressure is equal on both sides of the membrane, the air-pressure in the middle ear, which is normally equal to atmospheric pressure, may be determined, and air-pressures which are less than normal are detected. The tympanogram is normally defined in terms of *(i)* the height of the peak, *(ii)* the location of the peak in relation to atmospheric pressure, and *(iii)* the shape or 'gradient' of the peak.

The compliance instrument may also be used to detect the contraction of the stapedius muscle which occurs in response to loud sounds. This results in a change in the compliance of the tympanic membrane, which may be detected with the impedance instrument. The presence of the contraction very strongly contra-indicates the presence of SOM (Brooks 1982), since fluid in the middle ear impedes detection of the muscle contraction. Ideally, each of these measures should be evaluated, and the results considered as a whole. A number of studies have investigated the efficacy of acoustic impedance measures in the detection of SOM, and have consistently shown a higher rate of identification than using other methods. Brooks (1982), in a review of published studies investigating the use of impedance measures, found the sensitivity to range from 65 to 99 per cent, and the specificity to range from 45 to 100 per cent, which is higher than pneumatic otoscopy.

The suitability of impedance measures as a screening technique has been advocated by Renvall et al. (1975), Harker and van Wagoner (1974), Brooks (1973), Grosso and Rupp (1978), Paradise et al. (1977) and others. Use of impedance screening consistently results in a higher identification rate of middle-ear disorder than pure-tone audiometry (e.g. Brooks 1973) but can lead to over-referral. As with any other screening technique, criteria must be applied to the interpretation of the impedance data such that: conditions with an underlying medical disorder requiring treatment are identified; cases where the condition may deteriorate (for example, middle-ear pressure that is much less than atmospheric) are identified; and significant disturbances in speech perception are identified. The condition is so common that to establish the criteria that would achieve the second of these aims is difficult, and so a strict observation of adult norms for impedance tests, and the retesting of all failures some weeks after the first test, is probably the optimal solution.

Used with care, impedance measures would therefore seem to be a suitable method for identifying conductive hearing loss, by identifying the underlying middle-ear disorder rather than by attempting to measure hearing levels directly. Note that the technique does not give direct information on the extent of hearing loss.

Attempts have been made to use measurement of middle-ear function for predictions of hearing loss. This seems reasonable since, as the air in the middle-ear cavity is replaced by fluid, the greater viscosity presents greater resistance to the eardrum and ossicle, resulting in hearing loss. But it seems that the two measures are not simply related. Notable studies by Bennett and Mowat (1981), Fiellau-Nikolajsen (1983), Lildholdt et al. (1979) and Cooper et al. (1975) found very different degrees of predictability, possibly arising from the differing presentations of the middle-ear disease. The hearing-loss and middle-ear measures will reflect to differing extents the viscosity and the amount of middle-ear effusion, the extent to which the middle ear is obstructed, and the interference to ossicular movement, making it difficult to calculate a direct relationship. Additionally, recent evidence indicates that a mild depression of bone-conduction thresholds may be associated with middle-ear effusion, the degree and frequencies affected depending on the underlying mechanical changes in the inner and middle-ear systems (Kobayashi et al. 1988). This has been shown to be reversible following middle-ear surgery.

Impedance measures identify middle-ear disease, which represents a health problem and may cause a hearing handicap. This enables referral of abnormal cases for medical intervention and/or rehabilitation as necessary. In comparison, the pure tone sweep test, because of its ineffectiveness in identification of losses around 25 dB HL (the usual pass/fail level), is a weak screening test. The central question then becomes whether a pass at 25 dB HL is a sufficiently rigorous measure. It clearly will not detect all cases of middle-ear pathology, but furthermore it may not detect all cases of hearing difficulties.

If a child has a normal bone-conduction hearing level of say, 0 to -5 dB, and measured air-conduction threshold of 20 dB HL, then it will pass the screening procedure but will effectively have reduced hearing sensitivity. This child has a temporary air–bone gap of 25 dB which, although considered 'normal', would reflect a considerable change from the child's normal auditory environment. Even such a slight loss, particularly if it is fluctuating, may handicap the child in his learning processes and acquisition of language. When adults are given a temporary loss of as little as 20 dB, they experience some difficulty with discrimination of the weaker speech sounds, particularly in environments of competing noise. Further, by carrying out a screening test, and accrediting such a child with a 'pass' identification, it will be assumed that he or she is not having difficulties in hearing. Any subsequent psychoeducational problems will probably then be ascribed to other causes. We are not in a position to dismiss the effects of mild hearing loss as insignificant. Yet we do now realize that otitis media is an extremely prevalent condition in children.

Fluctuating conductive hearing loss and language development: theoretical considerations

There is widespread agreement that there is an association between repeated attacks of otitis media in childhood and the presence of language delay extending into the early school years. The extent to which the disease is the causal agent is, however, much less clear. Evidence has generally been sought from comparative studies of two populations, one containing children known to have repeated attacks of otitis media and a second, apparently free from the disorder. The former group has been shown to have a significant tendency to suffer delays in language. In a truly comparative study, it should be possible to ascertain which factor is causing the difference between the groups. While in the examples which will be considered later, otitis media is described as the causal agent, it has not been possible to make the groups identical in every other respect, so the test variable becomes confounded among others. From the data discussed in the preceding sections, it is clear that subject-matching is difficult. For example, children who frequently suffer from otitis media often have concomitant periods of ill-health. Also, there is a tendency for the condition to be more prevalent where environmental factors are also poor. Both of these may have effects on various aspects of a child's development and, later, on nursery and school attendance.

The precise interrelationship between auditory development and language development is not known; Sancho *et al.* (1988, p. 16) provide a useful picture of types of and routes to otitis media sequelae, using underlying factors, impoverished inputs, missed information and illness effects to describe the relationships between the following behavioural effects: (i) psychophysiological maturation; (ii) perception; (iii) language and speech; (iv) cognition and general intelligence; (v) educational attainment; and (vi) interpersonal behaviour. But it is clear that severe disturbances in auditory input are detrimental to normal language acquisition. This is apparent from our knowledge of the effects of sensorineural hearing loss. Disturbances to the auditory input caused by recurring attenuation of the speech signal to the cochlea (as in SOM) is also an attributed cause of language delay. Educational difficulties such as those of learning to read and spell are also tentatively associated with a history of persistent middle-ear problems (e.g. Zinkus and Gottlieb 1980). If this is so, whether these occur as a result of delayed language or are due to a more pervasive underlying auditory disability is a subject now under consideration.

In the following sections, the possible effects of fluctuating hearing loss on language acquisition will be considered within the context of our current knowledge of speech perception.

Conductive impairment versus sensorineural impairment

There are numerous reports of the damaging effects of severe sensorineural hearing loss on speech and language development (see Chapters 5 and 6). There is a rather smaller body of literature reporting on language in children with mild hearing impairment. Mild sensorineural hearing loss is usually located primarily in the high frequencies, resulting in reduced hearing in the frequencies which carry the consonantal information of speech, which are comparatively weak in energy and are important for comprehension of the message. Some of the early studies reporting on the effects of mild hearing loss have been described in Chapter 6. For example, Hardy et al. (1958) compared 20 normally hearing school-age children with 20 children of the same age who had a mean hearing loss of 42 dB (range 27–55 dB), on measures of intelligence, vocabulary, syntax, reading and speech intelligibility. Although the normally hearing children tended to score higher on each of these tests, the differences were not always significant, the overall finding being that the language of the hearing-impaired children was somewhat less complex than the hearing group. Confounding factors in this experiment, particularly subject selection, are such that the apparently small effects cannot be inferred from this study alone, but subsequent work supports the hypothesis that mild sensorineural hearing loss results in relatively small delays in language acquisition. Owrid's (1960) assessment of spoken-language skills in 300 hearing-impaired children led him to conclude that the deleterious effects of mild losses are small, and that language is delayed, rather than deviant.

Since mild and moderate degrees of bilateral sensorineural hearing loss tend to cause a child to experience some delays in language acquisition, we should be alert to the possibility that conductive losses may also result in language retardation. Recall however that, while conductive hearing loss due to secretory otitis media may be as severe as 50 dB, it is more commonly of the order of 25 dB and may be less. Furthermore, unlike sensorineural impairment, conductive loss of this kind usually affects hearing at all frequencies equally, or it may be slightly worse in the lower frequencies which are comparatively high in energy.

There are further differences between the two disorders. Conductive hearing loss due to otitis media is rarely present from birth and is not present continuously, so that there are periods when normal auditory input would seem to occur. The condition usually resolves entirely by about 10 years of age so that it is not, in itself, a permanent condition. Perhaps the most striking contrast between the two conditions is the nature of the resultant auditory processing. As described earlier, conductive hearing loss acts primarily to reduce the intensity of sounds reaching the cochlea. Although the condition may cause some nonlinearities at high intensities due to the abnormal functioning of the acoustic reflex mechanism, the coding of the features of the auditory signal is not disordered, as it is in cases of sensorineural loss. Perceptually, for some purposes, the effect of conductive hearing loss may be likened to occlusion of the external ear-canal with ear plugs. The sound intensity reaching the cochlea is reduced, so that normal peripheral coding of the (reduced) auditory input takes place; the resulting auditory effects seem uncomplicated. Results from speech audiometry further demonstrate this point. When this assessment is carried out on listeners who have conductive hearing losses, the resulting performance-intensity function (see Chapter 5) is similar to that for normals, in that the listener's maximum scores are of the order of 80–100 per cent correct, but the entire function is shifted to the right by an amount equal to the hearing loss. This finding supports the notion that as long as the signal is at a high enough intensity to overcome the middle-ear transmission loss, the cochlea will code the speech signal as normal.

Taken together, these factors might seem to indicate that a fluctuating condition would be less likely to cause delays in speech and language acquisition than would a congenital sensorineural hearing loss. However, there is a more negative view of the situation. First, a child subject to periods of otitis media may also belong to a subgroup of children at high risk for language delay due to other factors, perhaps associated with the disease. Secondly, the fluctuating nature of the condition may have a surprisingly adverse effect on speech and language development, in comparison with a sensorineural loss of the same, or even greater, degree. This fluctuation in the auditory input may impede efficient language learning by restricting the process of organizing and categorizing auditory information. Information to be categorized as part of the speech perception and learning process may be different at different times in the disease process, perhaps severely disadvantaging the child in this learning task. Thirdly, unless the hearing loss is entirely constant across frequencies, the normal relationships between the intensities of the sounds of speech will be altered. In evaluating the consequences of sensorineural loss on speech perception and language acquisition, psychoacoustic experiments may be carried out on adults, enabling a description of the limitations of the acoustic coding in the damaged cochlea to be made. Data from experiments of this kind have been used to broadly predict the information in the speech message which a child with a sensorineural loss may be receiving. While this is an imprecise approach, it gives a useful approach to understanding the difficulties that a child with a sensorineural loss may have in speech reception. There seem to be few useful parallel experiments that can be carried out on adults to predict the effect of a fluctuating conductive hearing loss in children. This presents a particular difficulty, since the extent of hearing loss alone is not sufficient to account for the apparent linguistic sequelae of recurrent otitis media.

It becomes apparent that, although in terms of pure-tone sensitivity the hearing loss caused by SOM may be little more than that experienced by an adult with a severe head cold, the functional auditory difficulties encountered by a child who repeatedly experiences middle-ear disease may be much more complex. For example, an adult is more likely to manipulate the situation – 'Sorry, what did you say?' – and retrieve missed information. An adult also possesses more mature processes of selective attention, resulting perhaps in less difficulty than a child in adverse listening conditions of competing stimuli. But most importantly, the child is still in the process of developing speech and language. As a result there is less of the intrinsic redundancy of a message available to fill in the 'gaps', and the implications of the instability of the auditory signal being processed may be severe.

From literature, it appears that some children are more affected than others. Many factors, known to influence a child's ability to develop spoken language at the normal rate, may be involved. For example, even the child's, and the parent's, personality will influence the situation. Compare two possible responses from a child who is called by name by his mother, and who is requested to carry out a task at a time when his hearing is dulled by otitis media:

Response A: 'What? – What, mummy?'
Response B: Child perhaps turns to name only.

A child responding as in (A) not only has the message presented a second time, but also draws attention to the nature of his or her difficulty–that of a problem in hearing rather than of behaviour. A child responding as in (B) may be interpreted as a child unwilling to follow instructions and does not so clearly demonstrate his hearing difficulty. This is reinforced by the inconsistent nature of the condition, so that sometimes he or she may appear to choose to carry out instructions. Thus the extent to which the child is affected may depend in part on the ability to manipulate the situation, and on the observation and understanding of his or her caregivers. The parent's ability to encourage language development in this situation is clearly important, and good parenting skills, difficult to evaluate from outside the family situation, except in the extreme, are probably of great importance in these cases. However, the hidden nature of the child's condition, who may be otherwise asymptomatic, means that parents are less likely to be aware of the need to provide compensatory stimulation. The ramifications of this may be diverse – cognitive and social development are closely related to language development, and to the parent/child relationship, which may be adversely affected by misinterpretation of the cause of apparent behaviour problems. Identification and parent education are thus of great importance.

Fluctuations in auditory sensitivity during the first years of life may provide the child with an inconsistent representation of the speech code. Rather than the periods of 'good hearing' enabling the child to 'catch up', the fluctuations are more likely to confuse the child in the formation of a framework for speech perception. One would perhaps expect the frequency of attacks, as much as the extent of the hearing loss incurred, to affect the child's spoken language development. The practice of issuing hearing aids to children awaiting surgical treatment for glue ear may, in this light, not be particularly helpful, since it is probably the inconsistency of the input rather than simple attenuation which causes a long-term problem. Since the extent of the hearing loss alone is not sufficient to account for the linguistic sequelae of this condition, an approach to hypothesizing the effect of repeated otitis media may be based on the effects of a fluctuation of the input on the development of speech perception. This view has previously been expressed by, for example, Holm and Kunze (1969). Sancho *et al.* (1988) argue that it is the overall *persistence* of the condition which relates to the degree of disability, on the grounds that persistence of the condition directly opposes 'catch-up opportunities'. The analogy with mild sensorineural hearing loss may argue against this view, however. As discussed above, study of the fluctuant effects provides an experimental problem. The consequences of sensorineural hearing loss on speech perception and language acquisition are studied by carrying out psychoacoustic experiments with adult subjects. This enables a description of the limitations to acoustic coding in the damaged cochlea to be made. Data from these experiments are extrapolated to predict the information in the speech message which a child with a sensorineural hearing loss may be receiving. A similar strategy cannot be employed to study the implications of fluctuating conductive hearing loss. Study of the perceptual effects has thus far been limited to simulation of a constant conductive hearing loss.

Simulation of the effects of conductive loss

Dobie and Berlin (1979) simulated a mild (20 dB) conductive loss in order to evaluate predictions on its effect on reception on the speech message. These authors demonstrated the degree to which the speech message would be degraded during periods of conductive loss. Normally speech is received at the cochlea at an average of 40–60 dB sound-pressure level; that is (bearing in mind the differential sensitivity of the ear to sounds of different frequencies), 10–50 dB above hearing thresholds. The mean hearing loss caused by otitis media is 25–30 dB. The loss is worse in the lower frequencies at first, when it is primarily a stiffening pathology, but as fluid accumulates the hearing loss affects perception at all frequencies. Some speech sounds reach the cochlea at about 10 dB, or less, above threshold. The speech sounds at the extremes of the frequency spectrum are weakest in intensity, and many of these sounds will be lost to the child with otitis media. The most vulnerable sounds are the stops, nasals and fricatives – the consonant sounds which carry much of the speech message. This situation would deteriorate further if the child were in a noisy environment, such as an open classroom in a school, where the signal-to-noise ratio is much worse.

Dobie and Berlin went on to simulate the conditions of a 20 dB conductive hearing loss on a 10-second recording of a reading test. The test consisted of eight simple sentences. The authors obtained a spectral analysis of the synthesis, and on this located and marked the onsets of each phonetic utterance. In other words, they hoped by visual inspection of the spectrographic analysis to identify the components of the speech message which would be lost, or weakened, by the presence of a 20 dB hearing loss. They found that brief utterances, of the type which are often elicited in connected speech such as *are* and *to*, were likely to be lost. High-frequency information was also susceptible to degradation. They suggested that plural endings and related final-position fricatives might not be heard. Temporal information and voicing information appeared robust. If the phonetic segments which are not perceived are also morphological markers, this imperception results in semantic ambiguity and may cause confusions to the child who is acquiring semantic knowledge. Dobie and Berlin also observed that some of these 'weaker' components of speech were inconsistently received. They suggest that formant transitions may be lost, or heard inconsistently depending on context. This leads to a wider consideration of the effects of hearing the phonetic units of speech inconsistently. The work of these authors is very useful in demonstrating which components of speech may be heard inconsistently both during attacks of otitis media and between attacks. The consequences of this will now be considered.

Areas 'at risk' in speech development

The principal mechanisms of speech perception, auditory attention and their development are not yet well established. The infant auditory system perceives some contrasts more easily than others, and some of these contrasts coincide with adult categories of phonemic perception (see Chapter 2). Cross-language studies show that the infant perceives contrasts which are later 'lost' if they are not present in his language environment. It appears that some kind of reinforcement is required for retention of the capability to perceive phonetic contrasts, and that adults perceive categorically only within their own language group. Largely then, the effect that we may predict a fluctuating hearing loss to have on language development depends on the way in which speech is perceived; on how speech perception relates to language development; and the extent to which auditory experience affects speech perception and language development.

Speech is made up of strings of phonemes, which are themselves context dependent. That is, their acoustic spectrum depends upon adjacent phonemes. To an adult with knowledge of language, the speech signal has high redundancy and the message can be derived even if it is considerably degraded. To a child developing this knowledge, more specific speech signals may be essential. A speech-perception-linked view of language acquisition would require the acoustic cues to be stored in long-term memory as phonemic segments, or words or familiar phrases, to build up a language referential system. Inconsistencies in the speech message caused by a fluctuating input may delay the acquisition of the reference structure for the perceptual units of speech. The units which will be most susceptible to the effects of a conductive loss, for example transitional endings, fricatives, and stops which are brief and weak in intensity, will be less easily accumulated in long-term memory store. These features are important, not just to develop age-appropriate lexical knowledge, but also for the development of a complex language structure. Deficiencies in detection of these transients may result in delayed acquisition of appropriate morphology and appreciably simplistic sentence structure.

Although the existence and identification of the basic unit of speech is still controversial, it is proposed that perception of acoustic events signalling phonetic segments is required during the early years of life to build a 'dictionary' unit in long-term memory. Inconsistent representations of the same phoneme due to hearing loss, rather than to context, may delay this acquisition. While a child may apparently 'catch up' to be described as having normal language, this may have a residual effect in tasks of selective attention. If the child acquires language competence, such that he can begin to use the intrinsic redundancy of language in speech perception, his performance on test tasks of, say, word identification may approach normal. But when the speech message is in competition with other auditory speech or nonspeech stimuli, the store may prove less robust. There appears to be a maturational factor in competing message tasks (Berlin *et al*. 1973). Studies on selective attention lead us to think that the ability to attend to a selected stimulus occurs above the level of linguistic processing. Paucity in inherent linguistic knowledge, while not apparent in 'good situations', may therefore be manifest in 'difficult' listening conditions.

Effect on binaural phenomena

Another dimension which should be considered is the effect of fluctuating conductive loss on binaural phenomena. Although otitis media is only truly unilateral in about 20 per cent of cases, the precise extent and time-course of the disease is unlikely to be identical in the two ears, causing inconsistences in binaural effects such as localization ability. Again, the dominant effect is probably due to inconsistencies in the situation. The advantages of binaural hearing were discussed in Chapter 1. The extent to which localization, the precedence effect, the phenomenon of release from masking, and auditory selectivity are 'learned' effects is not clear. However, if there is any learning component, we can expect a child to have a functional problem in difficult listening situations, even when he or she ceases to suffer attacks of middle-ear disease. For example, in classroom listening, where there may be considerable reverberation, the precedence effect enables fusion of the multiple images caused by sound reflections from surfaces. The major cue to auditory selectivity is probably the identification of the location of the sound in space. Difficulties in locating a sound quickly may impede a child in listening to the appropriate speaker in a noisy classroom. Theoretically, then, language delays and persisting difficulties in classroom learning may result from repeated bouts of conductive hearing loss in early childhood.

There is clearly considerable scope for careful experimental research into speech-perception skills in children with a history of fluctuating conductive hearing loss. It would be of value to investigate the ability of young children with this condition in tasks of categorical perception and retrieval of phonetic contrasts, perhaps using synthetic speech tasks of the type devised by Fourcin (1976).

Auditory deprivation

The preceding discussion is centred on an attempt to understand the effects of a fluctuating hearing loss on language processing and acquisition through its effect upon long-term memory. Some authors have proposed that even mild conductive losses, early in infancy, may cause persistent *auditory processing* problems. Evidence from animal studies has been used to show that periods of sensory deprivation, occurring during a time when the maturational processes of the auditory pathway are not complete, may result in abnormal development of these pathways. This evidence has taken the form of small but demonstrable neuro-anatomical differences in the brainstem from the normal (Webster and Webster 1979); abnormalities in the higher brainstem electrophysiological responses, as measured by auditory stimuli (Clopton and Silverman 1978); differences from the normal in auditory electrophysiological studies on binaural interaction and differences in the behavioural responses to complex sound stimuli (e.g. Tees 1967, Saunders *et al.* 1972). Typically, in these experiments the animal is given a known conductive hearing loss during a specified period after birth. Some of the effects seem to be reversible, depending whether or not the deprivation occurred during a critical time period. In general the effects would seem to be rather subtle. Tees (1967) used earplugs to cause a temporary conductive hearing loss in rats for the period of three to 60 days after birth. When the plugs were removed, comparison with a control group of rats showed the experimental group to have comparatively poor ability to discriminate sounds of different durations and frequency patterns. The period of sound deprivation did not affect the ability of the experimental groups to discriminate frequency and intensity. Tees suggested that early preconditioning is essential for complex auditory processing functions to develop normally. In a similar study, Clements and Kelly (1978) showed that a unilateral conductive loss in the first 10 days of life resulted in a markedly reduced ability to localize sounds. That is, there seemed to be disruption in basic binaural processes. From these and similar studies it is tempting to surmise that a mild transient conductive hearing loss, occurring in a critical period, may cause some auditory processing difficulties.

Continued maturational processes occurring in the first year of life can be monitored from studies of auditory brainstem electric response measures. The maturational changes do not relate to gross sensitivity measures which reach normal adult levels in the first few weeks of life, but may relate to the development of more subtle processing abilities. Downs (1977) links the animal studies on auditory deprivation to studies of maturational change in the human brainstem, and suggests that early otitis media may result in irreversible auditory processing problems. This in turn may adversely affect normal language development, or may later give rise to learning disabilities in the classroom where the nature of the problem may be difficult to assess. In other words, these authors attribute later delays in language acquisition not to the fluctuating auditory input in childhood and perception of inconsistent phonemic contrasts, but to an underlying disorder in auditory processing, resulting from the hearing loss early in infancy. Since the children who repeatedly undergo attacks of otitis media are usually the same children whose first attacks were in infancy, these theories are not easily separated. One promising approach involves the use of auditory electrophysiological procedures.

Since some auditory electric brainstem responses can be used to monitor the normal processes of maturation, detection of abnormal processes caused by auditory deprivation should be identifiable using this technique. Auditory brainstem electric responses, recorded from normal subjects, consist of a waveform with five principal peaks occurring within the first 7 milliseconds following a transient stimulus presentation. These peaks represent the synchronous electrical activity occurring in a subset of neurones within the auditory nerve and brainstem structures. The inter-peak latency intervals are reliable within and between subjects (standard deviations of the order of 0.2 ms) and as the responses can be recorded in sleep the technique is useful for examination of the integrity of the auditory brainstem pathways. Folsom *et al.* (1983) used brainstem recordings to compare recordings from children with histories of recurrent otitis media with recordings from normal-hearing children. These authors found that the interwave latencies were longer for the former group, suggesting some association between the pathology and 'central conduction time'. However, these studies have yet to be replicated (Mauldin and Jerger 1979).

The inferences which may be made with respect to the effects of early otitis media as a cause of auditory deprivation are highly speculative. There are disadvantages in the application of the results of animal studies to the developing human auditory system. For example, the description of the critical period during which the neural systems demonstrate plasticity cannot be directly transferred to human development. Although caution is required in interpreting these results, they have been discussed by authors attempting to interrelate auditory disabilities, learning disabilities and early onset of otitis media. These follow earlier attempts to relate the chronic condition to developmental delays in language, intelligence, psychological adjustment and scholastic performance. Recently, there have been a number of articles warning of the damaging effects on speech and language development, and on scholastic achievement of children, of repeated attacks of otitis media. It therefore becomes important that educational, rehabilitative and medical professionals can realistically evaluate the risk that this disorder carries in order to advise parents and plan intervention.

A fruitful approach to investigating the effects of a condition is to carry out retrospective studies on subjects sustaining it. In the case of sensorineural loss, the sensitivity deficit remains constant, generally, or deteriorates. There are no extended periods of remission or fluctuations in input. Studies on the effects of sensorineural loss may be made by evaluating hearing loss at the present time, and investigating language acquisition. Studies on the effect of a conductive loss, on the other hand, may be based on parental description of the history of the disease, which is quite different, and much less precise, since the extent of hearing loss in the stages of the disease process will probably not be known.

The effects of fluctuating conductive hearing loss on language skills

In the remainder of this chapter, the major experimental investigations which have been carried out to evaluate the effect of recurrent otitis media on various aspects of development will be reviewed. These studies are selected from among all the current available experimental evidence in this area.

Studies in this field originated in the 1930s. Bond, in 1935, in a study of New York school children, reported reading problems to be more common in children who had failed a pure-tone screening test. Other investigations found an association between verbal measures of IQ, academic ability and hearing loss.

These early studies generally involved performance measures on children who had failed a pure-tone screening test. Although the majority of this group would have middle ear problems, it was not identified *per se*. Neither was the history of the disease examined. Later investigations were more systematic, and include attempts to minimize confounding variables, and to identify children at high risk for language delay in the absence of otitis media. The studies share a number of features in common and may be conveniently described under various subheadings.

Primary nonhearing variables under study

1. Speech and language development (Holm and Kunze 1969, Owrid 1970, Lewis 1976, Lehmann *et al.*1977, Needleman 1977. Brandes and Ehinger 1981, Friel-Patti *et al.* 1982, Teele *et al.* 1984, Schlieper *et al.* 1985, Roberts *et al.* 1986, Brookhouse and Goldgar 1987, Rach *et al.* 1988).
2. Auditory abilities (Lewis 1976, Needleman 1977, Brandes and Ehinger 1981, Downs 1985).
3. Psychological development (Holm and Kunze 1969, Lewis 1976, Zinkus *et al.* 1978, Zinkus and Gottlieb 1980, Hutton 1983).
4. Educational abilities (Zinkus *et al.* 1978, Howie *et al.* 1979, Bennett *et al.* 1980, Zinkus and Gottlieb 1980, Roberts *et al.* 1986).

Whether the study examines

1. Children with histories of otitis media.
2. Children who have a hearing loss at the time of testing.
3. A combination of (1) and (2).

Whether the study

1. Compares the performance of children who either have or have had otitis media.
2. Examines a group showing a particular auditory or language delay or disorder (e.g. articulation), for incidence of middle-ear pathology or for histories of middle-ear problems, compared with a control group who do not exhibit the delay or disorder.

One of the earlier and most publicized studies was carried out by Holm and Kunze (1969), who looked primarily at the effect of fluctuating hearing loss on language and speech development. They compared two groups of children, aged 5 to 9 years, who were all attending the outpatients' department of a children's hospital. One group (the experimental group) comprised children who attended the ENT Clinic at the hospital for recurrent middle-ear disease and who had fluctuating hearing loss. The children in the control group did not have a documented history of middle-ear disease. The children were all Caucasians attending normal schools. The speech and language skills of the children were assessed by applying three standardized language measures (see later comments on standardization) at a time when their hearing loss was not 'sufficiently depressed to affect the test performance'. A measure of language development was also obtained by detailing the child's language skills as observed and reported by a parent. The data showed the experimental group to be significantly delayed in all but one of the tests requiring the processing of a verbal response. The children suffering repeated periods of conductive hearing loss were shown to be delayed in the acquisition of all the language skills tested.

Lewis (1976) used a somewhat better designed study in which he compared three groups of Australian children, aged 7–9 years: one group of Aboriginal children, who had SOM at the time of testing and a history of repeated middle-ear disease and associated fluctuating hearing loss, who had been identified by school screening; a second group of Aboriginal children who did not show any symptoms of ear disease; and a third group of European children who were attending a primary school in a low socioeconomic area. Comparisons of the means of pure-tone threshold-sensitivity tests showed the experimental group to have reduced thresholds, particularly in the low frequencies. Assessments included measures of speech discrimination in quiet and in noise; a same/different speech discrimination test; a test of phonemic synthesis; a dichotic measure of binaural separation ability; and measures of verbal (picture vocabulary) and non-verbal ('draw a man') ability.

Both Aboriginal groups were found to perform more poorly on the verbal intelligence scales than did the European children, but the group with a history of hearing loss achieved a significantly lower score than the Aboriginal control group. The experimental group also performed significantly less well on the auditory discrimination task and on the phonemic synthesis task. Results of factor analyses of the data prompted Lewis to suggest that one effect of repeated conductive loss was to distort the integration of mental abilities, and he likens this to a sensory deprivation-type phenomenon quoting Myklebust (1964).

Zinkus et al. (1978) and Zinkus and Gottlieb (1980) extended the investigation into the wider effects of repeated otitis media on language and psychoeducational variables. In their later study, they compared three groups of children, aged 7 to 11 years, two of which were described as having 'auditory processing difficulties' (this was not defined); children in one of these groups also had histories of chronic middle-ear infections (Group I), as ascertained from medical records and parent interviews. The third group (group III) comprised children apparently free of both disorders. All the subjects were required to have a full scale IQ of 85 or more. At the time of testing, the greatest hearing loss in Group I was 30 dB HL. The children in Group II were reported as having few if any middle-ear infections. The Revised Wechsler Intelligence Scale for Children (WISC-R) was administered to each child by an experimenter blind to the child's group classification. Results showed that children with a history of chronic otitis media performed more poorly than both Groups II and III on measures of verbal and full-scale IQ. These children also showed significant differences in comparison with children having no history of ear disease on two nonverbal subtests of the WISC, one of which would be described as combining visual, perceptual and language skills.

Receptive language and auditory processing skills were assessed using the Carrow test and the Illinois Test of Psycholinguistic Abilities (ITPA). The authors found receptive language skills and associated abilities related to symbolic language to be impaired. On the tests of auditory association, reception, phonemic synthesis and auditory sequential memory, the children with histories of otitis media scored similarly to the group described as having auditory processing problems, both groups being significantly worse than the control group. The rate of language acquisition was evaluated by parental interview, and the children with histories of chronic otitis media showed delays in speech and language, most marked in the delayed use of three-word phrases.

When the skills of reading, spelling and arithmetic were compared, the subjects with a history of chronic otitis media were significantly worse than the control subjects. Zinkus and Gottlieb ascribe this to auditory processing difficulties due to the similar results from the children in Group II. It is possible that delayed language at school entry results in a reading problem, and that the spelling problem reflects a classroom speech-perception problem with dictation. Unfortunately, the nature of the reading and spelling difficulties is not discussed.

Knowing the methodological problems besetting these early studies, the more recent studies have attempted to control for confounding variables more vigorously. A study with a slightly different emphasis and which specifically

Table 7.1 Selection of major studies which have examined the audiological, auditory, psychological and educational effects of fluctuating conductive hearing loss.

Authors	Population	Test procedure	Main observations
Holm and Kunze 1969	2 groups: ages 5–9 years; $n = 3$ (1) COM (2) asymptomatic	Language development: standard-ized measures of language and articulation; measures of verbal/nonverbal IQ	Test groups delayed on all language skills and on all tests relying on verbal processing
Kaplan et al. 1973	Eskimos; 3 groups: ages 5–7 years; $n = 489$ (1) COM since 0–24 months (2) COM since 2–10 years (3) asymptomatic	PTA; WISC: measures of non-verbal IQ	Test groups deficient in grade placement and verbal IQ Group 1 showed reduction in all verbal skills and scored less well on reading ability
Lewis 1976	Aboriginal: 3 groups: ages 7–9 years; $n = 30$ (1) current SOM and history of COM (2) asymptomatic (3) Europeans	Wepman Auditory Discrim. Test; auditory perceptual tests; measures of verbal and nonverbal IQ	Group 1 performed significantly worse on WADT, phoneme-synthesis test and verbal IQ
Needleman 1977	2 groups: $n = 40$ (1) history of SOM (2) asymptomatic	EPVT; 'draw a person'; evaluated productive and receptive phono-logy; syntactic discrimination and auditory discrimination	Group 1 performed more poorly on all tests except auditory
Zinkus et al. 1978	2 groups age 6–11 years $n = 40$, all with educ. delays (1) history of SOM (2) infrequent episodes of SOM	PTA; speech and language develop-ment; WISC: word-recognition, spelling and maths skills	Group 1 performed poorly on verbal IQ and word-recognition auditory processing tasks, and showed poor audiovisual integration
Lehmann et al. 1979	age = 9–5.4; $n = 47$ All had at least 3 episodes of SOM	Unspecified range of speech-language and auditory skills tests	Found expressive language and articulation to be delayed with respect to age norms

Study	Sample/Groups	Tests/Measures	Results
Howie et al. 1979	2 groups; n = 144 (1) 3 attacks SOM before 18 months (2) no attacks before 18 mo.	School tests of reading, language and maths	No significant difference between test results of two groups
Bennett et al. 1980	2 groups; ages 7–12 years; n = 109 (1) diagnosed learning-disabled (2) normal	PTA; tympanometry, otoscopy History of otitis media	Significantly more children in the learning-disordered group had middle-ear difficulties
Brandes and Ehinger 1981	2 groups; ages 7–8 years n = 30 (1) conductive loss and history of SOM (2) asymptomatic	12 auditory–perceptual tasks; measures of academic achievement; nonverbal IQ; visual perception	Group 1 performed significantly worse on auditory perceptual and visual perceptual measures
Hoffman-Lawless et al. 1981	4 groups; n = 40 Gps 1, 3: COM ages 7, 9 Gps 2, 4: asymptomatic, ages 7, 9	PTA tympanometry, speech audio; filtered speech test; speech in noise; SSW: auditory memory (ITPA) and phonemic synthesis (GFW)	Groups with SOM were significantly worse on filtered speech at 7 years but not by 9 years. No other significant differences
Sak and Ruben 1981	2 groups; ages 8–11 years n = 36 Gp 1: history of SOM Gp 2: asymptomatic	PTA: tympanometry, speech audio; WISC nonverbal IQ, ITPA, educational tests	Group 1 poorer in verbal ability, spelling and auditory decoding
Jerger et al. 1983	2 groups; ages 2–4 years n = 50 Gp 1: history of SOM Gp 2: asymptomatic	PTA, tympanometry, verbal skills, social maturity, speech intelligibility, nonverbal ability, home factors	Group 1 lagged Group 2 by 5–8 months in verbal skills, nonverbal ability and social maturity

Table 7.1 continued

Authors	Population	Test procedure	Main observations
Hutton 1983	2 groups, n = 48 ages 5–11 years (1) surgically treated for OM (2) asymptomatic	Slosson Intelligence Test; Peabody PVT; Block design of WISC; Spelling from WRAT; Spelling and reading from Peabody IAT and the GFW test of auditory discrimination	Group 1 showed comparatively poor results on Peabody PVT and Block Design of WISC only
Brookhouse and Goldgar 1987	3 groups; n = 480 ages 9–54 months (1) early onset SOM, no language delay (2) early onset SOM, language	PTA, tympanometry, ABR (some cases) environmental factors, speech and language measures, medical history, developmental examination, visual	Confirmed delays. Groups (1) and (2) showed language delay in detailed testing. Group 2 showed other developmental delays. Groups (1) and (2) only appeared to 'catch-up'
Rach et al. 1988	3 groups; n = 65 ages 2–4 years (1) persistent SOM (2) SOM 3–6 months duration (3) asymptomatic	Typanometry (serial tests); PTA (n = 20); Reynell DLS – Revised	Groups (1) and (2) showed reduction in expressive language, but not comprehension. Group (1) results significantly worse than Group (2)

PTA = pure-tone audiometry

*SOM = suppurative otitis media

COM = repeated attacks of otitis media (i.e. chronic)

examined the relationship of medical, hereditary and environmental factors affecting children with and without otitis media, and language delay, was carried out by Brookhouse and Goldgar (1987).

The studies we have discussed are representative of the experiments carried out in this area; a selection of the notable studies is summarized in Table 7.1. These studies are primarily addressed to the following two questions:

(i) Does repeated chronic otitis media cause delays in language acquisition, auditory processing problems, learning disabilities or any one of these?

(ii) How are the developmental sequelae of chronic otitis media influenced by the age at which it first occurs, and by the duration and frequency of successive attacks?

Methodological problems

In each study, a relationship between frequent occurrences of ear disease and either delayed language or poor performance on various measures of auditory or psychoeducational abilities is found. However, it has already been indicated that to identify definitively the language and other developmental delays as sequelae of otitis media, the nontest variables must be subject to rigorous control. This condition is rarely met in these studies.

Subject selection In a comparative design, subjects must be matched. Poor matching may allow an association to be inferred between, say, linguistic performance and frequent otitis media, but not a causal relationship. Other factors which have not been adequately matched may be the causal agent; for example, poor overall health, parental skills and influences, home environment and socioeconomic factors. Bennett et al. (1980) argue that poverty, overcrowding, poor parenting, poor teaching, poor schools, and undernutrition all contribute to handicap a child in schoolwork. Downs (1985) found language delay in a group of 'middle class' children with a history of repeated conductive hearing loss, in comparison with a similar group of asymptomatic children. The same test procedures showed no significant difference between disadvantaged children, with and without a history of recurrent conductive loss. The highest score in the underprivileged group was below the lowest score in the 'middle class' group, indicating a strong environmental effect. These factors should be considered before fluctuating hearing loss is identified as causal to learning disabilities in a particular child. The influences of health, hereditary, environmental and socioeconomic factors on the development of child language in children with otitis media was the subject of an investigation by Brookhouse and Goldgar (1987). These authors examined three groups of children who had been selected to minimize confounding variables, and in whom hearing acuity had been documented: one group with recurrent otitis media and language delay; a second group with an equally well documented otitis media history, but without language delay; and a third group with documented language delay in the absence of any known predisposing conditions, including early-onset otitis media. They found that among 329 children with positive histories of early otitis media, a significantly higher percentage of those with language delay were from homes in the lower socioeconomic category. Children with otitis media and language delay also showed articulation errors and borderline delays in other developmental areas compared with the otitis media children who were language age-appropriate. Their preliminary longitudinal data supported the notion that children with language delay due to otitis media 'catch up'. This was in contrast to results for the group with specific language disorder.

Selection of subject groups prone to attacks of otitis media has been carried out in the following ways:

(i)   Inspection of medical records (Holm and Kunze 1969, Zinkus et al. 1978, Howie et al. 1979).

(ii)   Parental questionnaire (Kaplan et al. 1973, Lewis 1976, Needleman 1977, Zinkus et al. 1978, Bennett et al. 1980).

(iii)   Pure-tone audiometry and/or tympanometry (Kaplan et al. 1973, Lewis 1976, Masters and Marsh 1978, Zinkus et al. 1978, Bennett et al. 1980, Friel-Patti et al. 1982, Silva et al. 1983, Schlieper et al. 1985, Rach et al. 1988).

(iv)   A combination of methods (Brookhouse and Goldgar 1987).

(v)   Longitudinal study of a high risk group (Friel-Patti et al. 1982, Roberts et al. 1986).

In method (i), selection of the experimental group is made from medical records, whereas control groups are usually assembled from children whose parents report them as not having had otitis media. Parents may not have sought medical advice, either because the condition has truly not occurred, or because attacks of otitis media have gone unnoticed. It is perhaps more realistic to think of the subjects as comprising not two groups but one, in which for some children the symptoms were distressingly overt and the parents alerted to the problem, and for others in whom the condition, if present at all, was mild. This is to some extent made explicit by Zinkus et al. (1978). These authors compared two groups of children who had been referred for educational underachievement with a group who were performing age-appropriately in scholastic skills. Medical records were available from birth for each of the children in the two experimental groups, and these two groups differed in the frequency and severity of attacks of otitis media, rather than in the presence or absence of the condition. They also consulted parents on the frequency of attacks and, although they do not statistically compare these methods, their subject group classification remained the same by either method. On this basis the control group was identified as symptom-free as a result of parental interview.

Subject selection, matching and experimental control provide the largest difficulty in studies of the effects of fluctuating hearing loss on development.

The preservation of scientific rigour is impeded by difficulties in obtaining accurate data retrospectively, or in providing truly matched groups in comparative studies.

Measurements of auditory sensitivity   Surprisingly, neither middle-ear status nor auditory sensitivity was assessed at the time of testing in any of the studies, although this is rarely overlooked in more recent work. Failure of a past school screening test does not give adequate information regarding a fluctuating condition. As we have seen, the hearing loss during an attack of otitis media can vary from negligible to 50 dB HL. In the studies where this was not evaluated (see examples in Table 7.1), the actual test conditions may have varied both between the subjects and between the groups, because of the different test stimulus sensation levels which may have resulted. Conclusions have been drawn on aspects such as auditory processing problems when the actual input to the cochlea is not known. Performance on all tests requiring normal auditory input for validity must be held in question.

In retrospective studies, where the longstanding nature of the disease was of most interest (e.g. Kaplan *et al.* 1973, Howie *et al.* 1979), data on the extent of the hearing loss over the full time-course were generally not available. There is no way of evaluating, from these studies, how severe the condition must be to exert an influence on language acquisition. This criticism can also be applied to consideration of the effects of early auditory deprivation.

Control for experimenter bias   A degree of experimenter bias must be expected when evaluative procedures are carried out by a tester who has full knowledge of whether the subject is a normally hearing subject, or one who has a history of middle-ear disease. Only a few studies have attempted to control for this (e.g. Schlieper *et al.* 1985).

Selection and application of test procedures   A wide range of psychoeducational tests have been used to examine the sequelae of otitis media. Ventry (1980), in an important critical review, draws attention to the importance of using standardized tests with the appropriate age groups. In a number of cases this requirement is not met.

Experimental evidence

Despite methodological flaws in many of the experiments in this area of study, they provide a wide sample of information regarding the effects of recurrent conductive hearing loss. Let us proceed to examine the findings in the light of the procedural and interpretive weaknesses that have been identified.

It is interesting that, superficially, only some of the children with histories of conductive hearing loss appear to have speech and language problems.

Measurements on vocabulary scales usually reveal vocabulary to be within normal limits (Owrid 1970), and the children probably have satisfied their parents and teachers that they are talking. A more detailed language evaluation may be required to reveal the extent of a child's problem: otherwise, where speech and language delays exist, they may escape detection until they are revealed later on as an educational problem. The studies mentioned in this chapter report reduced performance in measures of language production, and in assessments which require sophisticated verbal abilities.

There is no evidence to suggest that isolated or infrequent attacks of middle-ear disease give rise to delays in language acquisition. Rather, the evidence suggests that serious risk arises from chronic or recurrent periods of otitis media, even though the auditory sensitivity in these periods may be within 'normal limits', that is, better than 20 dB HL. Most of the studies reported here are cross-sectional comparisons, where the history of the disease is traced by parental interview or medical records. It is difficult to quantify the hearing loss which may have occurred in these periods, and there are few studies available relating extent of hearing loss to language delay.

The presence of otitis media in the first 3 years of life is thought to have the most deleterious effect on language development (e.g. Sak and Ruben 1981, Friel-Patti et al. 1982, Teele et al. 1984). This has theoretical appeal, since these years are known to be of paramount importance in language development. Most studies were carried out on older children who maintained recurrent bouts of otitis media into the early school years (e.g. Needleman 1977, Zinkus et al. 1978, Howie et al. 1979). The history of the disease, and in most cases also language development, was by parental interview. Results suggest that the effect may be progressive. For example, Jerger et al. (1983) found language to be delayed by 5–8 months by 3 years of age, and Ling (1972) found a delay of 1 year by school age. A range of more recent studies on younger children has been carried out. For example, Teele et al. (1984) prospectively followed 205 children from birth to the age of 3 years with otoscopic evaluation and speech and language assessments. Those children who had prolonged periods of middle-ear effusions, especially between the ages of 6 and 12 months, showed poor scores on the assessments. Early otitis media not only generally results in language delay, but also seems to predispose the child to further attacks, prolonging the time before a child is free to 'catch up'.

The relationship of the length or frequency of attack to language delay is uncertain. These data are not documented in most cases and in the retrospective studies would be, again, impossible to assess accurately. In any case, the duration for which fluid remains in the ear varies, being from 3 to 12 months in 30 per cent of children (Downs 1985). Zinkus and Gottlieb (1980) compared children 'in the extreme on the continuum of chronicity and severity' with children who had few attacks, or who were free from the problem. Although the group with the greater history of otitis media showed greater differences from the normal controls than children with few attacks, this latter group did not perform as well as the normals on some tests. The question of what degree of chronicity and severity of attacks may cause delays in language acquisition is unresolved. Kaplan *et al.* (1973) found a correlation between tests of verbal ability and the number of incidents of otitis media reported to have occurred in early life; but the score differences are small and may not represent significant functional differences. Further, it is still not clear to what extent intelligence, environment and personality may interact with the disease in affecting development of language.

The language delays reported are described either by reduced performance in comparison with normal children on various language-skill tests, such as the Reynell Development Scale (e.g. Rach *et al.* 1988), or by descriptions of language development based on guided parental interviews, such as the Vineland Scale (e.g. Jerger *et al.* 1983). Both methods show that age norms are not met, particularly in expressive language.

Delays in productive and receptive phonology have been reported (Needleman, 1977), and a tendency for a lack of syntactic sophistication, and use of comparatively simple constructions have been commonly reported (e.g. Lehmann *et al.* 1979, Rentscher *et al.* 1980, Jerger *et al.* 1983, Schlieper *et al.* 1985). Most studies report delays, rather than deviances in language (e.g. Silva *et al.* 1983). For example, Djupesland *et al.* (1981) found a high prevalence of children with middle-ear disorders in a cross-sectional study of children with immature phonology. Immature articulation has been reported by a number of authors as commonly occurring as a sequela of middle-ear disorders. Rentscher *et al.* (1980) studied a group of children attending a speech therapy clinic. Among their findings, they reported a higher prevalence of middle-ear disorders among children with fluency problems. This may be secondary to problems with language development, or may be related to difficulties with prosodic information due to changes in the acoustic input. There may, in addition, be other reasons to associate dysfluency with middle-ear disorder. For example, emotionally stressed children tend to show a higher incidence of physical illness (Haggerty 1980), and there is an association between emotional stress and the occurrence of dysfluency in children. This particular relationship emphasizes the importance of a broad-based developmental approach to the problem of the association between language development and middle-ear disease.

There are perhaps fewer pitfalls in assessing language development than some of the underlying prerequisite abilities such as speech perception. However, an element of caution must still be applied in the interpretation of test results. For example, Holm and Kunze (1969) used the Templin Darley Test of Articulation to demonstrate significant delays in a group of children with middle-ear disease, in comparison with a control group. Menyuk (1979) severely criticizes this test for its heavy reliance on lexical knowledge. If a feature of delayed language is a reduction in vocabulary size, then the test may be chiefly another reflection of language immaturity. The test tool used in the examination of particular language aspects is not always published, and this is an important omission in the light of Menyuk's comment. Subtests of the ITPA (Illinois Test of Psycholinguistic Abilities), where the child is required to generate verbal analogues, have been used in studies (Holm and Kunze 1969, Zinkus *et al.* 1978) to demonstrate immature language in children with middle-ear disease. This again taps lexical knowledge, which may be reduced because of the inconsistencies in the speech sounds available to the child with a fluctuating hearing loss. Menyuk (1979) compares the probable inconsistent input with that of a normally hearing child, who builds categories of speech sounds based on the fusion of the speech sounds heard with a concomitant visual–motor input. Integration of these simultaneous events provides the basis for the child's growing lexicon. A child with a mild sensorineural loss is able to employ the same strategy, but the child with a fluctuating hearing loss has inconsistencies in part of the input, impeding the acquisition of lexical knowledge.

Impoverished language skills also affect the results of tests of other areas of development; some of the studies in this chapter report verbal IQ to be lower for children with middle-ear disease than for their normally hearing counterparts. They also find verbal measures to be lower than nonverbal measures of IQ in these children. If there are any generalized cognitive delays resulting from fluctuating hearing loss, it seems to be a much less dominant problem than the effect on language. However, little experimental evidence is available directly relating to cognitive development. Horowitz and Leake (1980) note that measures of IQ are substituted, and there is little attempt to look at the interaction of an inconsistent auditory input, language development and cognitive development. They suggest that the development of language and cognition are simultaneously reinforcing, and hence we may expect some abnormal auditory experiences to affect cognitive development.

In summary, the pooled findings of a number of different types of study indicate that children who suffer recurrent periods of conductive hearing loss are generally delayed in their language development. Close inspection of the experiments reveals a number of confounding variables such as poorly documented history of the disease, parental and environmental influences, and periods of ill health, which perhaps give a poorer prognosis than is the case in more favourable conditions. However, there is sufficient evidence to consider a child who repeatedly has periods of otitis media as a high risk for language delay. Theoretically, it would appear possible to minimize this by appropriate intervention.

The effects of fluctuating conductive hearing loss on the development of hearing and auditory skills

There is a complicated and not fully understood relationship between language development on one hand and speech perception and its development on the other. Although the processes are related, we tend not to describe language development in terms of auditory skills. Yet we saw in Chapter 2 that the young have the ability to discriminate a wide range of acoustic contrasts in speech sounds, and we saw also that categorization of speech sounds is consistent with the infant's ability to distinguish some of the suprasegmental aspects of speech. At first sight, then, the processes of auditory development and language acquisition appear as somewhat independent, yet related, processes. It is certainly accepted that a degree of peripheral hearing is required for the speech-perception process: peripheral coding and adequate sensitivity is required at the entry point. Beyond this is an inadequately understood mechanism relating processing of acoustic events, perception of speech events and acquisition of language. In cases of sensorineural hearing loss, the peripheral coding mechanisms are disrupted: abnormalities in frequency and intensity coding cause a low-grade input to the remainder of the speech perception process. In cases of conductive loss, it would seem that the consequence is merely that a 'quieter' input is available for speech perception.

We have seen that disruptions in language development do occur as a result of fluctuating conductive loss, and some authors feel that this delay may not be entirely accounted for by fluctuations in hearing in the first years of life. For example, Downs (1977) hypothesizes that there must be a more pervasive underlying auditory disorder affecting central processing of sound, and some authors (e.g. Lewis 1976) claim that the test results of their studies support this.

It is not clear whether this process is reversible. Downs (1985) sees the fluctuating hearing levels in the early years as precluding the development of the necessary auditory strategies for speech perception, and strongly favours theories of auditory deprivation, leading to central auditory processing disorders. She feels that psychological deprivation, caused by a possible rift in the normal mother–infant bond may contribute to this developmental central disorder. Downs argues that this irreversible effect may not be noticeable at a superficial level, but may be revealed in the more difficult listening conditions of the classroom. Brandes and Ehinger (1981) lend support to this theory in showing poor results on test of central auditory function from children who have learning difficulties and histories of recurrent conductive hearing loss. The alternative theory for the occurrence of higher-level disorders in auditory processing is that neurophysiological changes leave an irreversible auditory deficit.

Some of the studies described in this chapter aim to examine the auditory abilities which they consider fundamental to the perception and development of speech, or necessary for classroom learning, and examine the hypothesis that fluctuating conductive loss causes irreversible auditory difficulties. The tests used to assess auditory abilities here overlap to some extent with the tests employed by audiologists for the evaluation of central auditory function (see Chapter 10). The tests of auditory skills commonly incorporate auditory discrimination (in quiet and in noise), auditory blending, sequencing, memory, closure and selective attention. A major criticism of these tests is that they are language-dependent, and that they are not therefore evaluations of fundamental skills requisite for language development. Rees (1981) goes so far as to suggest that the only true claim of such tests to be assessing auditory abilities is that they are presented by ear. If these skills are evaluated in isolation we do not know how they relate to language learning, and the application of these tests requires major assumptions to be made about how we perceive speech.

Auditory discrimination

We must consider first the effects of fluctuating conductive loss on auditory discrimination tasks. Published tests are used (e.g. Lewis 1976, Brandes and Ehinger 1981) where the child must complete a 'same/different' task, or identify a word from three or four choices, and deficiencies in auditory abilities are suggested on the basis of results of these tests. However the information pertaining to language skills which these tasks yield is not clear. We return to the question of the identity of the speech perception unit, and must ask whether we need language to be able to discriminate phonemes. If so, then auditory discrimination tasks will, at least in part, reflect linguistic development and not just auditory abilities. Since auditory discrimination improves with maturity, there is support for the notion that this is due to increasing language competence or to an increased ability to attend selectively. Poor ability on tasks of auditory discrimination has been shown to improve to normal after three months of language stimulation (Rees 1981). Unfortunately, the specific difficulties are rarely reported; the data are mostly in the form of mean results on standardized test patterns.

One of the few observations of specific problems was made by Jerger *et al.* (1983), who noted that the children did not have difficulty in the perception of any particular phonemes. This is in contrast to children with mild sensorineural hearing losses, which tend to be high-frequency, and to cause difficulties with weak consonants such as sibilants. The authors suggested that the lack of clustering in the data is due to the fluctuating nature of the hearing problem, which gives generalized difficulty in storing phonetic categories in long-term memory. Jerger and colleagues carried out an interesting cross-sectional study in which they examined the developmental function of the speech discrimination score in normal children, and in children with documented histories of recurrent otitis media; ages ranged from 24 to 36 months. Using their own word and sentence test, they measured performance/intensity functions over a range of suprathreshold intensity levels in conditions of quiet and background noise. Results from normal subjects showed that performance in noise developed more slowly than performance in quiet, and that performance for sentences developed more slowly than performance for single words (in competition with noise). This is not a surprising finding, since the sentence task relies more heavily on language development than does identification of single words. The most striking contrast between the two groups of children lay in the difference between the developmental functions for the speech materials presented in noise. The growth function of performance for word identification in noise was significantly slower for the experimental group. Performance increased by only about 10 per cent for the experimental group, compared with 60 per cent in the normally hearing children. The growth function for performance on sentence identification was not significantly different for the two groups, although the experimental group were slightly delayed in comparison to the normal group. Individual data on each subject did not reveal any correlation with verbal ability or current hearing levels.

The data suggest that the two groups did not differ significantly in the composition of skills required for the identification of sentence material, but that the children with histories of conductive loss showed comparative difficulty in carrying out tasks on isolated words in noisy conditions. Possibly the fluctuations in the auditory input cause disruptions to the categorization of the acoustic events used in speech perception, such that while isolated word recognition in quiet is unimpaired, when the task becomes more difficult the recognition process is not as robust as in the normal child. In tasks of selective attention, the child must attend to one channel of information, and possibly uses a central 'dictionary' or reference against which incoming signals are compared. The child who has less in the memory store, due to periods of inconsistent input, may perform less well in a competing task. Fluctuating conductive loss does not cause an underlying auditory disability as measured by simple auditory discrimination tasks. But there is a tendency for children with histories of the condition to score more poorly on tasks of speech discrimination where, for example, figure-ground or selective attention abilities are required. This may be caused by linguistic immaturity or a related deficit of familiar speech sounds in the child's long-term memory. The work of Jerger *et al.* (1983) suggests that in any case this deficit is reversible, and that the observed phenomena are delays resulting from inconsistent input, rather than more serious fundamental neurological abnormalities resulting from auditory deprivation.

Auditory memory

Another auditory ability tested in these studies is that of auditory memory span. This is usually tested by asking the child to recall a string of digits, phonemes or words. Again, language affects memory for linguistic processing; structured meaningful items are held more effectively in memory than strings of digits. To say that the ability to recall sequences of this kind is an auditory skill necessary for language development enforces the idea that word-order retains great significance. However, sense can be achieved by other means, and there is no natural precedence of word-order. Tests of auditory memory as used in these studies may not be representative of any function required for speech perception. The results are variable between studies, but performance on tasks of auditory memory is generally not worse for the experimental group, suggesting only that, if auditory memory is considered as a fundamental auditory skill (if indeed it is such a skill), children with histories of fluctuating hearing loss do not show a disability in this area.

Phoneme synthesis

A popular test battery applied in some studies is the Illinois Test of Psycholinguistic Abilities (ITPA). Another with some similar subtests is the Goldman–Fristoe–Woodcock test of auditory discrimination (GFW). One common subtest is that in which the child must synthesize a sequence of separate phonemes. This is known as a test of sound-blending or phonemic synthesis, and test performance is supposedly related to the abilities of reading and spelling. A number of authors (Holm and Kunze 1969, Brandes and Ehinger 1981, Zinkus and Gottlieb 1980) find poor performance on this task from children who have histories of conductive losses. Again, in some cases this is described as an *auditory* deficit, but it should perhaps be regarded rather as related simply to delayed language. The target word relies on lexical knowledge, and if the latter is impoverished, the child would be expected to experience difficulties.

The studies in Table 7.1 include data from tests which were designed to test auditory abilities, and results indicate that the subjects with histories of fluctuating conductive hearing loss often do not perform as well as normal-hearing subjects. In the preceding paragraphs, it has however been suggested that many of these tests are language-dependent, such that a child with a language delay would probably perform more poorly than a child with age-appropriate language. The authors have not necessarily identified underlying deficits in auditory skills which are prerequisite for language, but may have looked at more subtle and perhaps perceptual aspects of language delay. This does not mean that children with histories of fluctuating conductive losses do not have any auditory processing problems; but there is as yet no clear evidence to support this, and it is a field where careful experimentation is required. In the meantime, we should be aware that these children may have some difficulty with auditory skills, particularly for classroom listening.

The effects of fluctuating conductive hearing loss on scholastic skills

Recurrent attacks of otitis media have been suspected as a cause of language delay for some 50 years: while there has been some suggestion that specific difficulties with some aspects of education may occur, it is more recently that fluctuating hearing loss has been cited as a cause of both specific and generalized learning disabilities. Several authors agree that normal educational progress may be delayed indirectly by recurrent fluctuating hearing loss, but there is less agreement regarding the direct cause or the nature of the disability. Two questions may be asked. First, do educational difficulties occur as a result of the child entering school with delayed language? This language delay may then cause difficulties in reading, spelling and perhaps other skills where there is heavy reliance on spoken language as the teaching medium. Secondly, does the fluctuating auditory input, perhaps coupled with a situation analogous to auditory deprivation in infancy, cause an irreversible auditory perceptual deficit which is particularly disabling in classroom situations? The evidence is of an empirical nature, and reveals the presence of varying degrees of learning difficulties in these children, coupled with poor performance on tests of perceptive and productive language competence. For example, Bond (1935) found conductive hearing loss to be more common among children with reading delays. In 1956, the Scottish Council for Research in Education (quoted by Ling 1972) published results of a study on over 300 11- to 12-year-old children with histories of middle-ear disease, who showed evidence of significant educational retardation compared with children with histories of normal hearing.

Ling (1972) himself showed children with middle-ear disorders to be retarded by about one year in the skills of reading and mathematics. There is scant evidence from other studies to support the latter finding, but several other authors also found that these children had difficulties with learning to read. Masters and Marsh (1978) showed a high prevalence of middle-ear disease among children regarded as educationally retarded. Kaplan *et al.* (1973) found Eskimo children with conductive losses to be retarded in reading compared with their normally hearing peers. Children in both the control and experimental group in fact performed below chronological age, the recurrent hearing loss in this case appearing to be an additional problem in the child's already disadvantaged situation. Similar findings were made by Lewis (1976) comparing Aboriginal children, with and without middle-ear disease, and European children. Both the Aboriginal groups were delayed in reading with respect to the Europeans. Zinkus and Gottlieb (1980) found children with histories of recurrent loss to be delayed in reading skills, and to perform worse than normal controls on dictated spelling tests. In a sibling paradigm Sak and Ruben (1981) found recurrent conductive hearing loss to be reflected in spelling, but not reading, skills.

In contrast to these results, Howie *et al.* (1979) did not find significant differences between their experimental and control groups on the skills of reading, spelling or mathematics, although there was a tendency towards poorer performance by the children with histories of middle-ear disease reflected in a composite assessment score. The children in this study were matched for age, sex, father's occupation and school attended. Each child in the experimental group had three or more reported attacks of otitis media prior to 18 months of age.

There is then some evidence that learning difficulties may occur as a result of fluctuations in auditory sensitivity in the preschool and early school years. The authors quoted here support one or other of the hypotheses described earlier – that educational difficulties are caused as a secondary effect of delays of language, or as a secondary effect of subtle auditory disabilities. The former hypothesis has some appeal, partly because the evidence for language delay is more conclusive; if language is immature on entering school then the child may be less ready to learn to read than the child with age-appropriate language. The form of the reading difficulties encountered is not analysed in any of the studies reported here; neither is information available on the reading method taught. This information would be of interest, since one could then speculate as to any underlying deficiency. For example, an impoverished store of phonetic or lexical units in long-term memory may inhibit the reading process; the relative effects of one or the other may depend on the method used to teach reading.

Although there are reports of poor performance in spelling, in most cases the tests were presented as a dictation task. These results may therefore reflect either reduced lexicon or inadequate experience with perceptual contrasts, or even a problem with hearing the word. Where hearing was not checked on the day of testing, instances of reduced thresholds among a proportion of the children must be considered a possibility. Even a mild loss of 15–20 dB HL could invalidate the test stimuli in a spelling task. Similarly, the poor performance on mathematical tasks noted by some authors has been attributed to cognitive immaturity inhibiting the child in concrete operations of this kind (Zinkus and Gottlieb 1980), but could indirectly result from either impoverished language or some difficulties in auditory skills in the difficult conditions of the classroom. The contrasting results found by respective authors suggests that environmental factors affect performance.

The view that generalized auditory disabilities cause educational delays is supported by less experimental evidence. Even if these disabilities do exist, they are more likely to result in listening difficulties in classroom teaching than in delaying the acquisition of specific skills. No evidence is presented as to the types of teaching environment from which the children are drawn, but difficulty with discrimination of speech sounds in noise has been shown, and this may be a dominant functional disability in some classrooms. The children undergoing remedial teaching in the study of Brandes and Ehinger (1981) would not only have the benefit of additional language stimulation and help with specific skills, but would also presumably be taught in more favourable circumstances. Their study suggests that the prognosis for overcoming the underlying disability, however we choose to describe it, is favourable. This is in contrast to the suggestion of Downs (1977) that fluctuating conductive loss results in a syndrome-like condition, which she called an Irreversible Auditory Learning Disaster.

It has been shown that there is insufficient evidence to identify central auditory disabilities as a consequence of recurrent otitis media. However, in a rather different type of experimental paradigm, Tallal (1976) has shown specific auditory disabilities in a group of children with language disorder. Her subjects had difficulty in processing signals of brief duration, particularly when the stimuli occurred in rapid succession. Experiments with synthetic speech stimuli on the experimental group of children find them able to perceive steady-state stimuli of long duration such as vowel sounds, but to have difficulty with stimuli containing brief transitions. Important acoustic cues in consonant perception lie in the rapid transitions of the second and third formants, which occur over a period of about 50 milliseconds. It is not unreasonable to hypothesize this kind of perceptual difficulty resulting from a fluctuating auditory input. It would be interesting to apply Tallal's experiments to this group, as difficulty of processing the rapidly changing stimuli of the transitional elements of speech may result in language delays and perhaps learning disability.

Several of the general features of the child's background of the type described as affecting language development will further affect educational progress. If a child has a relatively impoverished or unhelpful home environment, this will probably exacerbate the problems encountered by a fluctuating hearing loss. Similarly, children who are frequently absent from school owing to poor health are disadvantaged in comparison to their healthier peers.

Few data are available on the effect of repeated attacks of otitis media on the development of selective attention, which is a necessary classroom skill. Speech perception in noise to some extent taps this skill, and as we have seen, Jerger *et al.*

(1983) found it to be delayed for children aged 2–3 years; however, there was evidence in their study that the children can 'catch up'. Intuitively, one might expect general attentiveness to be a susceptible skill. Lewis (1976), alone of these studies, attempts to correlate attention with other variables. Although his data suggest differences between the experimental and control groups, this was not confirmed statistically. Lewis suggests that the child develops inefficient listening strategies during the periods of conductive loss, which persist well beyond the episodes of active middle-ear disease and which affect levels of attention. If attention levels are affected by this condition, the nursery teacher, or parent, has a further feature to look out for, and should be aware of attributing poor attention *per se*, or behaviour, as the sole cause of a child 'appearing' not to hear or attend. A child may readily respond in easy listening conditions or when free from the disorder. Difficult listening conditions are not necessarily noted by the parent, who does not experience any great difficulty in perceiving speech when he is at a distance from the speaker or in a noisy room. A bright child may ask for a repetition of something not heard, but some children will simply guess, or not respond. In the context of instructions from a parent or teacher, the child may appear to be carrying out commands selectively, and their hearing deficiences may be mistaken for a behavioural problem.

Similarly, if listening strategies are inadequate, requiring considerable effort from the child, he may cease to attend at all. Wright (1984) describes an interesting case as follows: Wendy, now aged 7 and one of twins, had been receiving speech therapy intermittently for 3 years for language delay. She has a history of colds (thought to be accompanied by episodes of middle-ear disease) and over the last year has on several occasions shown a conductive loss of 25 dB HL. Her language is now described as age-appropriate, but she is still attending a speech therapy clinic because of her inability to direct her attention consistently. She appears to let her twin 'do the listening'. She uses her sister to interpret spoken messages and instructions, and rarely replies or interacts directly. While this may not be the result of the current hearing problems, difficulties in listening due to the middle-ear disease cannot be discounted.

Summary

In this chapter, a number of possible sequelae of fluctuating conductive hearing loss have been suggested and the evidence for them discussed, taking recurrent otitis media as the most common cause of this condition. It is concluded that children with this condition are at a high risk for sustaining delays in the acquisition of spoken language, and may be impeded in the acquisition of educational skills requiring age-appropriate linguistic competence. Despite some methodological flaws, there is an increasing body of data from increasingly better controlled studies, indicating that a significant relation exists between recurrent otitis media in the first 5 years of life, and subsequent problems in the acquisition of speech and language skills. Specific speech perception skills, particularly the ability to select the speech message from competing noise, may also be impaired for periods following the child's final episode of middle-ear disease. This disability is seen as a major cause of learning difficulties in the classroom, though some specific skills, such as reading, may be affected for other reasons. The experimental studies support the notion that children ultimately 'catch up', unless there is a language disorder underlying, not directly attributable to, recurrent otitis media. Evidence that permanent auditory perceptual deficits are sustained is questionable. Klein and Rapin (1988) argue that 'recurrent middle ear effusion in early childhood may affect language skills transiently, but is probably of limited significance for children with normal and above average IQs and with a school and home environment conducive to learning' (p. 108). With a slightly different emphasis, and more explicit, Sancho *et al.* (1988) conclude 'that there are genuine linguistic–educational sequelae of OME (otitis media with effusion); that they are not, however, very large; that they decrease with age (or, to be more precise, other factors, e.g. other illness, quality of home environment and schooling, come into play and swamp OME effects); and that they relate to early and persistent OME' (p. 17).

The current level of knowledge still leaves some important questions unanswered. Given the high prevalence of the condition, and given that it appears that only some of the children with recurrent, early-onset otitis media manifest delayed language development, it would be most helpful to establish a means of identifying those children who are at risk for delayed language development. It would similarly be useful to identify children with specific language disorders who also have recurrent otitis media.

Current methods of screening, and their implications in the detection and management of recurrent middle-ear disease have been discussed. The effects of even a hearing loss of 15–25 dB in early childhood, especially if it fluctuates, may interfere with the normal processes of language acquisition, and related areas of development. Awareness of the problem enables conservative intervention such as implementation of language-stimulation programmes and the structuring of home and classroom situations for easy listening. Professionals in the speech and hearing and related professions need to be aware of the importance of quality parent guidance in this area.

8

Reading disability in sensorineural hearing loss

Assessment of reading age in hearing-impaired children

Like intelligence quotient, 'reading age' (the common measure for reading tests) is a psychological construct limited and constrained by the nature of the measuring instrument; thus, 'reading tests measure what they measure'. Nevertheless, such constructs have considerable validity and utility in the early descriptive stages of investigation, and consequently reading age has been widely used as a measure of 'reading' in hearing-impaired children.

At this global level of assessment, the results have been extremely clear. In the great majority of cases, hearing impairment of at least a severe degree is accompanied by marked reading failure. In a survey of over 500 hearing-impaired children in schools throughout the USA and Canada, Wrightstone *et al.* (1963), using the Elementary Reading Test of the Metropolitan Achievement Tests, found that children aged 15;6–16;6 years had a mean reading age of about 9;6 years. That is to say, on this test the hearing-impaired children performed at the same level as the average hearing 9 year old. Furth (1966b) reported Wrightstone *et al.*'s data in more detail, and showed that only about 12 per cent of the children exhibited a reading age of 11 years or more. Additionally, reading age advanced by less than one year on average between 10 and 16 years of age.

Di Francesca (1972) used the Paragraph Meaning subtest of the Stanford Achievement Test to measure the reading ability of nearly 17 000 hearing-impaired children in the USA. The median reading grade for the 16-year-old children in the survey was 3.27, which translates into a reading age of just over 9 years. The particular test used measures the child's ability to understand connected prose. Despite the disadvantages associated with obtaining test results using a large number of different testers (necessitated by the scale of the survey), and with using a narrow-span test in which the tester has to judge which level of the test is likely to be most appropriate for a given child, the agreement between di Francesca's data and that of Wrightstone *et al.* suggests that the results are reasonably reliable. Jensema (1975) used the same test administered to 6871 hearing-impaired children, and found similar results. The data also showed that there was a marked decline in reading age as the degree of hearing impairment increased.

In Britain, Redgate (1972) used the Southgate Reading Test (Test 2) to assess the reading age of 698 hearing-impaired children from 23 different schools. The age range was 9 to 18 years. The Southgate test consists of a series of cue sentences of varying difficulty from each of which a single word is missing; the subject's task is to select the appropriate word to complete the sentence from a list of five given words. Thus, for example,

Careless driving leads to *happiness/cars/tractors/accidents/improvements*.

The results showed a gain of approximately one month in reading age for every year of education, culminating in a mean reading age of 7;8 (7 years 8 months) for children aged 15–15;11. Morris (1978) used the same test on 73 hearing-impaired children aged 9 to 16 years and found a mean reading age for school leavers of 7;6 years. Hamp (1972) devised a Picture Assisted Reading Test (PART) in which each of 55 individual stimulus words is presented with four pictures; the task for the child is to read the word and choose the picture corresponding to that word. Children aged 9 and 15 years and attending special schools for the Deaf or Partially Hearing were screened with the test. Mean reading age for the children aged 15 years was about 9 years; hearing age correlated significantly with degree of hearing loss and with a measure of intelligence.

In a series of comprehensive studies, Conrad (1977, 1979) studied a variety of verbal skills in 355 hearing-impaired children aged 15–16;6 years. The children were all 'prelingually' impaired (hearing-loss onset before the third birthday), were not multiply handicapped, and had English as a mother tongue. The chidren represented a near 100 per cent sample of the hearing-impaired school leavers from Special Schools for the Deaf and/or Partially Hearing in England and Wales. In his 1979 study Conrad discusses details of a sample of 109 children of similar age who were being educated in PHUs (Partial Hearing Units) attached to ordinary schools. Somewhat confusingly, he then proceeded to omit them from his analysis of reading ability. This is unfortuate, since it is likely that this subgroup will have rather better reading ability than those in Special Schools, if only because the criteria for placement in PHUs often (though not invariably) include literacy skills. He also chose not to study children with hearing impairments who were fully integrated into normal schools. Again, this may have biased the results somewhat towards the poorer end of the scale, since those chosen for integration would usually have been selected at that time on the basis of their ability to cope with normal school environment, and as such would have been likely to possess relatively good verbal skills. Nevertheless, the exclusion of such a subsample probably did not seriously affect the results of the survey, since at the time of testing integration was not a widespread policy (following the 1981 Education Act this has changed somewhat). Conrad's sample contained children with a wide range of peripheral hearing losses: the 359 Special School children were approximately equally divided amongst the five categories of less than 66, 66–85, 86–95, 96–105 and greater than 105 dB HL.

Conrad chose the Brimer Wide-span Reading Test (Brimer 1972) to assess the reading ability of the children in his sample. This test consists of 80 items of increasing difficulty which provide a range of reading ages (standardized on normally hearing children) of between 7 and 16 years. Each item consists of a pair of written sentences from one of which a word is missing. The testee's task is to choose a word from the other sentence which is appropriate to the incomplete sentence, and to write it in the space provided. The following are examples of test items (taken from Form B):-

3	He will sit on a big rock and look at the sea	Mothers often____their babies to sleep
9	Some are larger than others so try another if one doesn't fit	We should be kind to one____
13	He went across the path, through the orchard, and into the vineyard	The boys used to steal the apples that grew in the____behind the house
20	A small sum of money is paid as an entrance fee to visit the museum	Hospitably, her friends wrote to invite her to pay them a____
30	Its pendulum would vacillate and vibrate with the indeterminate sound of machinery that would reverberate around the house	When faced with making a commitment this indecisive man would____and temporize

In broad agreement with earlier studies, Conrad found that the median reading age of his sample 9;0 years. Analysis of covariance showed a highly significant effect of intelligence (measured with the Raven's Progressive Matrices) on reading age; and a highly significant effect of degree of hearing loss. With regard to the latter, there were no significant differences in reading age between the three hearing-loss categories above 85 dB loss, nor between the two categories below 85 dB. Thus the principal effect of hearing loss was between those children with a loss up to 85 dB and those with a greater loss. Correlations between reading age and intelligence ranged from 0.53 to 0.30 for different subgroups; and mean reading ages were 10;4 and 10;1 for the two hearing-loss categories below 85 dB loss, and 9;1, 8;11 and 8;3 for the three categories above 85 dB, with lower reading age associated with greater impairment. Considering only those children with hearing losses greater than 85 dB, almost 50 per cent failed to achieve the 'floor' level on the Brimer test of 7;0 years. For those children with hearing losses less than 85 dB, the corresponding figure is 25 per cent. However, of the less impaired, only 8 per cent achieved a reading age commensurate with chronological age; and a mere five children out of the 208 more severely impaired did likewise.

In the face of the foregoing data from this country and from North America, several authors have discussed the possibility that there is a plateau or ceiling of reading achievement for most hearing-impaired children. Conrad (1979) talks of 'a stage of reading in which many deaf children may remain trapped' (p. 163) and identifies it as that stage when the child is required not simply to identify a single word but to read for meaning and draw inferences from strings of words with syntactic structure. He does speculate that the plateau might reflect some functional level of literacy sufficient to cope with basic day-to-day (as opposed to strictly educational) needs. Although we have no independent measures of literacy levels required to extract meaning from everyday materials, the argument remains unconvincing, if only because hearing children do not stop at this 'functional' level; furthermore, massive effort is put into the task of teaching reading skills to the deaf, and it would seem unlikely that at a particular functional level of skill the children choose to resist these efforts.

Quigley and Kretschmer (1982) review the literature and conclude that reading scores 'tend to plateau at about third to fourth grade level at about age 13 to 14 years and change very little by age 19 years' (p. 76). Hammermeister (1971) studied the reading abilities of deaf adults up to 13 years after leaving school and found that, although vocabulary continued to improve slowly, comprehension did not. The notion of a plateau in the reading ability of hearing-impaired children is of theoretical relevance to issues discussed in earlier chapters, since it is posited not just as a matter of delayed development but as a cessation in the normal though delayed progression through the various stages of reading skill. Against this must be placed the data from Quigley and his co-workers which we examined in Chapter 6 (see Fig. 6.1, p. 142). This showed that deaf students' mastery of certain grammatical structures did continue to increase, albeit slowly, throughout adolescence.

Why do hearing-impaired children fail to progress on the Brimer and other tests of reading? It may be that these tests, designed and standardized as they are for hearing children with a rich and well-developed language base, are simply too insensitive to the slower and more fragile progress of hearing-impaired readers: 'faced with most test and reading materials he is simply overwhelmed linguistically and uses other strategies in order to proceed with the task' (Webster 1983, p. 87). As we have mentioned in earlier chapters, it is dangerous to assume that a deaf adolescent with a reading age of 9;0 years is behaving in the same manner as a hearing 9;0 year old with average reading ability. The deaf adolescent brings to the task quite different percepts, experience and cognitive abilities from those of the 9-year-old hearing child. Faced with reading tests which are designed for the hearing child and which may be linguistically too difficult, the older deaf child, in order to proceed with the task, may adopt other strategies which are too subtle to be picked up by such a global measure as reading age. Webster and his colleagues (Webster et al. 1981, Wood et al. 1981) used the traditional tests of Brimer and Southgate, and studied the error patterns in order to see if they could sift out any support for this notion. If the earlier reports of Conrad (1979) and others are to be believed, performance of the hearing-impaired on these tests reflects simple reading retardation, and should therefore be no different from the performance of average 9 year olds. If, however, linguistic deficit is involved (which cannot be the case with many poor readers with normal hearing) then one might expect that analysis of, for example, error patterns would reveal different performance strategies in use by the hearing-impaired. Webster et al. (1981) studied the performance of 60 prelingually hearing-impaired children age 15–16;6 years on the Brimer Wide-span Reading Test. Subjects were chosen post hoc, so as to fall into three groups of 20 subjects each with reading ages on the test of 7, 8 and 9 years. They were then matched for reading age, intelligence and sex with three groups of normally hearing children; in order to be included, the latter had to achieve reading-age scores commensurate with their chronological ages.

The Brimer test is open-ended in that the testee may attempt as many items as he wishes. Analysis of the errors made by the subjects in Webster et al.'s study showed that the deaf children made many more errors (for the same reading age) than the hearing children: mean deaf error rate was 33.1, compared with 8.9 for hearing children. Independent observers classified errors as linguistic (e.g. semantically acceptable but nevertheless incorrect, syntactically correct word-class but semantically inappropriate) and nonlinguistic (e.g. the response word chosen on the basis of same spatial position in the 'cue' sentence). It turned out that the deaf children overall made 902 linguistic errors and 1081 nonlinguistic errors; the hearing children made 391 linguistic and 142 nonlinguistic errors. Thus the hearing-impaired made more errors overall, but a significantly smaller proportion of their errors were linguistic in nature. The greater proportion of nonlinguistic errors in the deaf groups (most of which defied analysis in terms of the reasons why they might have been chosen, although a sizeable minority were of the 'spatial position' type) was not due to their greater tendency to attempt items well beyond their capacity. Analyses of the errors which occurred only up to the ceiling point (i.e. the point at which reading age was attained) showed a similar disproportionate number of nonlinguistic errors in the deaf children's responses. Finally, the results showed that those deaf children who achieved higher reading ages on the test make proportionally more linguistic errors than the poorer readers, indicating genuine linguistic improvement with increased reading age.

These results are interpreted by the authors as indicating that deaf adolescents are 'not only retarded in their reading ability but they obtain their test scores in different ways from hearing children . . . Reading age estimates of deaf children are not reliable guides to their functional linguistic skills. . . . They are likely not to indicate a similar delayed process but the outcome of quite different reading abilities' (Webster *et al*. 1981, pp. 145–6). They suggest that the wide-span test is insensitive to the linguistic limitations of the deaf and forces them, perhaps aided by a tendency to perseverance in the face of failure which may spring from their educational experience (Furth 1973), to adopt strategies which are unlikely to produce correct responses.

Weight was added to this interpretation by Wood *et al*. (1981). This parallel study examined the performance of the same 60 hearing and 60 hearing-impaired children matched for reading age on the Southgate reading test. Examination of the incorrect answers to items revealed that, unlike the hearing children, who did not converge on the same incorrect solution to difficult items, the deaf children tended to select the same answer. This indicated that they were using consistent strategies in their choice of (incorrect) answers. Post hoc examination of individual errors suggested that one such strategy might be word association, as revealed in this example in which *nests* was the most popular answer:

Birds are covered with____*trees/skirts/sky/nests/feathers*

Again, the authors conclude that 'hearing-referenced tests would seem to generate unreliable data and act as poor guides to the reading processes of deaf children'.

Beggs and Breslaw (1983) have presented data on the performance of 40 severely hearing-impaired children on Hamp's (1972) Picture Assisted Recognition Test.

Even this test, which has been standardized for hearing-impaired children, showed distinct results for their sample. Errors were not always random, and evidence was presented of both initial-letter similarity strategies (producing errors such as *telescope* for *treasure*) and strategies based simply upon picture 'saliency'. Furthermore, the authors noted, as have others, that deaf children with reading ages matched to hearing controls do not fail on the same items as the hearing children; in particular, they do not reach a clearly defined ceiling but continue through many quite advanced items, picking up correct items here and there. Finally, Beggs and Breslaw (1982), although able to confirm the usual relationship of clumsiness and poor reading ability for hearing children, failed to find any such relationship in their deaf subjects. The authors argue that either 'the underlying mechanism linking perceptual-motor skills to reading ability is not functioning in the deaf, or . . . reading test performance in deaf and hearing children are not equivalent' (p. 36). They conclude (along with the authors of the preceding studies in this section) that indeed the 'reading age' of a deaf child means something quite different from its meaning for a hearing child. The significance of this lies in the fact that reading age scores will be less likely to serve as a guide to useful reading materials for hearing-impaired children than for hearing children, and will be similarly unlikely to offer useful information as to the details of the hearing-impaired child's individual reading problems.

The nature of reading disability in hearing-impaired children

Thus, any intervention based upon reading age and materials designed for hearing children and applied to hearing-impaired children is unlikely to be particularly productive. The poor reading skills of hearing-impaired children are not simply a matter of delay; their performance is not directly analogous to younger hearing children. Simplification of the reading materials to take account of poorer control of vocabulary and syntactic structures may be helpful to a point, but it could be counterproductive if grammatical structure is made too simple. Howarth *et al.* (1981) studied video recordings of reading lessons given to deaf and hearing children, and it was clear that the lessons were used for different purposes for the two groups of children. Reading lessons for hearing-impaired children are used not only to explore and develop the relationship between spoken and written words, but as an opportunity for language learning itself. As such, they are characterized by much more frequent stops to rehearse articulation, practise vocabulary and the like. The ability to extract meaning from the syntactic and semantic constraints inherent in connected text is unlikely to develop when the reading lesson is being stopped every four words or less (Howarth *et al.* 1981).

If merely simplifying the reading material in order to take account of linguistic deficit is not enough to secure adequate progress, what then is the problem for the hearing-impaired child? To answer this fully we would need to know a great deal more than we do about the reading process in both beginning and mature hearing readers, and about the idiosyncratic language base, cognitive processes and strategies which any individual hearing-impaired child brings to bear in the task of reading. The hearing child approaches the task when he has already developed an extensive vocabulary and extensive command of language structure. By the time he begins to learn to read, the hearing child has already acquired sophisticated oral language (although it is worth pointing out that development of the finer points of language in hearing children continues well after the fifth birthday, and such children do not therefore come to the reading task with essentially complete language). At one level, the task for a hearing child is to learn a graphemic code for an already established phonemic code, such that meaning can be linked to graphemes. Clearly, the hearing-impaired child arrives at the task with a double problem: not only does he not know the coding principles of the written symbols, he does not have adequate command of the phonemic code and language structures into which he must decode these symbols. Simplifying the language of the written symbols to keep within his linguistic competence may be useful, but it is unlikely to be sufficient.

To regard reading as no more than translating a graphemic code into a phonemic one would be a gross oversimplification. Reading is a complex task requiring mastery of a whole range of subskills, from discrimination of letter shapes, extraction of salient invariant features from letter shapes, word identification, and word recognition in context, through to complex processing skills which optimize information from not only visual but phonemic, semantic and syntactic sources. According to Smith (1975), the fluent reader draws on prior knowledge about properties of language to generate his own hypotheses about what text means, and to look for rules and regulations in the written code to enable him to reject or confirm such hypotheses. Thus, 'the ability to comprehend depends to a large extent on knowing what you already know about what you're supposed to know' (Pearson and Johnson 1978, p. 27). Learning to read is not simply 'parasitic upon speech' (Baddeley 1982) but involves in addition a large number of skills at various levels of complexity, any or all of which could represent an area of difficulty for the hearing-impaired child. Which skills are implicated as problem areas is a difficult question, since we know so little about the reading process itself. However, some progress has been made.

Kyle (1980) examined the lower-order skills of letter identification, equivalence and discrimination in 7- to 9-year-old deaf children. Their performance on these tasks was, by 9 years of age, very similar to that of hearing children, and Kyle concludes that deaf children develop these lower-order skills in a relatively normal fashion. On the other hand, there are a number of studies which show visual perceptual dysfunctions in deaf children (Myklebust and Brutten 1952, van Zyl and Ives 1971, Pollard and Neumaier 1974, Cooper and Arnold 1981). Cooper and Arnold administered five subtests of the Frostig Developmental Test of Visual Perception to 19 partially hearing children (mean age 11;2 years). The subtests used were eye–hand coordination, figure–ground perception, constancy of perception, perception of position in space, and perception of spatial relationships. The results showed developmental deficit on all five tests, such that the hearing-impaired children performed at the same levels (or worse, on one subtest) as a group of hearing children who were 3;6 years younger on average. Despite Cooper and Arnold's assertion that therefore 'deficiency in reading may be due . . . to retardation on the development of visual perceptual skills' (1981, p. 47), it cannot be assumed that the relationship between these skills and poor reading in hearing-impaired children is causal. However, it does support the notion that a complete description of the causes of reading problems is not to be found in speech and linguistic deficiencies alone.

The underlying mechanism linking visual perceptual and perceptual–motor skills to reading ability is not known. Piaget has stressed the relationship of perceptual–motor skills to overall cognitive development. Others relate it to cortical functioning (Reed 1967), or to eye-movement control (Arnheim and Sinclair 1975). On the latter, Beggs et al. (1981) found that the eye-movements of deaf children while reading were unlike those of hearing children of matched reading ages. In some cases eye-movements were quite pathological – reading alternate lines in different directions, for example. Marcel (1974) found that hearing 11 year olds who were slow readers exhibited inadequate fixation and/ or scanning patterns. He examined the amount read from the second of two successive fixations of text presented via a tachistoscope, and found that faster readers benefited more from contextual constraint: the 'effective visual field' was enlarged. It seems that with greater contextual priming, less sampling of visual information is necessary for word recognition, allowing more capacity for visual processing on the periphery.

Cooley (1981) extended the investigation of visual field to young prelingually deafened adults. They, and a comparison group of hearing subjects, read aloud materials of varying amounts of grammatical constraint. When the reader's voice reached a preselected point, the text was removed; the reader continued to report any words that he had already seen, and the number of words correctly reported was called his eye-voice span. The mean eye-voice span of the deaf subjects was significantly poorer than that of the hearing readers. Both hearing and deaf subjects had longer eye-voice spans at positions of high grammatical constraint, and shorter at positions of low grammatical constraint. Deaf subjects with higher reading scores have corresponding longer eye-voice spans, and they were more likely therefore 'to use their knowledge of the grammar of sentences to group words into grammatical units during reading and to use these units as units of processing for efficient reading' (p. 360). This strategy was used by all deaf readers, but those with the lower reading abilities used it inconsistently and less efficiently. They were less able to 'chunk' words into correct grammatical units.

A number of studies have investigated cerebral dominance in hearing-impaired subjects. In normal adults the mechanisms implicated in the production and perception of speech and language appear to be lateralized in the dominant cerebral hemisphere (Kimura 1961), usually the left, at least in right-handed people (see also Chapter 10). Conrad (1979) and Boshoven et al. (1982) have reviewed the literature, and although there are a number of ambiguities and unresolved questions, the general picture emerges that hearing-impaired individuals tend to exhibit much less left-hemisphere dominance for words and letters than do hearing individuals (Marcotte and LaBarba 1985). In certain cases a right-hemisphere advantage has been shown (e.g. Phippard 1977). Conrad concludes that in general 'while lateralized cerebral function for speech develops during the earliest years of life of hearing children, possibly through a shift away from right-hemisphere involvement . . . this may not occur in the case of children who are hearing-impaired' (1979, p. 262). The age at which cerebral asymmetry is first exhibited by hearing individuals has been shown to be 5 years for girls and 7 years for boys (Buffery 1971), and Marcel *et al.* (1974) found differences clearly present at ages between 7;6 and 8;7. In their extensive review, Boshoven *et al.* (1982) relate their findings to the notion of the critical period for language acquisition (Lenneberg 1967) and suggest that lack of language stimulation affects hemispherical function as the critical period is passed.

The link between cerebral dominance and reading proficiency has been made for hearing children by Marcel *et al.* (1974). They presented five-letter words for short durations to the right or left of a fixation point. The duration was short enough to ensure that eye-movements could not be involved, and in this situation the visual stimulus presented to the right visual hemifield is transmitted only to the left cerebral hemisphere and vice versa. Interest then centred on the number of correctly identified words and letters as a function of right or left hemifield presentation. Subjects were boys and girls of 7–8 years of age, who were divided into subgroups of good and poor readers on the basis of their performance on a standard sentence-completion reading test. The results showed consistent right hemifield (left hemisphere) superiority for all subjects – but good readers exhibited significantly greater right hemifield superiority than did poor readers. The mean difference of the number of words/letters correct between hemifields was 6.5 words for good readers compared with 3.9 words for poor readers; and 29.65 letters for good readers compared with 13.85 letters for poor readers. Marcel *et al.* concluded that good and poor readers of the same age differ in the degree of lateralization in terms of cerebral hemispheric specialization of language function. But as with many of the behavioural correlates of poor reading ability (in hearing or hearing-impaired children) it is too early as yet to speculate about causal links.

The crucial question for understanding the development of reading in hearing-impaired children concerns the mediating processes involved in deriving meaning from print. It is argued that if an individual adopts a particular mediating system, then stimulus materials will be best dealt with when they are consistent with the individual's coding strategy. In a typical experiment (Chen 1976), hearing, moderately hearing-impaired and severely hearing-impaired students were given a passage to read and asked to mark out all the *e* letters as they read. Hearing subjects, and those with only moderate hearing losses, were much more likely to miss silent *es* (as in *bite*) than the severely impaired group. It was argued that if the words were being decoded via a speech code, then silent *es* would tend to be overlooked because there is no acoustic correlate in the word's pronunciation. The results therefore indicated that the hearing children and to some extent the moderately impaired children were using a speech code;

but the severely impaired children were not. Conrad (1970) used an immediate recall task to investigate error patterns of deaf and hearing children. Stimuli were strings of letters, five or six letters in length according to an individual's ability, which were chosen to be phonologically similar (B, C, T) or which had common visual features (K, X, Y, Z). The hearing subjects showed highly significant error confusions within the phonologically similar letter strings, but not within the visually similar strings. The deaf children fell into two distinct groups: one group, slightly more than half the sample, exhibited 'phonological' errors like the hearing children. The remaining deaf children made few errors with the phonological letter strings, but many errors with the letters which were chosen to be visually similar. Conrad argued that the first group were using a phonologically based memory code, while the other group were using some kind of visual coding.

In his 1979 survey of the literacy skills of hearing-impaired school leavers, Conrad extended this technique to the immediate recall of words which were chosen to be homophonous or nonhomophonous. The homophonous words sounded alike, but were visually dissimilar: *do, few, who, zoo, blue, true, screw, through*; the nonhomophonous words, on the other hand, were chosen to be visually similar but acoustically dissimilar: *bare, bean, door, furs, have, home, farm, lane*. Children in the study were asked to recall sets of between three and six words (according to ability, such that a reasonable error rate was achieved) selected from either the homophonous list or the nonhomophonous list. Some children found the homophonous words more difficult, as evidenced by their error rates, and such children were supposed to be using phonological coding. Conrad calls this 'internal speech', although the term should not be taken to imply that full articulation without sound is necessarily involved: auditory speech imagery as a purely inferred phenomenon without articulation is conceivable. Other children had more difficulty in memorizing the words which were nonhomophonous and were said to be using, therefore, alternative coding strategies, probably visual.

Conrad devised a measure called the Internal Speech Ratio (IS ratio) which reflected the degree to which a particular child appeared from the short-term memory task to be relying on phonological coding of written stimuli. Of 119 normally hearing children tested for comparison, 94 per cent used internal speech according to criteria based upon IS ratio. This proportion fell significantly to about 75 per cent for children with hearing losses up to 85 dB HL. But for the children with hearing losses of 86–95 dB and 96–105 dB, only about 45 per cent used internal speech, and of the most deaf group (106 + dB) less than 30 per cent used internal speech in the immediate recall task. Conrad then proceeded to examine the relationship between reading ability on the Brimer test and availability of internal speech. Those children with 'internal speech' had very significantly greater reading ages than those children without 'internal speech'. Although we must be cautious in assuming that just because a child uses phonological coding strategies – perhaps amongst other strategies – in the recall task he will always prefer the same strategy in reading, the results are nonetheless very striking. Analysis of covariance showed that intelligence, hearing loss and use of internal speech were all significantly associated with reading age, with hearing loss less important than the other two variables.

Conrad (1979) argued from his results that internal speech is the defining variable for the hearing-impaired child's success in lipreading, memory span, the intelligibility of his speech, and reading ability. Other workers have suggested that the lack of internal speech is a primary cause of the deaf child's deficiencies in reading and writing. Pattison (1983) compared good and poor hearing-impaired readers, and found that it was the good readers who showed evidence of internal phonology in short-term verbal memory tasks. Also, subjects who used internal phonology retained more information than those who did not. Thus a link was established between internal phonology and both good reading levels and better short-term verbal memory.

These studies and others provide support for a view of reading disability in hearing-impaired children which highlights processing problems rather than simply linguistic deficiency. Specifically, at the transition from naming words to reading sentences it may be that a hearing child uses the phonological information in words to give a version of language with which he is familiar, and thereby lessens the processing load needed to extract meaning. It is interesting to note that it is at the level of reading which most deaf children attain that hearing children begin to make use of grammatical structure to make their reading more fluent. Hung *et al.* (1981) go further than this, and bring into the discussion a distinction common in cognitive psychology between mechanistic processes that require attention, a resource that is in limited supply, and processes that do not, i.e. automaticity.

> If a person must devote attention to a low-level process, for example, identifying words in the sentence, fewer resources are available for high-level semantic processing. From this perspective, one of the reasons for deaf subjects' reading deficiency seems to lie in the fact that they have not developed automaticity for low-level skills such as letter decoding and word recognition. (Hung *et al.* 1981, p. 605.)

Results from a letter-decoding task in which subjects had to judge whether a pair of letters were identical or not (i.e. same/different task) showed that profoundly deaf 14 to 18 year olds performed in a similar fashion to hearing children, in that their reaction times were depressed in name-identity conditions (e.g. Aa) compared with physical identity conditions (e.g. AA); however, their reaction times in all conditions were much longer, consistent with the view that letter decoding processes are 'less automatic' in deaf children.

If some hearing-impaired children do have access to phonological coding, as Conrad's (1979) data and other studies suggest, why then do these children, although showing better reading skills than those who do not, not develop reading skills commensurate with their chronological ages? Conrad suggests that hearing-impaired children may use internal speech 'less incisively' than hearing children. Pattison (1983) argues more convincingly that hearing-impaired children may derive phonological codes from a variety of sources – auditory, articulatory, lipreading cues – and that different children rely to a greater or lesser extent on each, and with more or less skill. This suggests that those children who do not appear to use internal phonology may not be using a visual or even a finger-spelling code (Locke and Locke 1971) as had previously been supposed (Conrad 1979), but rather relying on an idiosyncratic and distorted form of English phonology.

Webster (1983) has pointed out that the view of internal phonology which derives from Conrad (1979) emphasizes its role in assisting the child to understand phoneme-grapheme correspondences and that this is a stage of reading which is indispensable. Nonetheless, internal speech within Conrad's explanation of the reading process has a fairly limited, low-order role. We have already noted the connection between performance on short-term memory tasks and access to internal phonology, and Webster (1983) attempts to upgrade the role of internal speech within current models which emphasize the importance of temporary storage systems.

Baddeley (1979, 1982; also Baddeley and Hitch 1974, Baddeley and Lewis 1981) has proposed a model of working memory which consists of a central executive and, *inter alia*, an articulatory loop slave system. The articulatory loop is regarded as responsible for the many speech-like characteristics of short-term memory, and it was proposed in order to account for the variety of results which suggest a close link between verbal coding and short-term memory. These include the phonological similarity effect (the more phonologically similar items are, the more difficult they are to recall) of Conrad (1970); the word-length effect (word duration rather than number of syllables is a crucial variable determining ease of recall); the unattended speech effect (recall of visually presented items is markedly impaired if irrelevant spoken material which must be speechlike is presented simultaneously; and articulatory suppression (if subjects are prevented from subvocal rehearsal of items by uttering irrelevant speech sounds, recall is impaired). Baddeley suggested the existence of a separate phonological memory store capable of holding spoken material. In the case of visually presented items, registration in this store would occur only if the subject subvocally articulates the material. In the case of auditory presentation, registration in the store is obligatory. By articulating visually presented items, the subject 'can supplement the visual store with a more durable phonological trace' (Baddeley 1982, 415). It should be noted that on this view there is no obligatory translation from grapheme to speech code for visually presented material, at least for fluent readers. Baddeley (1982) suggested, then, that phonological coding in reading is used sometimes but is in fact optional. However, he argued that in learning to read,

> a child must decode a series of visually presented letters, store and outcome of his decoding in some temporary systems, and subsequently blend the contents of his store to produce a word. We suggested that the articulatory loop system would be ideally designed to assist in this . . . . Each item, when decoded, is stored in the slave system, hence freeing the central executive to decode the next item, and subsequently blend and map the blend onto a real word. (Baddeley 1982, p. 416.)

Webster (1983) argues for the importance of higher-order, organizational factors for reading, and speculates that internal speech is more closely related to cognitive processes at this higher level. Information about the syntactic structure of a sentence, together with information about individual lexical items, must be retained long enough to derive semantic relationships between words in a sentence. There seems little doubt that the concept of internal speech is central in mediating between text and comprehension. Its role, however, may be less to do with grapheme–phoneme correspondences than with a more central implication in short-term memory and the articulatory loop which allows access to syntactic and semantic information. Wilkenfeld (1981) has pointed out that the presence of phonological coding in reading has been convincingly demonstrated, but the explanation that the effect results from a process of grapheme–phoneme conversion is falsified by evidence for phonetic coding in reading non-alphabetic orthographics (e.g. Tzeng *et al.* 1977). Wilkenfeld demonstrates experimentally that the phonetic representation in fluent readers embodies, amongst other things, suprasegmental linguistic properties such as word-stress and sentence prosody. This is evidence for a model of reading which has a strong dependency upon speech perception, but at distinctly higher-order levels. It is difficult to conceive of the influence of such higher-order processes without incorporating the notion of short-term memory and, in particular, an articulatory loop system. It may well be that the difficulties for hearing-impaired children in learning to read involve the lack of or a distorted system of internal speech which compromises their access to a temporary auditory storage system. This in turn degrades access to the syntactic, semantic and perhaps suprasegmental context of the text, and it is with this stage, so crucial to fluent reading, that hearing-impaired children learning to read apparently find particular difficulty.

9

Unilateral hearing loss

Unilateral hearing loss refers to the case where one ear exhibits pure-tone detection thresholds which are within normal limits, while thresholds in the other ear are elevated. Conductive hearing loss associated with fluctuating middle-ear pathologies are, as we have seen, common in young children, and a proportion of these will from time to time be unilateral. We are not concerned here with such transient cases. In this chapter we shall look at the effects of unilateral hearing losses which are sensorineural in origin; as such, they will be permanent, and they will often be more severe in terms of degree of threshold elevation than unilateral conductive losses.

Prevalence and aetiology

Epidemiological data on unilateral hearing loss is hard to find. Bess and Tharpe (1984) have estimated that close to 6.4 million Americans have some degree of unilateral hearing loss. The prevalence rate for school-age children with unilateral loss of 45 dB or more in the USA is said to be 3 per 1000, a figure which rises to perhaps 13 per 1000 if the milder losses are included (Berg 1976). Jordan and Eagles (1961) examined approximately 4000 5- to 10-year-old children and found 12 per cent with unilateral abnormalities (including conductive pathologies). Kessner et al. (1974, reported in Northern and Downs 1978) conducted audiometric studies on 1639 4- to 11-year-old children, and found that 4.5 per cent had unilateral pure-tone losses in the so-called speech range (500–2000 Hz) of over 15 dB HL. A further 7.6 per cent had unilateral hearing loss of over 15 dB in the nonspeech range of frequencies (note that the distinction between 'speech' and 'nonspeech' frequencies is a gross oversimplification; we use it only because the data are reported in this manner). Early data from a recent developmental survey in the UK of some 7000 children indicate a prevalence rate of about 2.5 per cent (S. Stewart-Brown, personal communication); this relatively high figure includes conductive impairments and mild degrees of loss. In a study of the effectiveness of the Auditory Response Cradle (Bennett and Wade 1980) at detecting hearing losses in children in a neonatal intensive care unit, McCormick et al. (1984) report a prevalence rate for these high-risk babies of seven per 1000 for bilateral losses, and 15 per 1000 for bilateral and unilateral losses. These losses are likely to be mostly sensorineural in origin, and as such they compare with a bilateral rate of about 0.7 – one per 1000 for the normal (i.e. non-ICU) neonatal population. Northern and Downs (1978) summarize by saying that 'unilateral deafness has always been common among children, and its prevalence does not appear to be lessening' (143).

Everberg (1960) sampled 122 cases of unilateral loss. There was a greater prevalence of affected males (62 per cent) than females (38 per cent). Aetiology was unknown in about half the cases, a figure in broad agreement with Tarkkanen and Aho (1966). Bess and Tharpe (1983) state that heredity is the most common congenital factor; however, it is widely thought that unilateral losses arise chiefly from postnatal conditions, in particular from viral infections (especially mumps) and meningitis. Of 60 unilaterally impaired children (hearing loss in the impaired ear greater than 45 dB HL) studied by Bess (1982), the aetiology was unknown in 51 per cent, viral complications in 26 per cent, meningitis in 13 per cent and head trauma in 8 per cent of the cases. Occasionally perinatal factors such as anoxia or jaundice have been known to cause unilateral rather than bilateral impairments. B. Davies (personal communication) has identified cytomegalovirus (CMV) as a frequent cause of unilateral impairments.

Unilateral hearing loss and auditory perception

We know that a listener's ability to perceive and organize his auditory environment depends partly on the use of two ears and the resulting neural interactions that occur between the binaural signals as they progress through the auditory pathways. During the past 30 years substantial progress has been made in the study of binaural interactions in normal listeners. This has been extensively reviewed (e.g. Durlach and Colburn 1978) and it is not our intention to repeat the task. There has been less work on binaural interactions in hearing-impaired listeners (both bilaterally and unilaterally impaired), but what there is has been reviewed in depth by Durlach et al. (1981). Information on the effect of unilateral hearing on aspects of auditory perception can come from two sources. First, from studies on normally hearing listeners who are rendered monaural either by presenting stimuli via one earphone only or, in the soundfield, by attenuating the input to one ear by means of an earplug and/or earmuff; all studies of binaural interactions in normal listeners employ such comparison conditions in order to quantify and elucidate the nature of the binaural effects. Secondly, from studies, fewer in number, which have directly examined the performance of subjects with unilateral hearing losses on tasks which are known to involve binaural interactions. Tasks which involve binaurality, and on which performance is therefore likely to suffer when there is a unilateral hearing loss, can be subsumed under the following headings (see Chapter 1): binaural summation, right-ear advantage, localization, the precedence effect, head-shadow effects, and binaural masking level differences.

Binaural summation

The pure-tone binaural threshold is some 3 dB better than the monaural threshold (e.g. Pollack 1948). This also applies at suprathreshold levels, such that binaural sounds are louder than monaural ones by 3–6 dB (e.g. Hirsh and Pollack 1948). These findings apply to speech discrimination tasks (e.g. Bocca 1955) as well as to the detection of non-speech stimuli. Binaural summation has been shown to occur to an extent even when the signal levels at the two ears differ by as much as 25–30 dB (Pollack and Pickett 1958). Although the binaural summation effect is unlikely to be of major importance for listeners with unilateral hearing loss, it has to be pointed out that if the speech intelligibility curve for connected speech rises as a rate of, say, 5 per cent dB, then a 3 dB deficit because of unilateral impairment would reduce the speech intelligibility score by 15 per cent.

Right-ear advantage

Broadhent (1958) showed that with a series of dichotically presented pairs of digits, normally hearing listeners preferentially recalled the items presented to the right ear. Kimura (1961) found a right-ear advantage for speech and a left-ear advantage for nonspeech stimuli such as melody. This effect, which is small and probably of little practical importance, was attributed to the prepotency of the contralateral pathways to the language-specialized left hemisphere. In the context of cerebral asymmetry and its relationship with verbal skills such as reading (see Chapter 8), it would be of interest to know whether severe unilateral hearing loss of prelingual onset shows any tendency to be associated with reduced degrees of cerebral asymmetry.

Localization

Localization refers to the ability to judge the direction and distance of a sound source. It allows the listener to bring his attention fully to bear on the stimulus, and this is likely to be of some importance in a variety of situations, from the infant beginning to communicate and interact with his mother to the child in the classroom who needs to switch attention rapidly from speaker to speaker. As we saw in Chapter 1, research has shown that interaural differences in intensity, time of arrival and phase provide the basis for the localization of sound in the horizontal plane. Individuals with a severe unilateral hearing loss would be deprived of these cues and might be expected therefore to have difficulty with locating sounds. Durlach et al. (1981) review the published studies, and despite difficulties in comparison and interpretation of data conclude that in general localization performance is indeed degraded by unilateral hearing loss.

Two studies by Bess and Newton confirm this conclusion (see also Bess et al. 1986). Bess (1982) examined the performance of 20 unilaterally impaired children (hearing thresholds no better than 45 dB HL in the impaired ear) aged 6–13 years on a localization task, in comparison with 20 normally hearing children. Pure-tone stimuli at 500 and 3000 Hz and of 0.5 s duration were presented randomly to one of 13 loudspeakers located in a 180° horizontal arc in front of the listener in a large anechoic chamber. Each trial was preceded by a visual warning signal and consisted of four tone-bursts presented to one of the loudspeakers. The loudspeakers had a separation of 15 degrees. The listener's task on each trial was to indicate from which loudspeaker the signal had been presented, and performance was measured in terms of the number of speakers from the correct source by which the subject was in error. A measure was devised (see Gardner and Gardner 1973) which varied from 1.0 for random guessing to 0.0 for perfect localization.

Results showed that the performance of the hearing-impaired subjects was considerably poorer than that of the normally hearing children. Mean error index for the latter was approximately 0.04 at 500 Hz and 0.14 for 3000 Hz. This was very similar to results in the same task for adult normally hearing listeners (Humes *et al.* 1980). The unilaterally impaired children, on the other hand, gave mean error indices of 0.66 at 500 Hz and 0.75 at 3000 Hz. Thus, both groups showed greater difficulty localizing a high-frequency stimulus than a low-frequency one, although the differences were small and probably not significant. There was much more variability among the hearing-impaired children, as evidenced by large standard deviations in the error indices. Viehweg and Campbell (1960) suggested that there might be a relationship between degree of hearing loss in the impaired ear and ability to localize; and if so, this would account of course for some of the variability. Bess (1982) did indeed find large and significant correlations between average hearing loss and error index: coefficients of 0.78 for 500 Hz and 0.51 for 3000 Hz signals. Newton (1983) speculates that the age at which a unilateral loss is acquired might be another source of variability between subjects. She suggests that if the loss is congenital or acquired early before a child has 'learnt to rely on binaural cues' (p. 197), then the child's ability to localize might be superior to those children who were impaired at a later age.

Newton (1983) points out that most previous studies have tended to use pure tones and low frequency stimuli. She used a similar situation to that used by Bess to measure localization ability, except that signals consisted of 5s bursts of either pure tone at 500 Hz, narrow-band noise centred at 500 Hz, or high-pass filtered noise with a filter cut-off at 3 kHz. In addition signals were presented from one loud-speaker which could be moved continuously through a 180 degree horizontal arc, and error was expressed in terms of degrees of deviation of subjects' responses from the actual position of the sound source. Subjects were 44 unilaterally impaired children aged 10–16 years with hearing losses of at least 70 dB HL, and 40 normally hearing listeners. These latter made small errors of (mean) 4.5 degrees for the pure-tone and 2.5 degrees for the noise stimuli. The hearing-impaired listeners, on the other hand, showed deviation errors of 30 degrees for the 500 Hz pure-tone, approximately 25 degrees for the low-pass noise and approximately 13 degrees for the high-pass noise. Why, in contrast to Bess's results, the localization of the high-frequency stimuli should be better than that of the low-frequency stimuli is not entirely clear. It has been suggested (Batteau 1967) that pinna effects are particularly involved for stimuli at 4000 Hz or above: Bess's pure-tones (3 kHz) would not have contained such frequencies, whereas Newton's high-pass noise would have. The variability of the hearing-impaired data in Newton's study was markedly greater than for the normal listeners; this was unlikely to be due to the variable influence of the impaired ear, since presentation level was 65 dB SPL, which was at or below threshold. There was some overlap of performance between the hearing-impaired and normal listeners on the high-pass noise signal, in that nine of the former were able to localize as accurately as those with normal hearing. When the pinnae on the good ears of a subgroup of 22 impaired children (including the nine with good high-pass noise performance) were covered, the performance of these nine subjects was depressed more than the remainder of the group, indicating that better use of pinnae information at high frequencies was an important factor in their superior performance.

The precedence effect

This effect refers to the phenomenon whereby, within certain limitations of time interval and spectral composition of the signals, successive signals are fused into a single percept. This is thought to depend upon binaural interactions, and is one of the ways in which normal-hearing listeners cope with signals and their echoes in reverberant environments (see Chapter 1). There has been little formal research on the effects of reverberation on listeners with hearing impairments (see, however, MacKeith and Coles 1971, Markides 1977), but on theoretical grounds we would expect them to find reverberant environments problematical, and this is certainly confirmed by subjective reports. Markides (1977) examined the ability of subjects with severe unilateral hearing loss to localize a speech signal, and found no significant differences between their performance in a reverberant and in a non-reverberant environment. On the other hand, reverberation had a detrimental effect upon speech discrimination as measured by a phoneme-scored word list presented in background noise. The detrimental effects of reverberation were more marked for subjects with asymmetrical hearing losses than for those with symmetrical (i.e. bilateral equal) hearing losses.

These results refer to patients wearing either one or two hearing aids (the chief purpose of Markides' extensive studies was to investigate the advantages of binaural hearing aids over monaural aid provision), but he also tested a group of listeners with severe unilateral losses, for whom a conventional hearing aid would not be appropriate. Irrespective of whether the speech was presented to the side of the good ear or the side of the bad ear (noise was always presented to the side opposite the speech signal), reverberation significantly and adversely affected these subjects' speech-discrimination performance. The difference in speech intelligibility score was of the order of 15 per cent at certain signal-to-noise ratios. Interestingly, although both conditions showed significant disadvantages of reverberation, the condition in which the speech signal was presented from the side of the good ear showed a greater effect of reverberation than when speech came from the side of the bad ear. In everyday listening conditions the unilaterally impaired child in, for example, a classroom would tend to face his good ear to the speech source. This is of course sensible, and will give him better speech perception than if the speech is to the bad ear (see head-shadow effect, below), but it is apparently particularly susceptible to reverberation.

Head-shadow effects

Signals coming from the right side of an individual will be louder in his right ear than in his left, and vice versa. This is due to the acoustic shadow cast by the head. Thresholds for pure tones on the ear contralateral to the sound source are depressed by a few dB, depending upon frequency: tones with longer wavelength (low frequencies) will bend round the head more easily than higher-frequency tones (e.g. Wiener 1947). The same effect applies not surprisingly to speech signals. Tillman *et al.* (1963) determined a reduction in speech-reception threshold for spondee* words of 6.4 dB due to head shadow, a figure which agrees well with data from other workers. When speech is presented in noise, the head-shadow effect may be even greater for a monaural listener: the head-shadow loss on the ear contralateral to the speech will translate into – 6 dB signal-to-noise ratio (assuming zero signal-to-noise ratio in the 'middle of the head' position); and if the positions of signal and noise sources are then reversed, the signal-to-noise ratio on the same ear will be + 6 dB. The masking effect of the noise on the speech will thus be some 12 dB less severe in one condition than in the other. For a unilaterally impaired listener, this means that if he is unfavourably placed with regard to the sound sources he will be 12 dB 'worse off' than in the favourable position. This was clearly demonstrated by Carhart (1965) using normal listeners rendered monaural – the difference between the two conditions for 50 per cent discrimination score was 13 dB. MacKeith and Coles (1971) performed a similar study, and found head-shadow effects in terms of change in speech-to-noise ratio for 50 per cent discrimination of up to 16 dB. In conditions where their (normally hearing) listeners were rendered only partly monaural, the same effect ranged from 2 to 9 dB.

Thus, the unilateral listener has marked difficulties when his good ear is on the far side of his head in relation to the wanted signal source. Of course, he could move to a favourable position in which the good ear is to the wanted signal and the bad ear to the unwanted noise signal, but there are circumstances (in the classroom, the theatre, a committee meeting) where this may not always be as easy as it might seem.

Binaural masking level differences (BMLD)

BMLD, also called 'binaural release from masking', occurs whenever the phase or intensity differences of the signal at the two ears are not the same as the phase or intensity differences of the masker at the two ears (see Chapter 1). Under these conditions the ability to detect and identify signals will be improved (e.g. Webster 1951, Gebhardt and Goldstein 1972). The phenomenon has been studied extensively, using headphones and apparatus which can independently alter the

---

* Spondee words: bisyllabic words with approximately equal stress on each syllable (e.g. *toothpaste*).

interaural relations of signal and of noise. To give a simple example, if two in-phase pure-tone signals of the same frequency are presented one to each ear, accompanied by noise from the same noise generator (so that it is interaurally identical), there will be certain masked threshold for the tone. If now the phase of the tone in one ear only is altered so that it is out of phase with the tone in the other ear, the masked-tone threshold will be improved by anything from 2 to 15 dB, depending upon the frequency of the tone and the phase difference applied. This 'binaural release from masking' has been demonstrated for complex tones, clicks and speech sounds as well as for pure tones. Studies of BMLD in patients with uni-lateral hearing losses (e.g. Schoeny and Carhart 1971, Bocca and Antonelli 1976) have shown in general less release from masking, compared to patients with symmetrical hearing losses and normally hearing listeners (again, see Durlach *et al*. 1981 for a thorough review).

Interaural relations in phase or intensity for the signal which are different from the interaural phase or intensity relations for the noise occur in the freefield only when the signal and noise sources are located in separate spatial positions. Thus the analogy of the earphone BMLD phenomenon in a soundfield is the dependence of performance (detection thresholds or discrimination scores) upon the position of signal and noise sources and the availability of one ear vs two ears. Carhart (1965) measured speech intelligibility for words in competing sentences for normally hearing subjects listening binaurally and listening monaurally with one ear occluded. In one condition the words were presented from 45 degrees to one side of the listener and the competing sentences from 45 degrees to the other side. Carhart found a binaural advantage over monaural near-ear listening (i.e. signal on the side of the 'good' ear) of 3 dB for 50 per cent discrimination. This is the soundfield equivalent of BMLD, and Carhart called it the 'squelch effect'. Note that the comparison of monaural near-ear listening with monaural far-ear listening gives a measure of head-shadow effects. A similar study by MacKeith and Coles showed a squelch effect of between 0 to 4 dB.

Since the squelch effect is clearly dependent upon adequate binaural interaction, one would expect the binaural advantage to be absent or reduced in patients with marked degrees of unilateral hearing loss. Tonning (1971, 1972 a and b) has investigated this and found it to be the case.

Language skills and unilateral impairment

In Chapter 5 we examined the auditory perceptual dysfunctions that are found in people with bilateral sensorineural hearing loss. The greatest proportion of the dis-ability suffered by such people is related to impaired peripheral processes, such as loss of auditory sensitivity, reduced dynamic range, and poor frequency and temporal resolving ability. In congenital onset this may lead not only to poor speech perception, but as a consequence to reduced central auditory skills, and to poorly developed speech and language skills. As far as reduced central auditory skills are concerned, these may be largely 'linguistic' – development of the phonetic mode, of phonological coding, of auditory memory; or largely 'auditory' and perhaps lower-level – binaural interactions of various kinds, for example. Thus, it should not be overlooked that the listening problems of the bilateral sensorineurally impaired person will be exacerbated in poor acoustic conditions. Localization, the squelch effect and the precedence effect are generally present, but to a less than normal extent in bilateral impairments; although it may not at first sight appear to be the main source of disability for such listeners, their task can be made markedly more difficult in poor acoustic environments. It is essential, there-fore, to educate bilaterally impaired children in conditions which are not unduly noisy, in which the speaker's spatial position remains clear, and in which reverberation is at a minimum.

The problem for the unilaterally impaired child is somewhat different. This child will have adequate peripheral auditory processing on the normal ear, and in broad terms at least the child will develop nearly normal speech and language skills. The focus of this child's disability is more subtle, since it results solely from the dis-advantages related to reduced or absent access to binaural interactions. Depending upon the degree of hearing loss and the details of the acoustic environment (degree of reverberation, position of sound sources etc.), such a child will have less than normal binaural summation, poor localization ability, extra problems with reverberation, susceptibility to the effects of head shadow, and reduced binaural squelch for signals which have to be listened to in background noise. Bess *et al.* (1986) have demonstrated poorer speech recognition ability of unilaterally impaired children in adverse listening conditions, particularly as the level of background noise increases. On the other hand, if listening conditions are near perfect (little reverberation, low ambient noise levels, listener facing the speaker etc.) the disadvantages of unilateral listening may be largely overlooked. Unfortunately, most normal classrooms do not satisfy these conditions, and it is here that children with severe unilateral losses may first begin to encounter real difficulties. Linguistic competence, therefore, may be normal, but linguistic performance – receptive performance skills in particular – will be adversely affected.

The more subtle effects of unilateral losses mean that this condition is often overlooked by parents and teachers, despite the evidence that it may give rise to feelings of embarrassment, annoyance and confusion (Giolas and Wark 1967). Northern and Downs (1978) point out that audiologists and otolaryngologists 'are not usually concerned over such deafness, other than to identify its etiology and assure the parents that there will be no handicap' (p. 143). Nevertheless, as they point out, the condition may be bewildering, and may be more traumatic to the child than the parents can appreciate. Not only are the effects of unilateral hearing losses often overlooked, but very often the condition is not even diagnosed until relatively late.

Bess (1982) studied the records of 60 children with unilateral losses, and showed that identification of the loss generally did not occur until school age. The children exhibited normal hearing sensitivity in their good ears, and losses of 45 dB HL or more (average over 500–2000 Hz) in the affected ears; they were of normal intel-ligence, and free from other significant medical problems (for example, there was no history of middle-ear effusions in the good ear). The mean age of identification of the hearing loss for these children was 5;7, and only 23 per cent of the children had their loss identified prior to 5 years of age. Of course, this relatively late identification may be partly accounted for by the fact that some of the children would have suffered late onset of the impairment; but at least some of the impairments were congenital in origin, and late onset is unlikely to have been the complete answer to late identification. The significance of the mean identification age of 5;7 is probably to be found in the age at which children begin their formal schooling. Prior to this, in the preschool years, the acoustic environment to be found in the home is often quite good: one to one, close communication, reasonable ambient noise levels, plenty of soft furnishings reducing reverberation, and so on. It is when formal schooling begins that the listening conditions for the children will be likely to point up the disability to surrounding adults; furthermore, it is then that school screening audiometry takes place.

Despite the existence of some early studies (e.g. Owrid 1970) which appeared to show quite favourable levels of verbal attainment by children with unilateral losses, recent data suggests a more cautious conclusion. Thus, Boyd (1974, reported by Bess 1982) found that 38 per cent of a group of unilaterally impaired children exhibited reading problems, 31 per cent had spelling problems, and 23 per cent had problems with arithmetic. Case-history information revealed that of Bess's (1982) 60 unilaterally impaired children, 35 per cent failed one or more grades in contrast to a normal failure rate of some 3.5 per cent (see also Bess and Tharpe 1986). If one added the children in Bess's group who needed extra resource help to those who had to repeat grades, the percentage rose from 35 to 48 per cent. The author comments:

> This finding was indeed surprising since it has long been assumed that children with unilateral hearing loss would have few, if any, problems in school. It thus appears that the listening difficulties imposed by a unilateral hearing-impairment often have an effect on the individual's classroom performance. Since all of the hearing-impaired children . . . were receiving preferential classroom seating, it can be concluded that greater efforts are needed to help them overcome the apparent listening difficulties they encounter in the educational setting. (Bess 1982, p. 137.)

Most of Bess's subjects exhibited severe hearing losses on the affected ear.

The failure of preferential seating completely to alleviate the disability even in good acoustic environments receives further confirmation from Bess's data on 17 of his children who were matched with a group of normally hearing children. They were tested for speech discrimination using the Nonsense Syllable Test (Levitt and Resnick 1978). This was presented in an acoustically treated room from one of two speakers located to the front at 45 degrees from the midline. Canteen noise was presented from the other speaker. Figure 9.1 shows the percentage correct scores as a function of the primary to secondary (i.e. signal to noise) ratio for normally hearing and unilaterally impaired listeners. Note that even when the signal was presented on the side of the good ear, the impaired children performed worse than the normally hearing children.

There have been too few studies of the effects of unilateral hearing loss in children. However, the recent data do suggest that such children experience more difficulty with communication, and with educational progress, than was previously supposed.

Rehabilitative strategies for the unilaterally impaired child

There are a number of points which should be observed with these cases. First assurance needs to be given to the child and/or parent that schooling and education

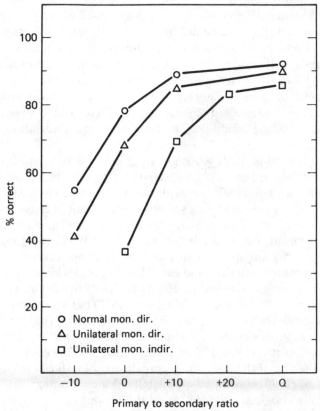

Figure 9.1 Mean percentage correct scores for the Nonsense Syllable Test presented in different amounts of noise for a group of normally hearing children ($n = 17$) and a matched group of unilaterally impaired children ($n = 17$). For the latter, presentation of the signal was either from the side of the good ear (monaural direct) or from the side of the affected ear (monaural indirect). (From Bess 1982, Fig. 5.)

ought to be able to proceed like that of any other normal child. Secondly, teachers, parents and child need to be fully aware of what can be done to help such a child: preferential seating in class and good acoustic conditions (as for all hearing-impaired children); use of visual cues and speechreading in general; and access to remedial or more intensive teaching programmes, if progress slows down. Thirdly, advice upon hearing conservation for the good ear should be given to the child and parents: thus, avoid loud noises; seek prompt medical treatment from an otologist for any ear infection, or any middle ear/external ear problem; avoid ototoxic drugs; and avoid putting anything into the ear canal.

Finally, advice on possible use of a hearing aid should be given. A small number of early studies suggested that, for those with 'aidable' residual hearing on the affected ear, a hearing aid could be beneficial (e.g. Malles 1963, Harford and Muskett 1964). On the other hand, Markides (1977) failed to find any significant improvement either in speech discrimination in noise or in the localization ability of 16 aidable unilaterally impaired adults when wearing an ear-level aid on the affected ear. Indeed, the mean differences he did find were in the other direction (i.e. poorer when aided), although the differences were not significant and there was much individual variability. Of course, as with all hearing aids, it will take time for the listener to adapt to his new-found 'binaurality', and to some extent this is borne out by the observations of some unilaterally impaired patients who clearly like their hearing aid. Whatever the effects of the aid, they are likely to be relatively small, very dependent upon acoustic conditions, and subject to much variability from patient to patient.

For those unilaterally impaired patients whose hearing loss is severe and for whom, given the existence of the good ear, a conventional hearing aid is likely to be of no use at all, a CROS aid is a possibility in particular circumstances. The CROS (Contralateral Routing of Signal) aid comes in a variety of forms, but in essence a hearing-aid microphone picks up sounds at the affected ear and sends them (via a small lead strung behind the head, via spectacles, or via FM signals) to the good ear. At the good ear the signals are amplified slightly and fed via an open earmould or simply through a piece of tubing into the good ear. This type of device is really for specialized use, primarily when head-shadow effects are likely to intrude and yet the listener cannot seek preferential seating. Markides (1977) has shown that, not unexpectedly, the CROS aid is helpful to speech discrimination when the signal is on the side of the poor ear (approximately 5 dB improvement in S:N ratio in non-reverberant conditions), but positively harmful when the signal is to the good ear and noise is presented on the side of the poor ear (approximately 13 dB change in S:N ratio). Kenworthy et al. (1990) confirmed and extended these findings with a small group of unilaterally impaired children, using three simulated listening conditions encountered in the classroom, two types of speech recognition tasks, and three types of audiological recommendations (unaided, CROS and a personal FM, or radio aid, system). Unaided and CROS conditions produced the expected results, depending upon listening conditions; but the FM system was the only recommendation to produce uniformly high speech recognition scores across all listening conditions with both types of speech materials. The authors conclude that perferential seating is not enough, and that 'a more aggressive audiological management approach may be warranted. The positive result with the FM system . . . was encouraging and should be explored further'.

10

Central auditory dysfunction

Professionals working in the disciplines of speech and hearing, and in education, now recognize that speech and language problems, together with classroom learning difficulties, may sometimes be caused by subtle difficulties in the processing of auditory signals. The approach to research studies in this area, and to the assessment and management of the individual cases has been quite different between these disciplines. In the last 10 years there has been increasing interest in, and rapid development of, the assessment of central auditory processing and its effect on language and learning difficulties. In the past, the speech therapist/pathologist has looked at the child's ability to carry out tasks in specific areas of language, so that remediation may be planned. This approach assumes that the normal ability to receive spoken language may be considered to be a composite of discrete abilities such as auditory discrimination, auditory sequencing and auditory memory. If a specific difficulty can be identified, then a remediation programme, aimed at training the child to overcome the difficulty, may be implemented. Test procedures used for this purpose are usually classified as tests of psycholinguistic abilities, and consist of a number of subtests designed to tap specific abilities. This approach has been widely criticized on the basis of the reliability and the validity of a number of the assessments (e.g. Rees 1981). Further, the assumption that training overcomes poor performance on these tests is also questionable (e.g. Hammill and Larsen 1974). The failure to test auditory sensitivity is an important omission in most of the psycholinguistic test batteries, but it is the realization that it is necessary to test the more complex aspects of auditory function, rather than to use uncontrolled acoustic stimuli to assess language related functions, that has led to increased criticism and research.

Central auditory dysfunction and learning disorders

A deficiency in a child's auditory–perceptual ability may restrict the child in a normal educational environment. When a child exhibits poor language and/or listening skills, and an academic performance below his estimated potential, the child has traditionally been referred for hearing sensitivity and speech language assessments. Increasing numbers of children are now referred to clinics, usually multi-disciplinary, for the investigation of learning disorders. Such investigations would include an assessment of central auditory function. It is now a widely held view (e.g. Willeford 1985, Ferre and Wilbur 1986, Jerger *et al.* 1988) that central auditory processing disorders are the cause of many cases of classroom learning difficulties. This provides a compelling reason to study further the central auditory pathway and its clinical assessment, the latter still being incompletely understood.

A range of tests of central auditory function has been devised, based on tests in which the emphasis was initially to assess the site of clinical lesion, rather than to provide information for remediation. The tests were originally used with adults and poor performance on various tests was shown to relate to known anatomical lesions in the central auditory pathways. For example, Willeford (1977) used a battery of tests on learning-disabled children, where the diagnostic value was apparently standardized on brain-damaged adults. He was one of the first to postulate that children with learning difficulties may have a minimal dysfunction of the central nervous system, unrevealed by standard neurological assessments, and that the locus of the dysfunction may be identified by generalizing from the adult data. This assumption has gained more recent support but, as yet, knowledge of how to apply information obtained in this way to remediation is lacking, and it is necessary to develop a more comprehensive approach.

Children who are suspected of classroom learning disorders are probably the group most commonly assessed for the presence of an underlying central auditory processing disorder. In this chapter, central auditory processing and the procedures currently in use for its assessment in children will be described and discussed, and some of the weaknesses currently besetting these procedures will be reviewed. Although there are many questions as yet unanswered, research from the last 10 years suggests that central auditory processing disorders in children are recognizable phenomena, and that inclusion of a central auditory assessment as part of a multi-disciplinary approach to investigation of classroom learning disorders is to be seriously considered. At the least it perhaps represents a more responsive attitude to the problem than the traditional situation, aptly described by Duchan and Katz (1983) in two case reports. These reports reflect the division between those who see normally developed auditory processing abilities as a prerequisite to normal learning abilities and normal language acquisition, and those who focus on the linguistic and cognitive aspects of language processing. In the latter case, auditory perceptual problems would be seen as related, but not causal. The negative aspects of inclusion of central auditory testing are the procedural and interpretive difficulties, to be described later in this chapter, and the rehabilitative implications which remain largely unformed. The following review will include a discussion of the auditory and language tasks drawn from the psycholinguistic and central auditory function test batteries.

Clinical presentation of central auditory dysfunction

Information on the epidemiology and incidence of central auditory dysfunction is inconclusive, and scarce. Differences in terminology and clinical description of the condition preclude meaningful comparison of most reports. However, it seems that children who are referred for assessment of central auditory function usually show aberrant behaviour in one of three general areas.

The first group consists of children with inconsistent listening and attention behaviour, where this cannot be related to an organic cause, such as fluctuating conductive hearing loss. Clinic populations probably vary widely according to the expectations of the local referring agencies. The group may be further subdivided into those who show deficient comprehension or retention of single words, or connected speech, or those where the problem is less specific. Willeford (1985) reports the observation of a psychologically damaging chain of events prior to clinical confirmation, which may lead to a diminished self-image, and a home and school management problem. Gascon et al. (1986) postulate a link between disorders of central auditory processing and attentional deficit disorder. Their work, and the earlier work of Ludlow et al. (1983), is important, since their findings indicate that it is the attentional deficit disorder which leads to poor results on test of central auditory processing, rather than vice versa, and that therapy directed at auditory processing may be misdirected, in these cases. This is one of many observations which indicate that extreme caution should be used in the application and interpretation of central auditory tests at this time.

The second group are those who are suspected of having a learning disability, where the concern may come from the parent or the classroom teacher. The manifestation and classification varies widely (Adelman 1971) and a clinic population may depend on the guidelines provided to local referring agencies. In general, a child who is performing below the level expected may be referred for central auditory testing. This is clearly open to wide interpretation.

The third group are children referred because of abnormal social behaviour. Willeford (1985) reports that these are children who are characteristically 'loners', or who tend to have friends only from a much younger age group.

Neuroanatomical basis of central auditory dysfunction

The central auditory system consists of a series of neuroanatomical connections from the cochlear neurone to the cerebral cortex (see Fig. 4.2, p. 73). The pathways are both crossed and uncrossed, but the majority of the complex array of pathways and synapses exciting the cochlear nucleus cross to the opposite superior olivary nucleus, and some groups of fibres decussate at each nucleus. Descriptions of the central auditory pathways are provided by Durrant and Lovrinic (1984), Noback (1985), Musiek and Baran (1986) and Musiek (1986), the latter two being comprehensive tutorial articles. Briefly, second-, third- and fourth-order contralateral and ipsilateral fibres synapse at the inferior colliculus, from which fibres pass to the medial geniculate body, and to the visual system's superior colliculus. Fibres from the superior olivary nucleus, the lateral leminiscus and perhaps the cochlear nucleus travel ipsilaterally and contralaterally to the geniculate body, from which the majority of the fibres project to the superior temporal lobes. There are further intersensory connections to the cerebellum and to the reticular formation, which interact with higher levels in the central nervous system. In parallel to the afferent system, efferent fibres descend caudally from the cortical regions to the two cochleas, enabling some higher brainstem control upon the neural activity of the auditory structures.

The pathways are complex, and have high intrinsic redundancy anatomically, physiologically and biochemically. This high redundancy is reflected in the hearing loss caused by a lesion. A very small lesion in the peripheral auditory system (say, in the cochlea) causes a much bigger hearing loss in comparison with a lesion of similar magnitude in the central auditory pathway. Characteristically, mild brainstem and temporal lobe lesions cause minor losses in pure-tone threshold sensitivity. A brainstem lesion of sufficient magnitude to cause a marked pure-tone sensitivity loss may result in other, more severe, neurological symptoms.

The neuroanatomical evidence suggests that the development of language closely parallels neurological maturation of the auditory system. This has been inferred from study of the developing brain, in conjunction with studies of language development (Young 1983). This in turn has led some investigators (Keith 1981) to look at central auditory function as a measure of maturation of the auditory pathways. Keith proposes that in immature pathways a plateau of language development is reached as the structural maturity begins to impose limitations, and he interprets measures of central auditory function in the light of this theory.

Assessment of central auditory function and auditory processing skills

There is an interdependence of signal and language processing which complicates assessment for site-of-lesion and remediation. In formulating assessments, it is a complex task to identify and isolate the fundamental auditory–perceptual and auditory–language comprehension abilities. The early tests of central auditory function assumed that, since speech perception is the highest auditory function, tests of central auditory function should be based on speech material. Since the auditory system has high intrinsic neurological redundancy and speech material itself has high redundancy, the latter (extrinsic redundancy) is reduced to provide a more difficult task. The earliest attempts to assess central auditory function using speech, with decreased message predictability, was carried out by Bocca et al. (1954). They used low-pass filtered speech to assess the integrity of the lower temporal lobes and found that discrimination of bisyllabic words, with information above 500 Hz removed, was poor in patients with a temporal lobe tumour on the side contralateral to the stimulated ear, regardless of the side of the lesion. Since the work of Bocca *et al.*, other authors have devised monaurally presented speech tasks to assess cortical lesions, notably time-compressed speech (Calearo and Lazzaroni 1957); low sensation level speech, where speech is presented at 5–10 dB SL (Jerger 1960); speech-in-noise (e.g. Noffsinger *et al.* 1972); and periodically interrupted speech (Bocca 1958). Clinical investigation on adults using these tests generally shows impaired results in the contralateral ear, or both ears, of patients with cortical lesions. More variable results have been found in patients with a variety of intracranial and brainstem lesions.

To evaluate auditory function in the brainstem, binaural speech tests have been developed. The most notable of these tests is named after its originator, the Matzker test (1959), and requires the binaural fusion of a speech message, split such that a low frequency (500–800 Hz) band of spectral energy is passed to one ear and a higher frequency (1815–2500 Hz) band is passed to the other simultaneously. This test has been carried out on a clinical population by several authors (e.g. Lynn *et al.* 1972) and the results suggest that the task is useful in detecting central auditory dysfunction and in differentiating brainstem from cortical lesions. Various other binaural speech tasks have been used in the assessment of central auditory function, though not primarily brainstem function. In all these tests, the auditory system is assumed to be taxed by the reduction of the extrinsic redundancy of the stimuli. Although speech perception is a higher-order process, and hence degraded speech material may be a suitable material for the assessment of central auditory processing in adults with normal language, it is important to identify the language and cognitive weighting implicit in the assessment of children with suspected central auditory dysfunction, classroom learning difficulties or language delay. This weighting may be a significant factor in the assessment and interpretation of the test result. Immature language, for example, may be said to be further decreasing the extrinsic redundancy of the speech material.

Of particular interest too is the effect of attention skills on the complex task of listening. The ability to attend selectively to a signal among competing tasks, auditory or otherwise, is of primary importance. Selective attention is required in dichotic listening tasks, where the listener may need to synthesize the signal from both inputs, and in competing message tasks where the listener must focus on one message and exclude the other. Strategies for focusing and dividing attention become increasingly sophisticated with increased maturity (Butler 1983). Furthermore, attention requires effort and this is a highly variable factor, partly dependent on the complexity of the task.

Functional measures of hemispherical specialization

Traditionally, the left hemisphere has been ascribed a role of language dominance, but the evidence from cerebral blood flow measurements indicates that the right hemisphere contributes to linguistic processing and that the traditional view should be treated with caution. Functionally, however, the cerebral hemispheres are thought to be cognitively and perceptually asymmetrical. The degree to which this occurs and the type of specialization are less clear. The left hemisphere is thought to be specialized for the identification of stop consonants (Beasley and Rintlemann 1979); stimuli of short duration, such as rapid formant transitions (Tallal and Newcombe 1978); verbal memory, conceptualization, grammar and temporal ordering (Young 1983). The right hemisphere has been thought to play a major role in vowel perception (Shankweiler and Studdert-Kennedy 1967); intonation and stress; and in the processing of melodic nonspeech information. It may be that there is a language supportive role for the right hemisphere in processing extralinguistic features of speech and nonverbal cues. There is some evidence for brain lateralization at or near birth; but most studies suggest that developmental lateralization changes continue until about 6–7 years of age (Buffery 1971, Moscovitch 1977). The clinical implication of this debate is the extent to which insult to the left cerebral hemisphere could cause permanent language dysfunction.

The roles ascribed above to the different hemispheres are now being seriously questioned, since it is felt that the majority of the functional evidence for hemispherical specialization has been confounded by task requirements (Haggard and Parkinson 1971, Berlin and McNeil 1976). A review by Efron (1985) outlines some of the experimental anomalies and misconceptions that have contributed to inappropriate deductions in this area. He particularly examines the erroneous conclusions which he postulates are drawn from dichotic listening experiments. His arguments are compelling, and he urges caution in the interpretation of the possible role of hemispherical specialization on central auditory processing. The clinical studies of Bocca *et al.* (1954) and Kimura (1961) add doubt to the interpretation of hemispherical specialization given above. Both authors used speech, or speech-like, sounds to demonstrate the reduced scores obtained from the side contralateral to the lesion. Efron questions whether the effect is caused by an auditory deficit or a speech deficit. His perspective of this topic should be considered in analysis of the results of central auditory assessment.

Assessment of central auditory function in children

Interpretation of central auditory test results has been based largely on comparison of patients with suspected central auditory dysfunction to results in subjects with known lesions of the central nervous system, the assumption being that the abnormality functions in the same way as a central nervous system lesion. Whilst there is some evidence for this (Musiek *et al.* 1984), there is controversy regarding the parity of test results of children with central auditory dysfunction and adults with central nervous system lesions. In a discussion of this topic, Jerger *et al.* (1988) report that several studies suggest that the cognitive deficits accompanying central nervous system lesions are less specific in children than in adults. In the auditory domain, this leads to the deduction that the auditory deficits in a young child with a central nervous system lesion may be more generalized than the ear-specific patterns of deficit seen in adults. Their review leads these authors to conclude that there is considerable evidence available to support the hypothesis that the immature brain is capable of some functional reorganization that tends to normalize perceptual function. However, they found an equally strong body of data supporting the notion that the behavioural auditory manifestations of childhood and adult brain lesions do not differ significantly. It is clear that further research is needed to clarify this important area of test result interpretation. The conflicting reports, commonly found in work in this area reflect differences in methodology (including the criteria applied to stimulus conditions), subject selection and interpretation of experimental data.

The relationship between auditory processing skills and the development and use of language is not precisely clear and is the subject of continuing study and debate. The mutual interdependence of auditory and linguistic processes complicates the interpretation of test results, and few studies have been addressed to examination of this point, despite the important consequences for the design of the remediation programme. A study by Jerger et al. (1988), in which they compared children having confirmed central nervous system lesions affecting the auditory centres of the brain, with children having confirmed central nervous system lesions affecting nonauditory areas is of interest. They used three measures only: pure-tone audiometry, acoustic reflex patterns, and the Pediatric Speech Intelligibility (PSI) Test (Jerger and Jerger 1984). Their results supported an auditory-specific basis for central auditory dysfunction.

It is desirable for test stimuli intended to assess auditory capabilities to be as free as possible from language bias. A list of criteria was formulated by Keith (1981), which he considered to be essential in designing a test of normal central auditory function. The test:

1. Should not be loaded with language comprehension items.
2. Should not require linguistic manipulation.
3. Should use nonlinguistic signals.
4. Should minimize cross-sensory input and response modalities.

The assessment is aimed at disclosing disturbances in the auditory modality, not children who become overloaded by multisensory inputs, nor children who have a visual disturbance or cross-modal disorder. However, it should be noted that it could be these more complex aspects which underlie a functional learning disorder in the classroom. Although it is commonly recognized that it is preferable to use nonlinguistic signals, speech sounds are commonly used as stimuli since they require higher-order processing. In some of the more recent studies there have been attempts to control for language bias in the selection of speech stimuli.

Design and selection of test procedures are incomplete in the absence of an understanding of the interpretation of test results. Used with children, the central auditory test assessments are generally aimed at revealing a functional disorder, rather than a site-of-lesion investigation. However, poor achievement scores cannot currently be readily converted into therapeutic measures. It is felt by many professionals in the field that there is value in identifying an auditory deficiency, and in demonstrating to parents and educators that a child has auditory skills which are less sophisticated than in the normal case. Objective support may be provided for the subjective parent and teacher suspicions, enabling a greater understanding of the child's needs. Keith (1981) describes tests within the framework of a neuromaturational level; poor test performance is said to reflect central auditory immaturity, which is in turn responsible for language delay. This stance too raises questions regarding the interrelationship of language maturity, auditory maturity, and attentional effects. Since Gascon and his colleagues (1986) were able to demonstrate the use of a central auditory test battery in the monitoring of central nervous system control of attentional deficit disorder, this implies a confounding effect of attention in the test battery.

The sensitivity of tests within a battery varies, and the pass/fail rate must be considered for each test and for the battery as a whole. As with any clinical test, careful consideration must be given to the false-positive rate, and this is of particular importance given the wide intersubject variability, the maturational effects involved, and the restrictive normal databases available. This leads some authors to recommend a test battery approach with a pass/fail criterion established. Ferre and Wilber (1986) found, with a battery of time- and frequency-altered central auditory tests, that children who performed below normal levels on more than half of the tests may be considered 'at risk' with respect to auditory perceptual dysfunction.

A selection of tests is described in the following pages. These are representative of the large number of central tests devised and are among those most commonly used with children. The tests to be described may be subdivided into tests of binaural fusion and integration; tests using dichotically presented stimuli; and tests using monotic stimuli, patterned or distorted. Only behavioural tests will be discussed in this chapter, since the current understanding of the interpretation of electrophysiological assessments has limited value in the functional assessment of central auditory dysfunction in children.

Binaural interaction

Speech and nonspeech tasks of binaural interaction, or synthesis, have been devised. In the normal auditory system, it is posible to transmit a message by providing a different portion of the information to each of the two ears. Tests using stimuli presented in this way are primarily devised to assess brainstem function.

Binaural fusion The speech signal presented to the subject is split in such a way that neither portion contains sufficient of the speech spectrum to allow recognition. When both portions are presented simultaneously, one to each ear, the message is 'fused' to give a representation of the whole. In Matzker's original 1959 report, he associated difficulty with fusion of the message with the presence of a brainstem lesion. A number of different versions of the test have been devised, with variations in stimulus type, width and frequency region of the pass-bands, and stimulus presentation levels. Changing these variables results in different findings with various test populations. For example, it has been found that increasing the cut-off frequency or widening filter bandwidths improves test performance and reduces the intersubject variability of groups of normal and learning-disabled children (Farrer and Keith 1981, Plakke *et al.* 1981, Ferre and Wilber 1986). The most popularly used version of this test today is that of Willeford and Ivey, with a low pass-band for the spondaic words of 500–700 Hz, and a high-pass band of 1900–2100 Hz (Tobin 1985). There are several reports of the use of this format with children with learning disabilities (Willeford 1976, 1977; Pinheiro 1977, 1978, Roush and Tait 1984). Willeford (1977) reports age norms for the task, presented at 30 dB SL. Results showed wide individual ranges, reducing the specificity of the test, particularly for young children. Clinical results also vary widely. Although there are numerous reports of children with confirmed brainstem lesions performing poorly on the test, reports of its sensitivity to central auditory function vary. The normative data for the Willeford Test Battery indicate it to be one of the more difficult tests, giving the lowest scores, and this finding is supported by other authors (Beasley *et al.* 1976, Windham *et al.* 1986). A recent study by Ferre and Wilber (1986) contradicts this finding. The test may be criticized by its use of symbolic material, which is dubious even for a test of functional ability, since it will be weighted by aspects of cognition and linguistic maturity.

Rapidly alternating speech test This test was included in Willeford's 1977 battery of tests for central auditory function, but he reports it more recently as being one of the less sensitive and useful tests in the detection of central auditory dysfunction. In this test, a speech message is switched alternately between the subject's two ears at rapid intervals. An apparent confounding variable in completing this task is the role of auditory memory. The implications of this for differential diagnosis are quite confusing, as a disruption in normal auditory memory would suggest a higher level disorder. A poor performance in this test as a measure solely of dichotic function would reflect a brainstem disorder, although recent studies (Efron and Crandall 1983, Efron 1985) of the diffuse perceptual effects of discrete lesions in the auditory system may partially explain this contradiction. As a theoretical compensation, Protti (1983) suggests that a test of auditory memory should be administered in conjunction with the rapidly alternating speech. However, both sorts of tests are influenced by linguistic maturity and it is doubtful whether measures of underlying auditory capabilities, as related to brainstem function, can be made in this way. The rapidly alternating sentence task itself requires mature processing of syntax in conjunction with an auditory memory load, making it primarily a test of language maturity.

Masking level differences (binaural release from masking)   The phenomenon of masking level difference is a binaural effect (see Chapter 1), which facilitates selective listening to a specified signal in a noise background. The phenomenon occurs when the phase relationship of a signal presented to the two ears is different to that of a noise simultaneously presented to the two ears. Tests of central auditory function have been devised using this phenomenon for both speech and nonspeech stimuli. Matkin and Hook (1983), and others, recommended its inclusion in test batteries of central auditory function, and these authors presented both a speech and a nonspeech version, the former using children's spondaic words. It is a test that is quick and easy to administer with children, and the results from site-of-lesion studies suggest that the test may have some diagnostic significance; but, as a functional measure in children, its value has yet to be established.

Dichotic speech tasks

Measures of binaural separation

The competing sentences test   This test, developed by Willeford (1977), and initially validated on adults with cortical lesions, has become widely used with children (e.g. Protti and Young 1980, Welsh *et al.* 1980, Musiek *et al.* 1982, Young 1983, Gascon *et al.* 1986, Windham *et al.* 1986). Dichotic sentences of similar length and semantic content are presented, usually with a message-to-competition ratio of −15 dB, where the subject is required to repeat the test (message) sentence. Willeford reports developmental norms from 5 to 10 years, with a right-ear dominance observed at the lower ages (Fig. 10.1). There is wide variability in the test norms, particularly for the weaker ear and the younger children, in common with many of the dichotic speech tasks, perhaps reflecting the weakness in the concept of ear advantage. There is also some ambiguity about the intended scoring technique; that is, whether it is the sense of the sentence that is to be recovered, or an exact repeat of the individual words used. The contamination of the task by linguistic capabilities is thus inferred. This test is probably most useful as a monitor of the attentional capabilities in children, although it may provide some comparative information on auditory neuromaturational levels where differences from the normal are marked.

Measures of binaural integration

The staggered spondaic word (SSW) test   This test, reported by Katz in 1962, is probably the best known and most widely used of the central tests. The SSW is composed of two spondaic words, presented one to each ear at 50 dB SL, with

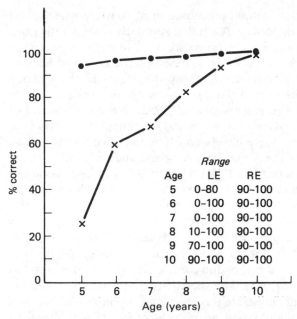

Figure 10.1   Mean percentage and range of correct scores obtained on normal children using a competing sentence test of binaural separation. (From Keith 1981, p.68.)

the words staggered so that the second syllable of one word is simultaneous with the first syllable of the other. For example:

left ear: up stairs
right ear: down town

In this example, the timing is such that *stairs* coincides with *down*. The test has been predominantly used with adults in the investigation of cortical lesions, with mixed results (Katz 1962, Katz *et al*. 1963, Lynn and Gilroy 1972, Jerger and Jerger 1975). The test is becoming more frequently used with children (see Arnst and Katz 1982, for a detailed presentation of selected studies). Results have been found to be more variable in brainstem cases. Although the test was originally designed as a site-of-lesion test, it is thought that several functional skills are assessed in it (Willeford 1985). In general, children show a superior performance to the stimuli presented to the right ear. Katz also describes a maturational effect. Children improve at the task between the ages of 6 and 11 years, and the test variability reduces with increasing subject age.

Dichotic digits and words   Dichotic recall tasks of digit strings, word lists, nonsense syllables and phonemes have been used to demonstrate right-ear advantage, and to relate speech-processing laterality to language problems. Musiek (1983) describes a common approach to digit presentation, which is quickly and easily administered. Two digits are presented to each ear simultaneously, at 50 dB SL, with a total presentation of 20 pairs. The subject recalls all the digits heard in any order. A similar approach is used with word presentations. These dichotic tasks were primarily used in the assessment of adult cortical and interhemispherical disorders, based on the model of Kimura (1961). This states that the contralateral pathway dominates in the dichotic situation, unless there is hemispherical damage to disrupt this pattern. There have been studies with children (e.g. Musiek *et al.* 1982), but interpretation of results is restricted due to the possibly inappropriate weighting of memory load on the task. Strong order effects have also been found in a dichotic digit task, indicating that attentional biases may exert a strong and enduring influence on ear asymmetry (Hiscock and Bergstrom 1982). Dermody *et al.* (1983) reviewed the literature on studies of recall of dichotic consonant-vowel syllables presented simultaneously to the two ears. Normal children appear to show a weak right-ear advantage in this task (Keith 1981).

The rationale behind dichotic listening tasks is that normally there is a right-ear advantage, or left-hemisphere dominance, for processing language, particularly for the information carrying the phonetic contrasts of speech; this view has been questioned recently (Efron 1985). The specificity of this laterality and the implications of an inability to demonstrate this specificity are not clear, but may be due to weakness in the methodology. Alternatively, or in addition, the right-ear advantage on a dichotic listening task may reflect a developmental process requiring the integration of several skills. Breakdown of any one of several areas may lead to poor performance, so that demonstration of left-ear or no-ear advantage is a measure of central nervous system immaturity. However, this may not be strictly auditory. Further research on these tests with greater control of the input stimuli is required.

It is vital to the validity of all of the dichotic tasks that acoustic (i.e. signal intensity, onset–offset alignment, signal-to-noise ratio) and phonetic factors are appropriately controlled, and it is felt that weakness in these areas has led to discrepancies between test results (Porter and Berlin 1975, Musiek and Pinheiro 1985). For example, if input asymmetries are allowed to occur in the test, ear advantage could be identified and falsely ascribed to hemispherical specialization (Teng 1981). It has been found that the presence of abrupt onsets determines lateralization for stop consonants, and that transition information, including duration, also contributes; this indicates a contribution from temporal processing and duration to demonstrable right-ear advantage (Dwyer *et al.* 1982). Efron (1985) further points out the scant attention that has been given to the very wide test result variability, with the exception of studies by Lauter (1982) and Speakes *et al.* (1982).

Monotic tasks employing assessment of resistance to distortion

Speech-in-noise (auditory figure-ground tasks)

Comparison of the discrimination of (monaurally presented) speech-in-quiet against discrimination of speech-in-noise (also monaurally presented) has been used by several authors in site-of-lesion assessments (e.g. Morales-Garcia and Poole 1972, Noffsinger *et al.* 1972). Poor discrimination in noise has been reported for patients with brainstem lesions. This effect is found both in the ear contralateral to a cortical lesion, and from either ear but, in the latter case, the results are more variable. In this task, a performance-intensity function for monosyllabic words or sentences is obtained by presenting material at different intensity levels. In the absence of a competing stimulus, speech material has been thought to be too highly redundant to reflect the presence of a central auditory dysfunction or lesion. When the task is made more difficult with the addition of noise, then the shape of the function may be abnormal, with a reduced maximum percentage score.

This test has been used to demonstrate the presence of central auditory dysfunction in children (Jerger 1981), but it is perhaps used more frequently to demonstrate the functional difficulty of hearing speech in background noise in cases of suspected classroom learning difficulties. Variants of the task are incorporated into the speech pathologist's test batteries of auditory skills, where it is usually described as a test of selective attention. An example of this is the Goldman–Fristoe–Woodcock (GFW) Auditory Skills Battery, which contains an auditory selective attention subtest, in which monosyllabic words are presented against a background of cafeteria noise, with a steadily increasing signal-to-noise ratio. It is not strictly accurate to describe this test as a task of selective attention, which should be regarded as a two-component task, where the first component is a brainstem-mediated process requiring a binaural input (the phenomenon of binaural advantage), as well as a higher-order task. Presented monaurally, with a signal/noise mix, only the latter component is assessed. However, the task is thought to give some idea of how easily a child can attend amid distractions (Dempsey 1983). In this context, the speech-in-noise test has less language bias than Willeford's Competing Sentence Test. The normal developmental trends on the task are shown in Fig. 10.2.

The speech-in-noise task is not free of the confounding effects of receptive language ability. Elliott (1979) clearly demonstrated the increasing proficiency of children aged 9–17 on speech-in-noise tasks, and the contaminating influence of receptive language levels on the task has been well reported (for example, Mills 1977). There have been more recent attempts to construct speech intelligibility tests for young children, notably the Pediatric Speech Intelligibility Test (PSI) of Jerger *et al.* (1980), using test materials that are as free as possible from the influence of developmental differences in receptive language skills in young children. The PSI is not sensitive enough for use with children over 6 years old (Jerger *et al.* 1983). The authors also recognize the nonauditory factors that may result from testing young children on a speech task of this kind. They have built in techniques in order to focus the child's attention more effectively, and they have attempted to reduce the load on echoic and short-term memory by some use of pictorial representation, and by listing what they consider to be meaningful, age-appropriate material that is easier to code, store and retrieve.

Speech-in-noise tasks are often not administered in appropriately controlled

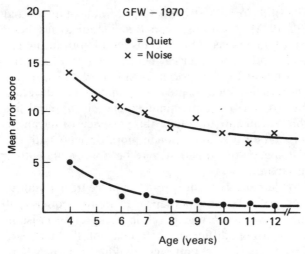

Figure 10.2 Mean error scores obtained by normal subjects on the quiet and noise subtest of the Goldman–Fristoe–Woodcock test auditory discrimination. (From Keith 1981, p.71.)

conditions, in terms of signal-to-noise ratio, type of speech stimuli and the noise competition used. Some are presented monaurally, through headphones and some binaurally, either under phones or in the soundfield. As described earlier, different auditory capabilities are assessed by the different techniques. These weaknesses are reflected in the data collection.

Filtered speech The natural intelligibility of speech is degraded by limiting its frequency content. Such stimuli are perceived with difficulty by listeners with temporal lobe lesions. This test is thus employed in the assessment of central auditory dysfunction. However, a strong maturational effect and widely varying individual scores have been reported (Willeford 1977). It is thus difficult to use this measure as a 'clean' measure of neuromaturational ability. Quantitative scores are only considered abnormal when the score for one or both ears falls below the range boundary for the child's age group, or where there is a marked difference in the score for the child's two ears. As the test is reported to be difficult for young children (Dempsey 1983), the Filtered Word Identification By Picture Test (WIPI, Willeford 1977) was developed. Young children find this test easier and, as a picture-pointing response is required, less tester bias is introduced than in the identification of the child's spoken response. However, visual motor skills are introduced as confounding variables in the test.

Time compressed speech In this task speech is 'speeded-up', but with the frequency factor held constant. In the time since it was devised in 1957 it has been found to be sensitive to disorders of the auditory pathway at all levels (Bocca and Calearo 1963). Tests of time-compressed speech show much less conclusive results with children, and studies have shown that, presented as part of a test battery, it is often the only test that a child fails, or conversely the only test that a child passes. However, the wide range of test results on children, which possibly reflect methodological differences between studies, limit the significance of this test in the assessment of central auditory dysfunction in children. Beasley *et al.* (1972) report results from 60 children, aged from 6 to 8 years; they found intelligibility decreased as a function of increasing time compression, and decreasing age and sensation level. This effect was more pronounced the more difficult the test material. Freeman and Beasley (1976) presented a time-compressed version of the WIPI test, in both a closed- and open-set response format, to children with and without readiing difficulties. The children with reading difficulties performed less well than the control group, on at least one test condition. The diagnostic implications of this test for children are uncertain. The test results are equivocal even as a measure of functional disability.

A more significant measure of auditory processing was identified by Tallal (1976), as the ability to perceive rapid transitions in acoustic signals. Tallal presented pairs of nonspeech and speech sound stimuli to dysphasic children of 6–9 years of age. The children were required to make a same/different judgement to stimuli presented with varying inter-stimulus intervals. Performance was affected by the size of the interval. A developmental effect was recognized and the dysphasic group required longer inter-stimulus intervals than even the youngest normal subjects. Tallal argued that this test demonstrates a primary inability to analyse the rapid stream of acoustic information that characterizes speech. She speculated that this is essential to normal speech perception and language development. Rees (1981), on the other hand, argues that since the test results demonstrated that phonetic distinctions could be discriminated, if the interval between the stimuli were long enough, then the child would have sufficient auditory processing skills to learn the distinction. Even though the precise relationship between difficulty with this task and the normal development of language is unclear, as a functional measure, which is the concern of this discussion, it leads to a prediction of difficulty in situations where rapid processing is essential – for example in reverberant acoustic conditions.

The brief review of a representative sample of the tests available for the attempted assessment of central auditory dysfunction reflects the difficulty in finding a task which sufficiently taxes the highly redundant central nervous system, without unduly loading the test with cognitive, attentional and linguistic factors. Particular care is also required in setting up the acoustic, temporal and phonetic characteristics of the tests. Interpretation of the test data and, in particular, determining the pass/fail criteria must also be carried out with caution. Lack of attention in any of these areas will result in test data which are of little value.

Assessment of auditory processing skills in children

The discussion has so far centred on the measures of central auditory function which are commonly encountered under the description of central auditory tests. There are other skills involved in the processing of speech and language which are usually part of the assessment of a child thought to have language, communication, or other learning difficulties. These auditory processing skills, in particular auditory memory and auditory sequencing, may be assessed as part of a perceptual skills battery but are sometimes incorporated into the central auditory test battery. It is appropriate, in either case, to discuss them in this chapter, which examines central auditory dysfunction in children. Children thus affected may show difficulties in these areas. They differ from the previously described tasks in being more complex skills, and may be the precursor to central auditory testing.

Auditory memory

Tests of auditory memory require a child to recall auditory stimuli in terms of number and sequence. Auditory memory is often described as if it is an intrinsic property. An individual is thought to have various levels of memory:

 (i) Echoic memory, from which any utterance can be immediately repro-
      duced. A visual analogy would be the after-image on the retina after
      seeing a bright light.
 (ii) Short-term memory, which may be regarded as a sort of short-term data
      store where several items may be retained for a short while.
(iii) Long-term memory, which may be thought of as a quasi-permanent store.
      This is thought to occupy a role in language development, in that phonetic
      representations are stored to give a library of references. Syntactic and
      lexical information will also be stored there.

Whatever view is taken of speech perception, it is evident that there must be some mechanism by which the units of language are stored and held in sequence. Intuitively, therefore, auditory memory appeals as an underlying component of the speech perception process. However, major problems with auditory memory tests arise in knowing just why a child fails to do well, as there are several stages involved in the process. For example, if we assume that it is a coded message which is stored, do difficulties arise in the encoding, storage or retrieval processes? So poor performance on a standard memory task of the type employed in many test batteries may identify a test difficulty, but not necessarily reveal an underlying skill deficit. For this reason, this type of test is best used as a first stage in the identification of a child at risk for central auditory difficulties.

Although it is appealing to assume storage of units for speech processing, it is not at all clear what these are, and hence identification of the most appropriate test item is difficult. Even if a unit of perception is selected, a test requiring recall of a nonmeaningful list of, for example, phonemes, does not give the same memory task as recall of a sentence containing the same number of phonemes. Rees (1981) notes that if an organization can be imposed on material, recall or retrieval usually improve, both for short- and long-term memory. Drawing from the work of Olsen (1973) she suggests that memory ability is so linked to organization that it is the child's ability to organize the input that imposes and defines the limits of ability. Language development and performance on tasks of auditory memory may be mutually dependent, which further indicates that this measure cannot be regarded as one of underlying auditory ability.

Auditory synthesis

Sound blending, phonemic synthesis and auditory synthesis are tasks in which a child is required to listen to words presented one phoneme at a time, with a silent interval between each. The rate of presentation varies between tests. The child is required to say the words (i.e. to blend the phonemes). Katz (1983) has been a major proponent of this test task. He relates difficulty with phoneme synthesis to specific lesions. He reasons that a deficit in this area of language may cause subtle difficulties not apparent during the years that speech is presented simply to a child, but becomes more obvious with increasing exposure to more complex language. Katz proposes that phonemic synthesis is a form of distorted speech, and hence taxes the auditory system. The distortions come from 'elongating the phonemes, inserting pauses between them, utilizing sounds with reduced contextual influence, decreasing formant transitions, greatly increasing the duration of the word, and forcing the listener to retain in storage rather unfamiliar and meaningless sounds'. This hardly appears as a unitary task of auditory function. Katz is correct in identifying it as a difficult task which will tax the auditory system, but the origin of the difficulties is complex. To complete this task, a degree of linguistic maturity is necessary, and the conclusion that this ability is an auditory process fundamental to language must be considered to rest on very little evidence. Phonemic synthesis has long been associated with reading and spelling: its study in this context should not be confused with the idea of regarding it as an auditory deficit. Children who show poor results in this assessment may perhaps be considered at risk for central auditory deficit, only, and more fundamental assessments carried out.

Training auditory skills

Considerable time and effort is expended by speech and hearing professionals in the training of what are thought to be fundamental auditory skills. In the case of auditory training of children or adults with peripheral hearing loss there is little hard evidence for any resulting improvement in discrimination skills (see

Bamford 1981 for a review). Nevertheless, there is an abundance of qualitative reports of the success of training which it would be hasty to discount. Furthermore, there is clear evidence from studies with normally hearing adults that discrimination can be improved with training. Peripheral sensitivity is not altered, but Bamford (1981, p. 77) proposes that: 'differences among similar things are not automatically perceived unless the perceiver's attention is alerted to the relevant distinctions. Thus, although the perceiver could discriminate the things, it is likely that he would not normally attend to them . . . Auditory training can be regarded as learning to attend, to "allocate cognitive resources".' The notion that auditory training can be used to improve listening skill and selective attention, is thus not far-fetched, although the quantitative effects of training remain to be shown.

With regard to speech therapy and speech/language production in children with normal peripheral sensitivity, there has been an assumed relationship between auditory perceptual functioning (specifically auditory memory and auditory discrimination) and linguistic skills. At one level this points to a relationship between auditory perceptual skills and phonological skills as reflected in articulation. This assumed relationship has resulted in therapy for children with delayed or deviant phonology being focused on improving auditory memory and discrimination. However, the evidence for such a connection is sparse. Supple (1983) reviewed a number of studies which examined the poor discrimination/poor articulation connection, and found a diversity of results that overall must remain inconclusive. Her own study of 60 children showed no significant relationship between discrimination errors and articulation errors.

The concept of underlying and basic auditory perceptual skills is part of the package of psycholinguistic principles which have generated a number of techniques used widely for both assessment and remediation of language. One such technique is the ITPA of Kirk *et al.* (1968). This test both measures specific psycholinguistic auditory abilities and provides a supposedly useful framework for language remediation. However, Hammill and Larsen (1974) reviewed the results of 38 studies which attempted to train children in those underlying skills and which used ITPA as the criterion of improvement. They concluded from their review that the effectiveness of such retraining has not been clearly demonstrated. Whether this is because the skills are untrainable, the training programmes inadequate, or whether the ITPA subtests are inappropriate measures of these abilities, the authors could not say at this time, but it does raise questions about the theoretical underpinning of some approaches to therapy.

Summary

There is sufficient evidence to support the view that delayed language and classroom learning difficulties are sometimes the result of an underlying central auditory dysfunction. It is therefore important to investigate the underlying mechanism which may be quite subtle, and yet may cause a child considerable difficulty in some listening situations, in particular that of background noise such as is present in the modern classroom. Existing tests of central auditory processing were initially for use in site-of-lesion investigation, and not for the definition of the degree and type of auditory dysfunction. Consider, for example, the treatment of normal data, within and between studies, where wide inter-subject variability is accepted as a feature of central auditory testing, but rarely investigated. Yet it is just this kind of information which is needed if we are to achieve an understanding of the underlying mechanism. Efron (1985) supplies a neat and provocative comment on this issue: 'If 20% to 30% of some species of animals failed to develop clinical signs of tubercle bacilli, it is unlikely that the importance of individual differences in host response would be so ignored.' Not only is it necessary to investigate the reason for the wide variability in the data, it is necessary to accumulate much more normative data, and to study epidemiological characteristics of the results of the central auditory assessments.

Jerger *et al.* (1988) suggest three priority areas of investigation for the future:

1. Establishing a database in children with confirmed lesions.
2. Establishing the relationship between this database and results in children with central auditory disorders.
3. Establishing the relation between a pattern of auditory results and functional deficit.

To this should be added an analysis of possible related external factors, such as auditory and language and living environment, learning environment, maturation, stress factors, emotional environment, fatigue levels, attention levels and personality effects. Each of these areas needs to be assessed in relation to the determination of possible underlying nonauditory influences on performance. In this area, determination of a simple pool of normal data is not adequate, given our current understanding of what is being tested. To varying degrees, the specificity and sensitivity of such tests with children leaves much to be desired. So-called auditory processing tasks (and some of the central auditory tests in use), which have been developed more specifically to identify perceptual problems, which result in language and learning difficulties, are frequently very language dependent. Auditory memory, for example, is a demonstrable phenomenon which is implemented in language development and learning, but the deeper implications of poor performance on this task are not easily accessed, and the underlying dysfunction may remain unknown.

There are severe limitations surrounding our current ability to carry out and interpret valid, sensitive and specific tests of central auditory dysfunction on children. If the current lines of assessment are to be pursued, it should be with an awareness of the research needs and the limits of their diagnostic capabilities. This view does not deny the existence of central auditory processing problems in children. Existing data indeed suggest that problems of this sort may underlie cases of classroom learning difficulties. But it is important that central auditory dysfunction does not become the scapegoat for other reasons for failure, particularly since there is very little available information on appropriate remediation in such cases. Diagnosis should be made in the knowledge of the remediation options available. From the earlier discussion, this is known to be limited.

It seems, in conclusion, that there are perceptual deficits which can cause delays in language, abnormal listening behaviour and learning disabilities. Considerable development in our knowledge of these processes and in the assessment procedures are required before we can begin to feel much confidence in the useful, practical and ethical application of these tests. Identification of the underlying skills and their dysfunctions is still incomplete. Since recent research seems to have raised more questions than are answered, it may be that a fresh approach to assessment procedures and, as has been suggested by some authors, away from the applied site-of-lesion testing is the solution.

Concluding remarks

It has always been known that hearing impairment in children can be extremely disruptive of the normal processes of language development, particularly if the impairment is permanent and of early onset. However, the precise nature and extent of the consequent language disability, and the underlying mechanisms of cause and effect, have until recently remained largely ignored. Early studies of the effect of hearing impairment upon language were global and descriptive in nature, and took little note of individual differences. Along with this, attempts at assessment and remediation were left largely to the efforts of parents and specialized teachers. Even among the latter, however, there were deep differences of opinion of the best ways to promote language development in hearing-impaired children. Indeed, these differences are still much in evidence: correspondence in the *Journal of the British Association of Teachers of the Deaf* (1984) has continued to argue around the issue of whether the failure of hearing-impaired children to learn language efficiently is in part due to the language they are presented with by teachers being too complex, or being too elementary and undemanding.

A number of recent developments have begun to break this mould, and to force us to look more questioningly at what is happening to hearing-impaired children's language, and why. Resources are in short supply, and political pressure is on to monitor results in order to guide future investment in services. Parents – and children – are more aware of their rights and are more demanding of society. Disabled people have found more effective pressure groups to further their interests. Society itself is less prepared than in the past to tolerate the discriminations in education, job opportunities, personal growth and a dozen other things with which disabled people have had to manage. Changes in educational practice have brought children with disabilities much more into mainstream schooling than previously. Family doctors, teachers in mainstream education, and community-based primary health care teams are being made much more aware of the consequences of hearing impairment in childhood, are being asked to refer to other agencies quickly, and are therefore demanding more information. The concept of the multiprofessional team and multiprofessional assessments is no longer innovative but a part of good practice at many centres. Thus professionals other than the specialist teachers are demanding to know more about hearing impairment and its consequences. Speech pathologists are becoming more involved in the assessment and remediation of children with sensorineural hearing loss, in addition to the contact they have always had with children who have suffered fluctuating conductive hearing loss. Graduate audiologists are playing an important role in specialist paediatric audiology centres, and the drive for early diagnosis of sensorineural hearing loss involves them in considerations of auditory and language development in order for them to fulfil this role. Old barriers – between audiologists, teachers, speech pathologists, ENT doctors, parents – are beginning to be broken down, requiring a wider understanding of disciplines other than those only most central to their particular profession.

Considerations such as these lie behind the production of this book. The aim has been to provide an up-to-date review of our current understanding of the effects of hearing impairment upon language disability, and to present this knowledge in the context of audiology and auditory perception in an attempt to trace the causal links. There is, as we have said, no such thing as 'the language of the deaf'. There are group trends, and these are important to know, but there is also great individual variability, and until we can understand the causes of this variability the success of remediation programmes will be limited. We are still a long way from understanding the causal relationships, and the extent to which hearing impairment is associated with language disability depends among other things on

- –the degree of impairment; not simply pure-tone hearing loss, but other more complex perceptual processes
- – the way in which speech is perceived
- – how speech perception relates to language development
- – the extent to which auditory experience affects speech perception and language development
- – aspects of parental care, personality and educational practice
- – the extent to which we can diagnose hearing loss at an early age and undertake early intervention.

Our understanding of these issues is still limited, but a variety of professionals in fields such as psychology, speech pathology, audiology and education are beginning to push our knowledge into more promising areas than has been the case in the past. Such advances raise new questions, of course. Thus, for example, the assumption of the need for early diagnosis of congenital hearing loss raises issues such as

- –do we need to begin therapy for deaf children before they are 4 months old?
- –what is the nature of early intervention for hearing-impaired children and their families?
- –how is early communication facilitated?
- –what early assessment procedures are required? how are they to be interpreted, and what contingent decisions about early intervention do they allow?
- –how can very early identification of hearing loss in babies be achieved?
- – is there still, therefore, a place for a later screening programme, and if so who is it aimed at and what form should it take?

– what are the consequences of early diagnosis for parent–child relationships and for parent counselling programmes?

– do audiologists, speech pathologists, teachers and others have the necessary expertise and training?

In its review of the subject, this book raises many such questions and leaves them necessarily unanswered. But it has been timely to review current knowledge and in so doing to draw together audiology, auditory perception and language development in a form which is accessible to the professional groups who find themselves more and more involved with children with hearing impairments.

This fruitful area is now looking to advances in audiology and hearing aid technology, and in auditory perception (impaired and normal) and its interface with speech and language development to move us forward further still. A paper by Bard and Anderson (1984) points to the crucial importance of understanding the nature of children's speech perception. Their study followed an earlier one by Pollack and Pickett (1963) in which it was shown that words from conversational speech are more difficult for listeners to understand when they are presented in isolation. Bard and Anderson set out to protect current language acquisition theories by demonstrating that for the linguistically naïve language learner, the same effect did not apply. They took samples of parental speech to young children which, one might suppose, would be easy to decipher when presented word for word, in isolation. To their evident surprise, they showed quite clearly that parental speech was not easier to decipher, word for word, than ordinary conversational speech, but very much harder to decipher. They found that even adults who have fully mastered the vocabulary used were able to recognize the tokens from speech to children only 30 per cent of the time. They were forced to conclude that 'words spoken to children are largely unintelligible' (p. 290). It was clear that the words used in speech to children were more predictable from the linguistic context than words in speech to adults (hence the importance of giving the listener messages that are understood), but with listeners who have yet to master the linguistic constraints of the language it is difficult to see how this can help much. Bard and Anderson speculate that extra-linguistic context may therefore have to carry the burden of comprehension. Alternatively, it may be that children's speech perception is radically different from adults' such that they are able to recognize tokens with little support from linguistic context, and in such a way as to counteract the evident unintelligibility of parental speech (unintelligible to adult listeners, that is). This study points to our lack of knowledge of speech perception in children and its relationship to language acquisition.

We have approached the even more intractable problem of language disability in hearing-impaired children from both ends. While much of the first four chapters of this book provide the background to audiology, auditory perception, and to auditory and language development, the remainder is given over to these two approaches. Firstly we have discussed what audiologists and psychologists can tell us about the nature of the perceptual impairment in hearing-impaired children, and attempted to draw that knowledge towards factors that we presume must be involved in speech perception. We have shown that pure-tone hearing loss – that most ubiquitous measure of hearing impairment – is of limited utility for predicting the disability of hearing for speech. In order to understand the distorting effects of sensorineural hearing loss, account must be taken of other auditory perceptual impairments – frequency resolution, intensity coding, and so on – and their possible effects upon speech perception. Similar considerations apply to unilateral hearing losses and to fluctuating conductive losses, the consequences of neither of which are well predicted by simple pure tone detection.

Secondly, we have discussed what is the final outcome for language development in children with bilateral sensorineural hearing loss and for children with unilateral and fluctuating conductive hearing loss. We have attempted to close the gap between our auditory perceptual knowledge and our knowledge of the language disability, but the gap remains large. The gap is large for children with hearing impairments, since not only are words even less perceptually salient for such children, because of their perceptual impairment, than for normally hearing children (and Bard and Anderson's study points to the perceptual problems in speech for normally hearing children, let alone those with impaired auditory perceptual processes); but hearing-impaired children have less access to linguistic context since the complex relationships which underlie many function words are less accessible to them. It may take a dozen years or more for a normally hearing child to master all the aspects of deixis, for example, and the hearing-impaired child with poor auditory memory may be expected to find such function words extraordinarily difficult.

Nevertheless, progress is being made. The involvement of a wider range of professionals in the identification, diagnosis, assessment and remediation of children's hearing impairments and language disabilities is providing a new impetus to these problems. We have to understand the auditory perceptual processes of these children, how these affect speech perception, and how this affects language development. We have to design more appropriate hearing aids, perhaps signal processing aids, and more appropriate remedial intervention in order to be able to counteract these effects in a variety of ways tailored to individual children.

Currently in the UK there is more interest and a greater effort being put into these fields by various research and clinical groups than we have seen for a long time. The training courses for the various professionals involved with hearing-impaired children remain, however, less than optimum. Improvements in these courses so as to produce audiologists, speech pathologists, teachers and others with a greater degree of expertise and professionalism would undoubtedly improve the prospects for future generations of hearing-impaired children still further.

References

ADELMAN, H. 1971: The not so specific learning disabled population. *Exceptional Child* 37, 528–37.

ALEGRIA, J. and NOIROT, E. 1978: Neonatal orientation behaviour towards human voice. *International Journal of Behavioural Development* 1, 291–312.

ARNHEIM, D.D. and SINCLAIR, W.A. 1975: *The clumsy child*. St. Louis: Mosby.

ARNOLD, P. 1982: Oralism and the deaf child's brain: a reply to Dr Conrad. *International Journal of Pediatric Otorhinolaryngology* 4, 275–86.

ARNST, D. and KATZ, J. 1982: *Central Auditory Assessment: The SSW Test – Development and Clinical Use*. San Diego, College Hill Press.

ASLIN, R.N., PISONI, D.B., HENNESSY, B.L. and PERREY, A.J. 1981: Discrimination of voice onset time by human infants: New findings and implications for the effect of early experience. *Child Development* 52, 1135–45.

ASLIN, R.N., PISONI, D.B. and JUSCZYK, P.W. 1983: Auditory development and speech perception in infancy. In Haith, M.M. and Campos, J.J. (eds.), *Infancy and the biology of development* Vol. II of *Carmichael's Manual of Child Psychology* 4th edn. (New York: Wiley).

BADDELEY, A.D. 1979: Working memory and reading. In Kolers, P.A., Wrolstad, M.E. and Boursma, H. (eds.), *Processing of visible language* (New York: Plenum Press), 355–70.

BADDELEY, A.D. 1982: Reading and working memory. *Bulletin of the British Psychological Society* 35, 414–17.

BADDELEY, A.D. and HITCH, G. 1974: Working memory. In Bower, G. (ed.), *Recent advances in learning and motivation* (London: Academic Press), 47–89.

BADDELEY, A.D. and LEWIS, V.J. 1981: Inner active processes in reading: the inner voice, the inner ear and the inner eye. In Lesgold, A.M. and Perfetti, C.A. (eds.), *Interactive processes in reading* (Hillsdale, NJ: Lawrence Erlbaum, 107–29.)

BAMFORD, J.M. 1981: Auditory training. What is it, what is it supposed to do, and does it do it? *British Journal of Audiology* 15, 75–8.

BAMFORD, J.M. and MENTZ, D.L. 1979: The spoken language of hearing-impaired children: grammar. In Bench, J. and Bamford, J.M. (eds.), *Speech-hearing tests and the spoken language of hearing-impaired children* (London: Academic Press, 381–471.

BAMFORD, J.M., WILSON, I.M., ATKINSON, D. and BENCH, J. 1981: Pure tone audiograms from hearing-impaired children: predicting speech-hearing from the audiogram. *British Journal of Audiology* 15, 3–10.

BARD, E.G. and ANDERSON, A.H. 1984: The intelligibility of speech to children.

Journal of Child Language 10, 265–92.

BARGEN, D.H. Von 1983: Infant heart rate: a review of research methodology. *Merrill Palmer Quarterly* 29, 115–49.

BATOD, 1981: Recommendations for nomenclature of degree of hearing loss. *Journal of the British Association of Teachers of the Deaf* 5.

BATTEAU, D.W. 1967: The role of the pinna in human localization. *Proceedings of the Royal Society* B 168, 158–80.

BAX, M., HART, E. and JENKINS, S. 1983: The behaviour, development and health of the young child: implications for care. *British Medical Journal* 286, 1793–6.

BEASLEY, D.S. and RINTLEMANN, A.K. 1979: Central auditory processing. In *Hearing assessment*, Rintlemann, W.F. (ed.), (Baltimore: University Park Press, 321–49).

BEASLEY, D.S., SCHWIMMER, S. and RINTLEMANN, W.F. 1972: Intelligibility of time compressed CVC monosyllables. *Journal of Speech and Hearing Research* 15, 340–50.

BEASLEY, D., MAKJ, J. and ORCHIK, D. 1976: Childrens perception of time-compressed speech using two measures of speech discrimination. *Journal of Speech and Hearing Disorders* 41, 216–25.

BEATTIE, G.W. 1979: Planning units in spontaneous speech: some evidence from hesitation in speech and speaker gaze direction in conversation. *Linguistics* 17, 61–78.

BEATTIE, R.C., EDGERTON, B.J. and GAGER, D.W. 1979: Effects of speech materials on the loudness discomfort level. *Journal of Speech and Hearing Research* 44, 435–58.

BEGGS, W.D.A. and BRESLAW, P.I. 1982: Reading, clumsiness and the deaf child. *American Annals of the Deaf* 127, 32–7.

BEGGS, W.D.A. and BRESLAW, P.I. 1983: Reading retardation or linguistic deficit? III: A further examination of response strategies in a reading test completed by hearing-impaired children. *Journal of Research in Reading* 6, 19–28.

BEGGS, W.D.A., BRESLAW, P.I. and WILKINSON, P.I. 1981: Eye movements and reading achievements in deaf children. In Groner, R. and Fraisse, P. (eds.), *Cognition and eye movements*. (Amsterdam: North Holland Publishing).

BÉKÉSY, G. VON 1960: *Experiments in hearing*. New York: Wiley.

BENCH, J. 1969: Audio frequency and audio intensity discrimination in the human neonate. *International Audiology* 8, 615–25.

BENCH, J. 1979a: Auditory deprivation – an intrinsic or extrinsic problem. Some comments on Kyle (1978). *British Journal of Audiology* 13, 51–2.

BENCH, J. 1979b: Introductory review. In Bench, J. and Bamford, J.M. (eds.) *Speech-hearing tests and the spoken language of hearing-impaired children* 25–72, (London and New York: Academic Press).

BENCH, J. and BAMFORD, J. (eds.) 1979: *Speech hearing tests and the spoken language of hearing-impaired children*. London: Academic Press.

BENCH, J. and MENTZ, L. 1975: Stimulus complexity, state and infants' auditory behavioural responses. *British Journal of Communication Disorders* 10, 52–60.

BENCH, J., COLLYER, Y., MENTZ, L., and WILSON, I. 1976a: Studies in infant behavioural audiometry I. Neonates. *Audiology* 15, 85–105.

BENCH, J., COLLYER, Y., MENTZ, L. and WILSON, I. 1976b: Studies in infant behavioural audiometry, II. Six-week-old infants. *Audiology* 15, 302–14.

BENCH, J., COLLYER, Y., MENTZ, L. and WILSON, I. 1976c: Studies in infant behavioural audiometry, III. Six-month-old infants *Audiology* 15, 384–94.

BENEDICT, H. 1979: Early lexical development: comprehension and production. *Journal of Child Language* 6, 183–200.

BENNETT, F.C., RUNSKA, S.A. and SHERMAN, R. 1980: Middle-ear infection in learning disabled children. *Pediatrics* 66, 254–9.

BENNETT, M.J. and MOWAT, L. 1981: Validity of impedance measurements and referral criteria in school hearing screening programmes. *British Journal of Audiology* 15, 147–50.

BENNETT, M.J. and WADE, H.K. 1980: Automated newborn screening using the auditory response cradle. In Taylor, I.G. and Markides, A. (eds.), *Disorders of auditory function III* (London: Academic Press, 59–68).

BERG, F.S. 1976: *Educational audiology: hearing and speech management.* New York: Grune and Stratton.

BERG, K.M. and SMITH, M.C. 1983: Behavioural thresholds for tones during infancy. *Journal of Experimental Child Psychology* 35, 409–25.

BERG, W.K. 1972: Habituation and dishabituation of cardiac responses in four-month-old alert infants. *Journal Experimental Child Psychology* 14, 92–107.

BERKO, J. 1958: The child's learning of English morphology. *Word* 14, 150–77.

BERLIN, C. and McNEIL, M. 1976: Dichotic listening In Lass, N. (ed.), *Contemporary issues in experimental phonetics* (N.Y.: Academic Press Inc.).

BERLIN, C.I., LOWE-BELL, S., HUGHES, L. and BERLIN, H. 1973: Dichotic right ear advantage in children 5 to 13. *Cortex* 9, 394–402.

BERLIN, C., WEXLER, K.F., JERGER, J.F., HALPERIN, H.R., and SMITH, S. 1976: Superior ultra-audiometric hearing: a new type of hearing loss which correlates highly with unusually good speech in the 'profoundly deaf'. *Otolaryngology* 86, 111–16.

BESS, F.H. 1982: Children with unilateral hearing loss. *Journal of the Academy of Rehabilitative Audiology* 15, 131–44.

BESS, F.H. and THORPE, A.M. 1984: Unilateral hearing impairment in children. *Pediatrics* 74, 206–16.

BESS, F.H. and THORPE, A.M. 1986: Case-history data on unilaterally hearing-impaired children. *Ear and Hearing* 7, 14–19.

BESS, F.H., THORPE, A.M. and GIBLER, A.M. 1986: Auditory performance of children with unilateral sensorineural hearing loss. *Ear and Hearing* 7, 20–6.

BEVER, T.G. 1970: The cognitive basis for linguistic structures. In Hayes, J.R. (ed.) *Cognition and the development of language* (New York: Wiley, 331–59).

BILGER, R.C. and WANG, M.D. 1976: Consonant confusions in patients with sensorineural hearing loss. *Journal of Speech and Hearing Research* 19, 718–48.

BLOOM, L. 1973: *One word at a time.* The Hague: Mouton.

BLUESTONE, C.D. and CANTEKIN, E.J. 1980: Design factors in the characterization and identification of otitis media and certain related conditions. *Am. Otol. Rhinol. Laryngol. Suppl.* 89, 13–27, Suppl. 68.

BLUESTONE, C.D., BERRY, Q.C. and PARADISE, J.L. 1973: Audiometry and tympanometry in relation to middle-ear effusion in children. *Laryngoscope 83*, 595–604.

BOCCA, E. 1955: Binaural hearing: another approach. *Laryngoscope 65*, 572–8.

BOCCA, E. 1958: Clinical aspects of cortical deafness. *Laryngoscope 68*, 301–9.

BOCCA, E. and ANTONELLI, A. 1976: Masking level difference: another tool for the evaluation of peripheral and cortical defects. *Audiology 15*, 480–7.

BOCCA, E. and CALEARO, C. 1963: Central hearing processes. In Jerger, J. (ed.), *Modern Developments in Audiology* (New York and London: Academic Press, 337–70).

BOCCA, E., CALEARO, C. and CASSIMARI, V. 1954: A new method for testing hearing in temporal lobe tumours. *Acta Otolaryngologica 44*, 219–21.

BOND, G.L. 1935: Auditory and speech characteristics of poor readers. New York, Teachers College, Columbia University Teachers Contribution to Education No. 657.

BOND, Z.S., PETROSINO, L. and DEAN, C.R. 1982: The emergence of vowels: 17 to 26 months. *Journal of Phonetics* 10, 417–22.

BONDING, P. 1979: Critical bandwidth in loudness summation in sensorineural hearing loss. *British Journal of Audiology* 13, 23–30.

BOOTHMAN, R. and ORR, N. 1978: Value of screening in the first year of life. *Archives of Diseases in Childhood* 53, 570–3.

BOOTHROYD, A. 1978: Speech perception and sensorineural hearing loss. In Ross, M. and Giolas, T.G. (eds.), *Auditory management of hearing-impaired children* (Baltimore: University Park Press, 117–44).

BOSHOVEN, M.M., McNEIL, M.R. and HARVEY, L.O. 1982: Hemispheric specialization for the processing of linguistic and non-linguistic stimuli in congenitally deaf and hearing adults: a review and contribution. *Audiology 21*, 509–30.

BOWER, T.C. 1974: *Development in Infancy*. San Francisco: W.H. Freeman.

BOWERMAN, M. 1974: Discussion summary – development of concepts underlying language. In R.L. Schiefelbusch, Z.L.L. Lloyd (eds.) *Language perspectives – Acquisition, retardation and intervention.* (Baltimore: University Park Press, 191–201).

BOWERMAN, M. 1981: Beyond communicative adequacy: from piecemeal knowledge to an integrated system in the child's acquisition of language. *PRCLD* 20, 1–24.

BRAINE, M. 1963: The ontogeny of English phrase structure: the first phrase. *Language* 39, 1–13.

BRANDES, P.J. and EHINGER, D.M. 1981: The effects of early middle ear pathology on auditory perception and academic achievement. *Journal of Speech and Hearing Disorders*, 46, 301–7.

BRANNON, J.B. 1968: Linguistic word classes in the spoken language of normal, hard-of-hearing and deaf children. *Journal of Speech and Hearing Research*

11, 279-87.

BRANNON, J.B. and MURRY, T. 1966: The spoken syntax of normal, hard-of-hearing, and deaf children. *Journal of Speech and Hearing Research* 9, 604-10.

BREGMAN, A.S. 1978: The formation of auditory streams. In Requin, J. (ed.), *Attention and Performance VII* (Hillsdale, N.J.: Lawrence Erlbaum, 63-75).

BREGMAN, A.S. and CAMPBELL, J.L. 1971: Primary auditory stream segregation and perception of order in rapid sequencies of tonnes. *Journal of Experimental Psychology* 89, 244-9.

BREGMAN, A.S. and DANNENBRING, G.L. 1973: The effect of continuity on auditory stream segregation. *Perception and psychophysics* 13, 308-12.

BRIMER, A. 1972: *Wide-span reading test*. London: Nelson.

BRINICH, P.M. 1980: Childhood deafness and maternal control. *Journal of Communication Disorders* 13, 75-81.

BROADBENT, D.E. 1958: *Perception and communication*. London: Pergamon Press.

BROADBENT, D.E. and LADEFOGED, P. 1957: On the fusion of sounds reaching different sense organs. *Journal of the Acoustical Society of America* 29, 708-10.

BROOKHOUSE, P.E. and GOLDGAR, D.E. 1987: Medical profile of the language delayed child: otitis-prone versus otitis free. *International Journal of Pediatric Otorhinolaryngology* 12, 237-71.

BROOKS, D.N. 1973: Hearing screening — a comparative study of an impedance method and pure tone screening. *Scandinavian Audiology* 2, 62-72.

BROOKS, D.N. 1982: Acoustic impedance studies on otitis media with effusion. *International Journal of Pediatric Otorhinolaryngology* 4, 89-94.

BROOKS, D.N., WOOLEY, H. and KANJILAL, G.C. 1972: Hearing loss and middle-ear disorders in patients with Down's syndrome. *Journal of Mental Deficiency Research* 16, 21-9.

BROWN, R. 1973: *A first language*. London: Allen and Unwin.

BRUNER, J.S. 1975: The ontogenesis of speech acts. *Journal of Child Language* 2, 1-19.

BUFFERY, A.W.H. 1971: Sex differences in the development of hemispheric asymmetry of function in the human brain. *Brain Research* 31, 364-5.

BUNCH, G.O. 1979: Degree and manner of acquisition of written English rules by the deaf. *American Annals of the Deaf* 124, 10-15.

BUNCH, G.O. and CLARKE, B.R. 1978: The deaf child's learning of English morphology. *Audiology and Hearing Education* 4, 12-24.

BURNS, E.M. and WARD, N.D. 1978: Categorical perception – phenomenon or epiphenomenon: Evidence from experiments in the perception of muscial intervals. *Journal of the Acoustical Society of America* 63, 456-68.

BURROUGHS, G.E.R. 1957: *A study of the vocabulary of young children*. Edinburgh: Oliver and Boyd.

BUSBY, P.A., TONG, Y.C. and CLARK, G.M. 1982: The perception of vowels by hearing-impaired children. *Australian Journal of Audiology* Supplement 1, 4.

BUTLER, K.G. 1981: Language processing disorders: factors in diagnosis and remediation. In Keith, R.W. (ed.), *Central auditory and language processing disorders in children*. (San Diego: College Hill Press).

BUTLER, K.G. 1983: Language processing: selective attention and mnemonic strategies. In *Central auditory processing disorders*, Lasky, E.Z. and Katz, J. eds., (Baltimore: University Park Press).

BUTLER, R.A. and ALBRITE, J.P. 1957: The pitch discrimination function of the pathological ear. *Archives of Otolaryngology* 63, 411–18.

BUTTERWORTH, G. and CASTILLO, M. 1976: Co-ordination of auditory visual space in newborn human infants. *Perception* 5, 155–60.

BYRNE, D. 1979: Hearing aid selection: an analysis and a point of view. *Archives of Otolaryngology* 105, 519–25.

CALEARO, C. and ANTONELLI, A.R.1968: Audiometric findings in brainstem lesions. *Acta Otolaryngologica* 66, 305–19.

CALEARO, C. and LAZZARONI, A. 1957: Speech intelligibility in relation to the speed of the message. *Laryngoscope* 67, 410–19.

CARHART, R. 1965: Monaural and binaural discrimination against competing sentences. *International Audiology* 4, 5–10.

CARHART, R., TILLMAN, T.W. and JOHNSON, K.R. 1968: Effects of interaural time delays on masking by two competing signals. *Journal of the Acoustical Society of America* 43, 1223–30.

CAZDEN, C.B. 1972: *Child language and education*. London: Holt Rinehart and Winston.

CHABON, S.S., KENT-UDOLF, L. and EGOLF, O.B. 1982: The temporal reliability of Brown's MLU-M measure with post-Stage V children. *Journal of Speech and Hearing Research* 25, 117–24.

CHARROW, V.R. 1975: A psycholinguistic analysis of 'Deaf English'. *Sign Language Studies* 7, 139–50.

CHEN, K. 1976: Acoustic image in visual detection for deaf and hearing college students. *Journal of General Psychology* 94, 243–6.

CHERRY, E.C. 1953: On the recognition of speech with one, and with two ears. *Journal of the Acoustical Society of America* 25, 975–79.

CHESKIN, A. 1981: The verbal environment provided by hearing mothers for their young deaf children. *Journal of Communication Disorders* 14, 485–96.

CHOMSKY, N. 1959: Review of B.F. Skinner, verbal behaviour. *Language* 35, 26–58.

CHOMSKY, N. 1965: *Aspects of the theory of syntax*, Cambridge, Mass.: MIT Press.

CLEMENTS, M. and KELLY, J.B. 1978: Auditory spatial responses of young guinea-pigs during and after ear blocking. *J. Comp. Physiol. Psychol.* 92, 24–44.

CLIFTON, R.K., MORRONGIELLO, B., KULIG, J. and DOWD, J. 1981: Developmental changes in auditory localization in infancy. In Aslin, R., Alberts, J. and Peterson, M., (eds.), *The development of perception: psychobiological per-*

spectives. Vol. 1: Audition, Somatic Perception and the Chemical Senses (N.Y.: Academic Press).

CLOPTON, B.M. and SILVERMAN, M.S. 1978: Changes in latency and duration of neural responding following developmental auditory deprivation. *Exp. Brain Research* 32, 39–47.

COHEN, D. and SADE, J. 1972: Hearing in secretory otitis media. *Canadian Journal of Otolaryngology*, 1, 27–9.

COLLINS, M.J. and CULLEN, J.K. 1978: Temporal integration of tone glides. *Journal of the Acoustical Society of America* 63, 469–73.

CONRAD, R. 1970: Short term memory processes in the deaf. *British Journal of Psychology* 61, 179–95.

CONRAD, R. 1977: The reading ability of deaf school-leavers. *British Journal of Educational Psychology* 47, 138–48.

CONRAD, R. 1979: *The deaf school child*. London: Harper and Row.

CONRAD, R. 1980: Let the children choose. *International Journal of Pediatric Otorhinolaryngology* 1, 317–29.

COOLEY, J.D. 1981: Use of grammatical constraints in reading by young deaf adults as reflected in eye–voice span. *Language and Speech* 24, 349–62.

COOPER, C. and ARNOLD, P. 1981: Hearing impairment and visual perceptual processes in reading. *British Journal of Disorders of Communication* 16, 43–9.

COOPER, J.C., LANGLEY, L.R. and MEYERHOFF, W.L. 1975: An abbreviated impedance bridge for school screening. *Journal of Speech and Hearing Research* 40, 260–7.

COOPER, R.L. 1967: The ability of deaf and hearing children to apply morphological rules. *Journal of Speech and Hearing Research* 10, 77–86.

COOPER, R.L. and ROSENSTEIN, J. 1966: Language acquisition of deaf children. *Volta Review* 68, 46–56.

CORRIGAN, R. 1978. Language development as related to Stage 6 object permanence development. *Journal of Child Language* 5, 173–89.

CROWDER, R.G. and MORTON, J. 1969: Precategorical acoustic storage. *Perception and Psychophysics* 5, 365–73.

CRUTTENDEN, A. 1979: *Language in infancy and childhood*. Manchester: Manchester University Press.

CRYSTAL, D. 1979a: Prosodic development. In Fletcher, P. and Garman, M. (eds.), *Language acquisition* (Cambridge: Cambridge University Press, 33–48).

CRYSTAL, D. 1979b: *Working with LARSP*. London: Edward Arnold.

CRYSTAL, D. 1981: *Clinical linguistics*. New York: Springer.

CRYSTAL, D., FLETCHER, P. and GARMAN, M. 1976: *The grammatical analysis of language disability*. London: Edward Arnold.

CULLEN, J.K. and COLLINS, M.J. 1982: Audibility of short-duration tone-glides as a function of rate of frequency change. *Hearing Research* 7, 115–25.

CURTISS, S. 1977: *Genie: a psycholinguistic study of a modern day 'wild child'*. New York: Academic Press.

CUTTING, J.E. 1978: There may be nothing peculiar to perceiving in a speech mode.

In Requin, J. (ed.), *Attention and performance VII* (Hillsdale, N.J.: Lawrence Erlbaum, 229–43).

CUTTING, J.E. and ROSNER, B.S. 1974: Categories and boundaries in speech and music. *Perception and Psychophysics* 16 (3), 564–70.

DALE, P.S. 1976: *Language development.* New York: Holt, Rinehart and Winston.

DALLOS, P., RYAN, A., HARRIS, D., McGEE, T. and ODZAMAR, O. 1977: Cochlear frequency selectivity in the presence of hair cell damage. In Evans, E.F. and Wilson, J.P. (eds.) *Psychophysics and Physiology of hearing* (London and New York: Academic Press, 249–58).

DALZELL, J. and OWRID, H.L. 1976: Children with conductive deafness: a follow-up study. *British Journal Audiology* 10, 87–90.

DANAHER, E.M. and PICKETT, J.M. 1975: Some masking effects produced by low-frequency vowel formants in persons with sensorineural hearing loss. *Journal of Speech and Hearing Research* 18, 261–71.

DANAHER, E.M., OSBERGER, M.J. and PICKETT, J.M. 1973: Discrimination of formant frequency transition in synthetic vowels. *Journal of Speech and Hearing Research* 16, 439–51.

DARWIN, C.J. 1971: Ear differences in the recall of fricatives and vowels. *Quarterly Journal of Experimental Psychology* 23, 46–62.

DARWIN, C.J. 1981: Perceptual grouping of speech components differing in fundamental frequency and onset-time. *Quarterly Journal of Experimental Psychology* 33, 185–207.

DARWIN, C.J. and BETHELL-FOX, C.E. 1977: Pitch continuity and speech source attribution. *Journal of Experimental Psychology: Human Perception and Performance* 3, 665–72.

DAVIS, A. 1990: Neonatal hearing screening: part of an integrated advance in audiological health services for the 1990s. *British Association of Audiological Scientists Newsletter* no. 17.

DAVISON, F.M. 1977: The written language of deaf children. Unpublished thesis, University of Reading.

DAWSON, E. 1981: Psycholinguistic processes in prelingually deaf adolescents. In Woll, B., Kyle, J. and Deuchar, M. (eds.), *Perspectives on British sign language and deafness* (London: Croom Helm, 43–70).

DAYAL, V.S., TARANTINO, L. and SWISHER, L.P. 1966: Neuro-otologic studies in multiple sclerosis. *Laryngoscope* 76, 1798–1809.

De BOER, E. 1959 Measurements of the critical bandwidth in cases of perception deafness. In Cremer, L. (ed.), *Proceedings of the third international congress on acoustics* (Amsterdam: Elsevier, 100–2).

De BOER, E. and BOUWMEESTER, J. 1974: Critical bands and sensorineural hearing loss. *Audiology* 13, 236–59.

De VILLIERS, J.G. and De VILLIERS, P.A. 1978: *Language acquisition.* Cambridge, Mass.: Harvard University Press.

DEMPSEY, C. 1983: Selecting tests of auditory function in children. In Lasky, E.J. and Katz, J. (eds.) *Central auditory processing disorders* (Baltimore:

University Park Press).

DEMPSEY, J.J. and MAXON, B. 1982: Temporal integration functions in hearing-impaired children. *Ear and Hearing* 3, 271–73.

DERMODY, P., KATSCH, R. and MACKIE, K. 1983: Auditory processing limitations in low verbal children: evidence from a two-response dichotic listening task. *Ear and Hearing* 4, 272–7.

DERWING, B.L. and BAKER, W.J. 1979: Recent research on the acquisition of English morphology. In Fletcher, P. and Garman, M. (eds.), *Language acquisition* (Cambridge: Cambridge University Press, 209–24).

DI CARLO, L.M. 1962: Some relationships between frequency discrimination and speech reception. *Journal of Auditory Research* 2, 37–49.

DI FRANCESCA, S. 1972: *Academic achievement test results of a national testing program for hearing impaired students – United States: Spring 1971.* Series D, Number 9. Washington, D.C.: Gallaudet College, Office of Demographic Studies.

DJUPESLAND, G., NICKLASSON, B., HELLAND, S. and HEMSEN, E. 1981: Hearing threshold level and middle ear pressure in children with phonetic/phoneme disability. *Scandinavian Audiology* Supplement 16, 73–9.

DOBIE, R.A. and BERLIN, C.I. 1979: Influence of otitis media on hearing and development. *Ann. Otol. Rhinol. Laryngol.* Suppl. 60, 48–53.

DONALDSON, M.C. 1978: *Children's minds.* Glasgow: Fontana/Collins.

DORAN, E.W. 1907: A study of vocabularies. *Pedagogic seminars* 14, 401–38.

DORE, J., FRANKLIN, M.B., MILLER, R.T. and RAMER, A.L.H. 1976: Transitional phenomena in early language acquisition. *Journal of Child Language* 3, 13–28.

DOWNS, M.P. 1976: Hearing loss: definition, epidemiology and prevention. *Public Health Report* 4, 255–62.

DOWNS, M.P. 1977: The expanding imperatives of early identification. In Bess, F. (ed.), *Childhood Deafness: causation, assessment and management* (New York: Grune and Stratton, 95–106).

DOWNS, M.P. 1985: Effects of mild hearing loss on auditory processing. *Otolaryngologic Clinics of North America* 18, 337–44.

DRESCHLER, W.A. 1982: Phonemic confusions in quiet and noise for hearing-impaired subjects. *International Association of Audiological Physicians Bulletin* 3, 19.

DRESCHLER, W.A. and PLOMP, R. 1980: Relation between psychophysical data and speech perception for hearing-impaired subjects. *Journal of the Acoustical Society of America* 68, 1608–15.

DUCHAN, J.F. and KATZ, J. 1983: Language and auditory processing. In Lasky, E.Z. and Katz, J. (eds.), *Central auditory processing disorders* (Baltimore: University Park Press).

DURLACH, N.I. and COLBURN, J.S. 1978: Binaural phenomena. In Carterette, E.C. and Friedman, M.P. (eds.), *Handbook of perception* (New York: Academic Press, 365–466).

DURLACH, N.I., THOMPSON, C.L. and COLBURN, H.S. 1981: Binaural interaction in impaired listeners. *Audiology* 20, 181–211.

DURRANT, J.D. and LOVRINIC, J.H. 1984: *Bases of hearing science* 2nd edn, Williams & Wilkins: Baltimore.

DWYER, J., BLUMSTEIN, L.E. and RYALLS, J. 1982: The role of duration and rapid temporal processing on the lateral perception of consonants and vowels. *Brain and Language* 17, 272–86.

EAGLES, E.L. 1972: Selected findings from the Pittsburg study. *Trans Am. Acad. Opthalmol. Otolaryngol.* 76, 343–8.

EFRON, R. 1985: The central auditory system and issues related to hemispheric specialization. In Pinheiro, M.L. and Musiek, F.E. (eds.) *Assessment of central auditory dysfunction* (Baltimore, MD: Williams & Wilkins) 143–54.

EFRON, R. and CRANDALL, P.H. 1983: Central auditory processing effects of anterior temporal lobectomy. *Brain and Language* 19, 237–53.

EGOLF, D.B., RHODES, R.C. and CURREY, E.T. 1970: Phoneme discrimination differences between hypacusics and normals. *Journal of Auditory Research* 10, 176–9.

EILERS, R.E. 1977: Context-sensitive perception of naturally produced stop and fricative consonants by infants. *Journal of the Acoustical Society of America* 61, 1321–36.

EILERS, R.E. and MINIFIE, F.D. 1975: Fricative discrimination in early infancy. *Journal of Speech and Hearing Research* 18, 158–67.

EILERS, R.E. and OLLER, D. 1976: The role of speech discrimination in developmental sound substitutions. *Journal of Child Language* 3, 319–30.

EILERS, R.E., GAVIN, W. and WILSON, W. 1979: Linguistic experience and phonemic perception in infancy: a crosslinguistic study. *Child Development* 50, 14–18.

EILERS, R.E., GAVIN, W.J. and OLLER, D.K. 1982: Cross-linguistic perception in infancy: early effects of linguistic experience. *Journal of Child Language* 9, 289–302.

EILERS, R.E., OLLER, D.K., BULL, D.H. and GAVIN, W.J. 1984: Linguistic experience and infant speech perception: a reply to Jusczyk, Shea and Aslin, 1984. *Journal of Child Language* 11, 467–75.

EILERS, R.E., WILSON, W.R. and MOORE, J.M. 1977: Development changes in speech discrimination in infants. *Journal of Speech and Hearing Research* 20, 766–80.

EILERS, R.E., WILSON, W.R. and MOORE, J.M. 1979: Speech discrimination in the language-innocent and the language-wise. A study in the perception of voice onset time. *Journal of Child Language* 6, 1–18.

EIMAS, P.D. 1974: Auditory and linguistic processing of cues for place of articulation by infants. *Perception and Psychophysics* 16, 513–21.

EIMAS, P.D. 1975a: Speech perception in early infancy. In Cohen, L. and Salapatek, P. *Infant perception* (eds.) (London: Academic Press 193–231.)

EIMAS, P.D. 1975b: Auditory and phonetic coding of the cues for speech. Discrimination of the [r-1] distinction by young infants. *Perception and Psychophysics* 18, 341–7.

EIMAS, P.D. and KAVFANAGH, J.F. 1986: Otitis media, hearing loss, and child development: a NICHD conference summary. *Public Health Report* 101, 289–93.

EIMAS, P.D., SIQUELAND, E.R., JUSCZYK, P.W. and VIGORITO, J. 1971: Speech perception in infants. *Science* 171, 303–6.

EISENBERG, R.B. 1965: Auditory behaviour in the human neonate. *Int. Audiol.* 4, 65–8.

EISENBERG, R.B. 1976: *Auditory competence in early life. The roots of communicative behaviour.* Baltimore: University Park Press.

EISENSON, J. 1968: Developmental aphasia (dyslogia): a postulation of a unitary concept of the disorder. *Cortex* 4, 184–200.

ELLIOTT, L.L. 1979: Performance of children 9 to 17 years on a test of speech intelligibility in noise using sentence material with controlled word predictability. *Journal of the Acoustical Society of America,* 66, 651–3.

ELLIOTT, L.L., HIRSH, I.J. and SIMMONS, A.A. 1967: Language of young hearing-impaired children. *Language and Speech* 10, 141–58.

ERBER, N.P. 1974: Pure-tone thresholds and word recognition abilities of hearing-impaired children. *Journal of Speech and Hearing Research* 17, 194–202.

EVANS, E.F. 1972: The frequency response and other properties of single fibres in the guinea-pig cochlear nerve. *Journal of Physiology* 226, 262–87.

EVANS, E.F. 1975a: The sharpening of cochlear frequency selectivity in the normal and abnormal cochlea. *Audiology* 14, 419–42.

EVANS, E.F. 1975b: Normal and abnormal functioning of the cochlear nerve. In Bench, J. and Pye, A. (eds.), *Sound reception in mammals* (London: Academic Press, 133–65).

EVANS, E.F. 1976: The effective bandwidths of individual cochlear nerve fibres from pathological cochleas in the cat. In Stephens, S.D.G. (ed.), *Disorders of auditory function* (London: Academic Press, 99–110).

EVANS, E.F. and HARRISON, R.V. 1976: Correlation between outer hair cell damage and deterioration of cochlear nerve turning properties in the guinea-pig. *Journal of Physiology* 256, 43–4.

EVANS, E.F. and WILSON, J.P. 1973: Frequency selectivity of the cochlea. In Moller, A.R. (ed.), *Basic mechanisms of hearing* (New York: Academic Press, 519–51).

EVANS, E.F. and WILSON, J.P. 1975: Cochlear tuning properties: concurrent basilar membrane and single nerve fibre measurements. *Science* 190, 1218–21.

EVANS, E.F., AINSWORTH, W.A., DARWIN, C.J., FANT, G.C.M., FOURCIN, A.J., GOLDSTEIN, J.L., KLINKE, R., LEITNER, H., MILLER, J.D., MILNER, B.A., NEFF, W.D, RISBERG, A. and TALLAL, P.A. 1977: Disorders of hearing and language: Understanding, diagnosis, rehabilitation seminar report. In Bullock, T.A. (ed.), *Recognition of complex acoustic signals* (Berlin: Dahlem Konferenzen, 367–86).

EVERBERG, G. 1960: Etiology of unilateral total deafness. *Annals of Otology, Rhinology and Laryngology* 69, 711–30.

EWERTSEN, H.W. and BIRK NIELSON H. 1973: Social hearing handicap index. *Audiology* 12, 180–7.

EWING, I. and EWING, A. 1944: The ascertainment of deafness in infancy and childhood. *Journal of Laryngology and Otology* 59, 309–33.

EWING, I. and EWING, A. 1947: Opportunity and the deaf child, London: University of London Press.

FANT, C.G.M. 1960: *Acoustic theory of speech production*. The Hague: Mouton.

FARRER, S. and KEITH, R. 1981: Filtered word testing in the assessment of children's central auditory abilities. *Ear and Hearing* 2, 267–9.

FERGUSON, C.A. 1978: Learning to pronounce: the earliest stages of phonological development in the child. In Minifie, F.D. and Lloyd, L.L. (eds.), *Communicative and cognitive abilities – early behavioural assessment* (Baltimore: University Park Press, 273–97).

FERRE, J.M. and WILBER, L.A. 1986: Normal and learning disabled children's central auditory processing skills: an experimental test battery. *Ear and Hearing* 7, 336–43.

FESTEN, J.M. and PLOMP, R. 1983: Relations between auditory functions in impaired hearing. *Journal of the Acoustical Society of America* 73, 652–62.

FIELD, J., MUIR, D., PISON, F., SINCLAIR, M. and DODWELL, P. 1980: Infant's orientation to lateral sounds from birth to three months. *Child Development* 51, 295–98.

FIELLAU-NIKOLAJSEN, M. 1983: Tympanometric prediction of the magnitude of hearing loss in preschool children with secretary otitis media. *Scandinavian Audiology Supplement*, 17, 68–72.

FITZGIBBONS, P.J. and WIGHTMAN, F.L. 1982: Gap detection in normal and hearing-impaired listeners. *Journal of the Acoustical Society of America* 72, 761–5.

FLAVELL, J.H. 1963: *The developmental psychology of Jean Piaget*. Princeton, N.J.: Van Nostrand Reinhold.

FLETCHER, H. 1929: *Speech and hearing*. New York: Van Nostrand.

FLETCHER, H. 1940: Auditory patterns. *Reviews in Modern Physiology* 12, 47–65.

FLETCHER, P. and GARMAN, M. (eds.) 1979: *Language acquisition*. Cambridge: Cambridge University Press.

FLORENTINE, M., BUUS, S., SCHARF, B. and ZWICHER, E. 1980: Frequency selectivity in normally hearing and hearing impaired observers. *Journal of Speech and Hearing Research* 23, 646–69.

FOLSOM, R.C., WEBER, B.A. and THOMPSON, G. 1983: Auditory brainstem responses in children with early recurrent middle-ear disease. *Ann. Otol. Rhinol. Laryngol.* 92, 249–53.

FOSTER, J.R. and HAGGARD, M.P. 1979: FAAF – An efficient test of speech perception. *Proceedings of the Institute of Acoustics*.

FOURCIN, A.F. 1976: Speech pattern tests for deaf children. In Stephens, S.D.G. (ed.), *Disorders of auditory function* (London: Academic Press, 197–208).

FRANKS, J.R. and DANILOFF, R.G. 1973: A review of audiological implications of testing vowel perception. *Journal of Auditory Research* 13, 355–68.

FREEDMAN, S.J. and FISHER, H.G. 1968: The role of the pinna in auditory localization. In Freedman, S.J. (ed.), *Neuropsychology of spatially oriented behav-*

iour (Illinois: Dorsey Press, 135–52).

FREEMAN, B.A. and BEASLEY, D.S. 1976: Lead and lag effects associated with the Staggered Spondaic Word Test. *Journal of Speech and Hearing Research* 19, 572–7.

FRIEL-PATTI, S., FINITZO-HIEBER, T., CONTI, G. and BROWN, K.C. 1982: Language delay in infants associated with middle ear disease and mild fluctuating hearing impairment. *Pediatric Infectious Diseases* 1, 104–9.

FRIES, C. 1952: *The Structure of English*. New York: Harcourt Brace Jovanovitch.

FROMKIN, V., KRASHEN, S., CURTISS, S., RIGLER, D. and RIGLER, M. 1974: The development of language in Genie: a case of language acquisition beyond the 'critical period'. *Brain and Language* 1, 81–107.

FRY, D.B., ABRAMSON, A.S., EIMAS, P.D. and LIBERMAN, A.M. 1962: The identification and discrimination of synthetic vowels. *Language and Speech* 5, 171–89.

FURTH, H. 1964: Research with the deaf: implications for language and cognition. *Psychological Bulletin* 62, 145–64.

FURTH, H. 1966a: *Thinking without language*. New York: Free Press.

FURTH, H.G. 1966b: A comparison of reading test norms of deaf and hearing children. *American Annals of the Deaf* 111, 461–2.

FURTH, H. 1973: *Deafness and learning: a psychosocial approach*. California: Wadsworth.

FURAKAWA, C.T. 1983: Conductive hearing loss and speech development. *Journal of Allergy and Clinical Immunology* 81, 1015–19.

FUSFELD, I.S. 1955: The academic program of schools for the deaf. *Volta Review* 57, 63–70.

GAGNE, 1982: Upward spread of masking among listeners with sensorineural hearing loss. *Periodic Progress Report* (Central Institute for the Deaf) 25, 2.

GALAMBOS, R., HICKS, G. and WILSON, M.J. 1982: Hearing loss in graduates of a tertiary intensive care nursery. *Ear and Hearing* 3, 87–90.

GARDNER, M. and GARDNER, R. 1973: Problem of localization in the median plane: effect of pinnae cavity occlusion. *Journal of the Acoustical Society of America* 53, 400–8.

GARDNER, R. and WILSON, J.P. 1979: Evidence for direction-specific channels in the processing of frequency modulation. *Journal of the Acoustical Society of America* 66, 704–9.

GARMAN, M. 1979: Early grammatical development. In Fletcher, P. and Garman, M. (eds.) *Language acquisition* (Cambridge: Cambridge University Press, 177–208).

GARVEY, C. and HOGAN, R. 1973: Social speech and social interaction: egocentrism revisited. *Child Development* 44, 562–8.

GASCON, G.G., JOHNSON, R. and BURD, L. 1986: Central auditory processing and attention deficit disorders. *Journal of Child Neurology* 1, 27–33.

GEBHARDT, C.J. and GOLDSTEIN, D.P. 1972: Frequency discrimination and the masking level difference. *Journal of the Acoustical Society of America* 51, 1228–32.

GENGEL, R.W. and WATSON, C.S. 1971: Temporal integration; I. Clinical implications of a laboratory study; II. Additional data from hearing-impaired subjects. *Journal of Speech and Hearing Disorders* 36, 213–14.

GERBER, S.E. and BAUER, B.B. 1974: Loudness. In Gerber, S.E. (ed.), *Introductory hearing science* (Philadelphia: W.B. Saunders, 151–71).

GIMSING, S. and BERGHOLTZ, L.M. 1983: Audiologic screening of seven- and ten-year-old children. *Scandinavian Audiology* 12, 171–7.

GINZEL, A., PEDERSEN, C.B. SPLIID, P.E. and ANDERSEN, E. 1982: The effect of age and hearing loss on the identification of synthetic /b, d, g/ stimuli. *Scandinavian Audiology* 11, 103–12.

GIOLAS, T.G. and WARK, D.J. 1967: Communication problems associated with unilateral hearing loss. *Journal of Speech and Hearing Disorders* 41, 336–43.

GIRAUDI-PERRY, D.M., SALVI, R.J. and HENDERSON, D. 1982: Gap-detection in hearing-impaired chinchillas. *Journal of the Acoustical Society of America* 72, 1387–93.

GLANVILLE, B., BEST, C. and LEVENSON, R. 1977: A cardiac measure of cerebral asymmetries in infant auditory perception. *Developmental Psychology* 13, 54–9.

GLASBERG, B.R. and MOORE, B.C.J. 1989: Psychoacoustic abilities of subjects with unilateral and bilateral cochlear hearing impairments and their relationship to understand speech. *Scandinavian Auditory Supplement* 32, 1–25.

GLEITMAN, L.R. and ROZIN, P. 1973: Teaching reading by use of a syllabary. *Reading research quarterly* 8, 447–83.

GODA, S. 1964: Spoken syntax of normal, deaf, and retarded adolescents. *Journal of Verbal Learning and Verbal Behaviour* 3, 401–5.

GODFREY, J.J. and MILLAY, K.K. 1978: Perception of rapid spectral change in speech by listeners with mild and moderate sensorineural hearing loss. *Journal of the American Auditory Society* 3, 200–8.

GODFREY, J.J. and MILLAY, K.K. 1980: Perception of synthetic speech sounds by hearing-impaired listeners. *Journal of Auditory Research* 20, 187–203.

GOLDIN-MEADOW, S., SELIGMAN, M.E.P. and GELMAN, R. 1976: Language in the two-year-old. *Cognition* 4, 189–202.

GOLDSTEIN, J.L. 1973: An optimum processor theory for the central formation of the pitch of complex tones. *Journal of the Acoustical Society of America* 55, 1496–1516.

GOODHILL, V. 1958: The relation of auditory response to the viscosity of tympanic fluids. *Acta Otolaryngologica* 49, 38–46.

GORDON-SALANT, S.M. and WIGHTMAN, F.L. 1983: Speech competition effects on synthetic stop-vowel perception by normal and hearing-impaired listeners. *Journal of the Acoustical Society of America* 73, 1756–65.

GREGG, C., CLIFTON, S.K. and HAITH, M. 1976: A possible explanation for the frequent failure to find cardiac orienting in the newborn infant. *Developmental Psychology* 12, 75–6.

GREGORY, S. and MOGFORD, K. 1981: Early language development in deaf children.

In Woll, B. Kyle, J. and Deuchar, M. (eds.), *Perspectives on British sign language and deafness* (London: Croom Helm, 218-37).

GREGORY, S., MOGFORD, K. and BISHOP, J. 1979: Mothers' speech to young hearing-impaired children. *Teacher of the Deaf* 3, 42-3.

GRIBBEN, KAY L. 1981: Psychoacoustic tuning curves in normal and impaired hearing. MSc Dissertation, ISVR, University of Southampton.

GROSS, R. 1970: Language used by mothers of deaf children and mothers of hearing children. *American Annals of the Deaf* 115, 93-6.

GROSSO, P. and RUPP, R.R. 1978: Pure tone and tympanometric screening: an ideal pair in identification audiometry. *Journal of the American Auditory Society* 4, 11-15.

GRUNWELL, P. 1981: The development of phonology. *First Language* 3, 161-91.

HAGGARD, M.P. and PARKINSON, A. 1971: Stimulus task factors as determinants of ear advantages. *Quarterly Journal of Experimental Psychology* 23, 168-77.

HAGGARD, M.P., GATEHOUSE, S. and DAVIS, S. 1981: The high prevalence of hearing disorders and its implications for services in the UK. *British Journal of Audiology* 15, 241-51.

HAGGERTY, R. 1980: Life stress: illness and social support. *Dev. Med. Child Neurol.* 391-400.

HAMMERMEISTER, F.K. 1971: Reading achievements in deaf adults. *American Annals of the Deaf* 116, 25-8.

HAMMILL, D.D. and LARSEN, S.C. 1974: The effectiveness of psycholinguistic training. *Exceptional Children,* 41, 5-14.

HAMP, N.W. 1972: Reading attainment and some associated factors in deaf and partially hearing children. *The Teacher of the Deaf* 70, 203-15.

HARBERT, F, YOUNG, I.M. and MENDUKE, H. 1970: Audiological findings in serous otitis media. *ENT Monograph.* 49, 409-11.

HARDY, W.G., PAULS, M.D. and HASKINS, H.L. 1958: An analysis of language development in children with impaired hearing. *Acta Otolaryngologica* supplementum 141, 1-51.

HARFORD, E. and MUSKETT, C.N. 1964: Binaural hearing with one hearing aid. *Journal of Speech and Hearing Disorders* 29, 133-46.

HARKER, L.A. and WAGONER, R. Van 1974: Application of impedance audiometry as a screening instrument. *Acta Otolaryngologica* 77, 198-201.

HARRIS, J.D., HAINES, H.L. and MYERS, C.K. 1956: A new formula for using the audiogram to predict speech hearing loss. *Archives of Otolaryngology* 63, 158-76.

HARRIS, J.D. and SERGEANT, R.L. 1971: Monaural/binaural minimum audible angles for a moving sound source. *Journal of Speech and Hearing Research* 14, 618-29.

HARY, J.M. and MASSARO, D.W. 1982: Categorical results do not imply categorical perception. *Perception and Psychophysics* 32, 409-18.

HECOX, K. 1975: Electrophysiological correlates of human auditory development. In Cohen, L. and Salapatek, P. (eds.), *Infant perception* Vol. II (London: Academic Press, 151-91).

HECOX, K. and GALAMBOS, R. 1974: Brainstem auditory-evoked responses in human infants and adults. *Archives of Otolaryngology* 99, 30–3.

HEIDER, F. and HEIDER, G.M. 1940: A comparison of sentence structure of deaf and hearing children. *Psychological Monographs* 52, 42–103.

HELMHOLTZ, H.L.F. 1863: *Die Lehre von den Tonempfindungen als physiologische Grundlage fur die Theorie der Musik*. English Translation by Ellis, A.J.: *On the sensations of tone*, 1875. London: Longman.

HIRSH, I.J. 1971: Masking of speech and auditory localization. *Audiology* 10, 110–14.

HIRSH, I.J. and POLLACK, I. 1948: The role of interaural phase in loudness. *Journal of the Acoustical Society of America* 20, 761–6.

HISCOCK, M. and BERGSTROM, K.J. 1982: The lengthy persistence of priming effects in dichotic listening. *Neuropsychologia* 20, 43–53.

HITCHINGS, V. and HAGGARD, M.P. 1983: Incorporation of parental suspicious in screening infants' hearing. *British Journal of Audiology* 17, 71–6.

HOEKSTRA, A. and RITSMA, R.J. 1977: Perceptive hearing loss and frequency selectivity. In Evans, E.F. and Wilson, J.P. (eds.), *Psychophysics and physiology of hearing loss* (London: Academic Press, 263–71).

HOFFMAN-LAWLESS, F., KEITH, R.W. and COTTEN, R.T. 1981: Auditory processing abilities in children with previous middle ear effusion. *Ann. Otol. Rhinol. Laryngol.* 90, 543–5.

HOLM, V.A. and KUNZE, L.H. 1969: Effect of chronic otitis media on language and speech development. *Pediatrics* 43, 833–9.

HORN, E. 1925: The commonest words in the spoken vocabulary of children up to and including six years of age. *National Society for Study of Education Yearbook* 24, 185–98.

HOUTSMA, A.J.M. and GOLDSTEIN, J.L. 1972: The central origin of the pitch of complex tones: evidence from musical interval recognition. *Journal of the Acoustical Society of America* 51, 520–9.

HOWARTH, S.P., WOOD, D.J., GRIFFITHS, A.J. and HOWARTH, C.I. 1981: A comparative study of the reading lessons of deaf and hearing primary school children. *British Journal of Educational Psychology* 51, 156–62.

HOWIE, V.M., JENSEN, N.J., FLEMING, J.W., PEELER, M.B. and MEIGS, S. 1979: The effect of early onset of otitis media on educational achievement. *International Journal of Pediatric Otorhinolaryngology* 1, 151–5.

HUGGINS, A.W.F. 1981: Speech perception and auditory processing. In Getty, D.J. and Howard, J.H. (eds.), *Auditory and visual pattern recognition* (Hillsdale, N.J.: Lawrence Erlbaum, 79–91).

HUGHES, M.E. 1983: Verbal interaction between mothers and their young hearing-impaired children. *Journal of the British Association of Teachers of the Deaf* 7, 18–23.

HUMES, L.E., ALLEN, S.K. and BESS, F.H. 1980: Horizontal sound localization skills of unilaterally hearing-impaired children. *Audiology* 19, 508–18.

HUNG, D.L., TZENG, O.J.L. and WARREN, D.H. 1981: A chronometric study of sentence processing in deaf children. *Cognitive Psychology* 13, 583–610.

HUTTON, J.B. 1983: Effect of middle ear pathology on selected psycho-educational measures following surgical treatment. *Perceptual and Motor Skills* 57, 1095–100.

INGRAM, D. 1976: *Phonological disability in children.* London: Edward Arnold.

IVIMEY, G.P. 1976: The written syntax of an English deaf child: an exploration in method. *British Journal of Disorders of Communication* 11, 103–20.

IVIMEY, G.P. 1982: Assessing the language skills of hearing-impaired children – a critical review. *Journal òf the British Association of Teachers of the Deaf* 5, 133–44.

IVIMEY, G.P. and LACHTERMAN, D.H. 1980: The written language of young English deaf children. *Language and Speech* 23, 351–75.

IWASAKI, S. 1981: Automatic noise suppression in hearing aids. *Hearing Aid Journal* 34, 10–11, 40.

JENSEMA, C.J. 1975: *The relationship between academic achievement and the demographic characteristics of hearing-impaired children and youth.* Series R, Number 2. Washington, D.C.: Gallaudet College, Office of Demographic Studies.

JERGER, J. 1960: Observations on auditory behaviour in lesions of the central auditory pathways. *Archives of Otolaryngology* 71, 797–806.

JERGER, J. and JERGER, S. 1975: Clinical validity of central auditory tests. *Scandinavian Audiology* 4, 147–63.

JERGER, J., WICKERS, N.J., SHARBROUGH, F.W. and JERGER, S. 1969: Bilateral lesions of the temporal lobe. *Acta Otolaryngologica* Supp. 258.

JERGER, S. 1981: Evaluation of central auditory function in children. In Keith, R.W. (ed.), *Central auditory and language disorders in children.* (San Diego: College Hill Press, 30–60).

JERGER, S. and JERGER, J. 1984: *Pediatric speech intelligibility test: Manual for administration* (St Louis, Auditec).

JERGER, S., LEWIS, S., HAWKINS, J. and JERGER, J. 1980: Pediatric speech intelligibility test. I. Generation of test materials. *International Journal of Pediatric Otorhinologyngology* 2, 217–30.

JERGER, S., JERGER, J., ALFORD, B.R. and ABRAMS, S. 1983: Development of speech intelligibility in children with recurrent otitis media. *Ear and Hearing* 4, 138–45.

JERGER, S., JOHNSON, K. and LOISELLE, L. 1988: Pediatric central auditory dysfunction. *American Journal of Otolaryngology* 9 (Suppl.), 63–70.

JESTEADT, W., BILGER, R.C., GREEN, D.M. and PATTERSON, J.H. 1976: Temporal acuity in listeners with sensorineural hearing loss. *Journal of Speech and Hearing Research* 19, 357–70.

JORDAN, R.E. and EAGLES, E.L. 1961: The relation of air conduction audiometry to otologic abnormalities. *Annals of Otology, Rhinology and Otolaryngology* 70, 819–27.

JUSCZYK, P.W. 1977: Perception of syllable final stop consonants by two-month-old infants. *Perception and Psychophysics* 21, 450–4.

JUSCZYK, P.W. 1981: Infant speech perception: a critical appraisal. In Eimas, P.D.

and Miller, J.L., (eds.) *Perspectives on the study of speech* (Hillsdale: Erlbaum Ass., 113–64).

JUSCZYK, P.W., ROSNER, B.S., CUTTING, J.E., FOARD, C.F. and SMITH, L.P. 1977: Categorical perception of non-speech sounds by two-month-old infants. *Perception and Psychophysics* 21, 50–4.

JUSCZYK, P.W., MURRAY, J. and BAYLY, J. 1979: Perception of place of articulation in fricatives and stops by infants. Paper to Society for Research in Child Development, San Francisco.

JUSCZYK, P.W., SHEA, S.L. and ASLIN, R.N. 1984: Linguistic experience and infant speech perception: a re-examination of Eilers, Gavin and Oller, 1982. *Journal of Child Language* 11, 453–66.

KAPLAN, E.L. 1970: Intonation and language acquisition. *Stanford Papers and Reports on Child Language Development* 1, 1–21.

KAPLAN, G.L., FLESHMAN, J.K., BONDER, T.R., BAUM, C. and CLARK, P.S. 1973: Long term effects of otitis media: A ten-year cohort study of Alaskan Eskimo children. *Pediatrics* 52, 577–85.

KARLAN, M.S., TONNDORF, J. and KHANNA, S.M. 1972: Dual origin of cochlear microphonics: inner and outer hair cells. *Annals of Otology, Rhinology and Laryngology* 81, 696–705.

KARMILOFF-SMITH, A. 1979: Language development after five. In Fletcher, P. and Garman, M. (eds.), *Language acquisition* (Cambridge: Cambridge University Press, 307–23).

KARZON, N. 1980: Consonants embedded in a multisyllabic sequence: discrimination by infants from 1–4 months of age. *Central Institute for the Deaf Perception Progress Report no. 24.*

KATSUKI, Y., SUGA, N. and KANNO, Y. 1962: Neural mechanism of the peripheral and central auditory system in monkeys. *Journal Acoustical Society of America* 34, 1396–1410.

KATZ, J. 1962: The use of staggered spondaic words for assessing the integrity of the central auditory neurons system. *Journal of Auditory Research* 2, 327–37.

KATZ, J. 1983: Phonemic synthesis. In Lasky, E.Z. and Katz, J. (eds.) *Central auditory processing disorders* (Baltimore: University Park Press, 269–95).

KATZ, J., BASIL, R.A. and SMITH, J.M. 1963: A staggered spondaic word test for detecting central auditory lesions. *Annals of Otology, Rhinology and Laryngology* 72, 906–17.

KEARSLEY, R.B. 1973: The newborn's responses to auditory stimulation: a demonstration of orienting and defensive behaviours. *Child Development* 44, 582–90.

KEITH, R.W. 1981: Audiological and auditory-language tests of central auditory function. In Keith, R.W. (ed.), *Central auditory and language disorders in children* (San Diego: College Hill Press).

KENWORTHY, O.T., KLEE, T. and THORPE, A.M. 1990: Speech recognition ability of children with unilateral sensorineural hearing loss as a function of amplification, Speech stimuli and listening condition. *Ear and Hearing* 11.

KERSLEY, J.A. and WICKHAM, H. 1966: Exudative otitis media in children. *J.*

Laryngol. and Otol. 80, 26–41.

KIANG, N.Y. 1968: A survey of recent developments in the study of auditory physiology. *Annals of Otology, Rhinology and Laryngology* 77, 657–75.

KIANG, N.Y., MOXON, E.C. and LEVINE, R.A. 1970: Auditory nerve activity in cats with normal and abnormal cochleas. In Wolstenholme, G. and Knight, J. (eds.), *Sensorineural hearing loss* (London: Churchill, 241–68).

KIANG, N.Y., WATANABE, T., THOMAS, E.C. and CLARK, L.F. 1965: Discharge patterns of single fibres in the cat's auditory nerve. *Research Monograph*, No. 35. Cambridge, Mass: MIT Press.

KIMURA, D. 1961: Some effects of temporal lobe damage on auditory perception. *Canadian Journal of Psychology* 15, 156–65.

KIMURA, D. 1964: Left-right differences in the perception of melodies. *Quarterly Journal of Experimental Psychology* 16, 355–8.

KIRK, S.A., MCCARTHY, J.J. and KIRK, W.D. 1968: *Illinois Test of Psycholinguistic Abilities*. Urbana: University of Illinois Press.

KLEIN, J.O. 1978: Epidemiology of otitis media. In Harford, E.R., Bess F.H., Bluestone, C.D. and Klein, J.O. (eds.) *Impedance screening for middle ear disease in children* (New York: Grune and Stratton, 11–16).

KLEIN, S.K. and RAPIN, I. 1988: Intermittent conductive hearing loss and language development. In Bishop, D.V.M. and Mogford, K. (eds.) *Language development in exceptional circumstances* (London: Churchill Livingstone).

KLUMPP, R.G. and EADY, H.R. 1956: Some measurements of interaural time difference thresholds. *Journal of the Acoustical Society of America* 28, 859–960.

KOBAYASHI, K., KODAMA, H., TAKEZAWA, H., SUZIKI, T. and KATAURA, A. 1988: Elevation of bone conduction threshold in children with middle ear effusion. *International Journal of Pediatric Otorhinolaryngology* 16, 95–100.

KOGAN, K.L., WIMBERGER, H.C. and BOBBITT, R.A. 1969: Analysis of mother–child interactions in young mental retardates. *Child Development* 40, 799–812.

KOKKO, E. 1975: Chronic secretory otitis media in children. *Acta Otol.* Supplement 327.

KRETSCHMER, R.E. and KRETSCHMER, L. 1978: *Language development and intervention with the hearing impaired*. Baltimore: University Park Press.

KRYTER, K.D., WILLIAMS, C. and GREEN, D.M. 1962: Auditory acuity and the perception of speech. *Journal of the Acoustical Society of America* 34, 1217–23.

KUHL, P.K. 1986: Reflections on infants' perception and representation of speech. In Perkell, J.S. and Klatt, D.H. (eds.) *Invariance and variability in speech processes*. (Hillside, NJ: Erlbaum).

KUHL, P.K. and MILLER, J.D. 1982: Discrimination of auditory target dimensions in the presence or absence of variation in a second dimension by infants. *Perception and Psychophysics* 31, 279–92.

KYLE, J.G. 1978: The study of auditory deprivation from birth. *British Journal of Audiology* 12, 37–9.

KYLE, J.G. 1980: Reading development of deaf children. *Journal of Research in*

Reading 3, 86–97.

LASKY, R., SYRDAZ-LASKY, A. and KLEIN, D. 1975: Vowel discrimination by 4 to 6 month old infants from Spanish environment. *Journal of Experimental Child Psychology* 20, 215–25.

LAUTER, J. 1982: Dichotic identification of complex sounds: absolute and relative ear advantage. *Journal of the Acoustical Society of America* 21, 701–7.

LAWRENCE, M. and YANTIS, P.A. 1956: Thresholds of overload in normal and pathological ears. *Archives of Otolaryngology* 63, 67–77.

LEAVITT, L.A., BROWN, J.W., MORSE, P.A. and GRAHAM, F.K. 1976: Cardiac orienting and auditory discrimination in six-week infants. *Development Psychology* 12, 514–23.

LEE, L.L. 1969: *The Northwestern Syntax Screening Test*. Evanston, Ill.: Northwestern University Press.

LEE, L.L. and CANTER, S.M. 1971: Development sentence scoring: a clinical procedure for estimating syntax development in children's spontaneous speech. *Journal of Speech and Hearing Disorders* 36, 315–40.

LEHMANN, M.D., CHARRON, K., KUMMER, A. and KEITH, R.W. 1979: The effect of chronic middle-ear effusion on speech and language development: a descriptive study. *Int. J. of Paediatric Otorhinolarynogology* 1, 137–44.

LENNEBERG, E.H. 1967: *The biological foundations of language*, New York: Wiley.

LEONARD, L.B., NEWHOFF, M. and MESSALAM, L. 1980: Individual differences in early child phonology. *Journal of Applied Psycholinguistics* 1, 7–30.

LESHOWITZ, B. and LINDSTROM, R. 1977: Measurement of non-linearities in listeners with sensorineural hearing loss. In Evans, E.F. and Wilson, J.P. (eds.) *Psychophysics and physiology of hearing* (London: Academic Press, 283–92).

LEVENTHAL, A.S. and LIPSITT, L.P. 1964: Adaptation, pitch discrimination and sound localisation in the neonate. *Child Development* 35, 759–67.

LEVITT, H. and RESNICK, S.B. 1978: Speech reception by the hearing impaired: methods of testing and the development of new tests. In Ludzingen, C. and Barfod, J. (eds.), *Sensorineural hearing impairment and hearing aids, Scandinavian Audiology* Supplement 6, 107–30.

LEWIS, M. 1971: Individual differences in the measurement of early cognitive growth. In Hellmuth, J. (ed.) *Exceptional Infant Vol. 2 Studies in abnormalities* (N.Y. Brunner/Mazel, 172–210).

LEWIS, N. 1976: Otitis media and linguistic incompetence. *Annals Otol.* 102, 387–90.

LIBERMAN, A.M. 1981: On finding that speech in special. *Haskins Laboratories: Status Report on Speech Research* SR-67/68, 107–43.

LIBERMAN, A.M., DELATTRE, P.C. and COOPER, F.S. 1952: The role of selected stimulus variables in the perception of the unvoiced stop consonants. *American Journal of Psychology* 65, 497–516.

LIBERMAN, A.M., HARRIS, K.S., HOFFMAN, H.S. and GRIFFITH, B.C. 1957: The discrimination of speech sounds within and across phoneme boundaries.

Journal of Experimental Psychology 54, 358–68.

LIBERMAN, A.M., INGEMANN, F., LISKER, L., DELATTRE, P. and COOPER, F.S. 1959: Minimal rules for synthesizing speech. *Journal of the Acoustical Society of America* 31, 1490–9.

LIBERMAN, A.M., COOPER, F.S., SHANKWEILER, D.P. and STUDDERT-KENNEDY, M. 1967: Perception of the speech code. *Psychological Review* 74, 431–61.

LIBERMAN, M.C. and KIANG, N. 1978: Acoustic trauma in cats. *Acta Otolaryngologica* Supplement 358, 1–63.

LICKLIDER, J.C.F. 1954: Periodicity pitch and place pitch. *Journal of the Acoustical Society of America* 26, 945.

LILDHOLDT, T., COURTOIS, J., KORTHOLM, B., SCHOU, J.W. and WARRER, H. 1979: The correlation between negative middle-ear pressure and the corresponding conductive hearing loss in children. *Scandinavian Audiology* 8, 117–20.

LING, D. 1968: Three experiments on frequency transposition. *American Annals of the Deaf* 113, 283–94.

LING, D. 1972: Rehabilitation of cases with deafness secondary to otitis media. In Glorig, A., Gerwin, K.S. (eds.) *Otitis media proceedings of the national conference*, (Springfield, Ill: Charles C. Thomas, 249–53).

LISKER, L. and ABRAMSON, A.S. 1964: A cross-language study of voicing in initial stops: acoustical measurements. *Word* 20, 384–422.

LISKER, L. and ABRAMSON, A.S. 1970: The voicing dimension: some experiments in comparative phonetics. In *Proceedings of the 6th international congress of phonetic science*, (Prague: Academia, 563–7).

LOCKE, J.L. and LOCKE, V.L. 1971: Deaf children's phonetic, visual and dactylic coding in a grapheme recall task. *Journal of Experimental Psychology* 89, 142–6.

LOWE, J.F., BAMFORTH, J.S. and PRACY, R. 1963: Acute otitis media: one year in a general practice. *Lancet* 1129–33.

LUDLOW, C.L., CUDAHY, E.A., BASSICH, C. *et al.* 1983: Auditory processing skills of hyperactive, language-impaired, and reading disabled boys. In Lasky, E.Z. and Katz, J. (eds.) *Central auditory processing disorders* (Baltimore, MD: University Park Press) 163–84.

LYNN, G. and GILROY, J. 1972: Neuroaudiological abnormalities in patients with temporal lobe tumors. *Journal of Neurological Science* 17, 167–72.

LYNN, G.E., BENITEZ, J.T., EISENBREY, A.B., GILROY, J. and WILNER, H.T. 1972: Neuroaudiological correlates in cerebral hemisphere lesions. *Audiology* 7, 66–75.

MACGINITIE, W.H. 1964: Ability of deaf children to use different word classes. *Journal of Speech and Hearing Research* 7, 141–50.

MACKAIN, K.S. 1982: Assessing the role of experience on infants' speech discrimination. *Journal of Child Language* 9, 527–42.

MACKEITH, N.W. and COLES, R.R.A. 1971: Binaural advantages in hearing of speech. *Journal of Laryngology and Otology* 85, 213–32.

MACRAE, J.H. and BRIGDEN, D.N. 1973: Auditory threshold impairment and everyday speech reception. *Audiology* 12, 272–90.

MALLES, I. 1963: Hearing aid effect in unilateral conductive deafness. *Archives of Otolaryngology* 77, 406–8.

MANN, V.A., MADDEN, J. RUSSELL, J.M. and LIBERMAN, A.M. 1981: Further investigation into the influence of preceeding liquids on stop consonant perception. *Journal of the Acoustical Society of America* 69, Supplement 1 (abstract).

MARCEL, A.J. 1974: The effective visual field and the use of context in fast and slow readers of two ages. *British Journal of Psychology* 65, 479–92.

MARCEL, A.J., KATZ, L. and SMITH, M. 1974: Laterality and reading proficiency. *Neuropsychologia* 12, 131–9.

MARCELLINO, G.R. 1981: Neonatal hearing screening utilizing microprocessor technology – a progress report. *Hearing Instruments* 32, 12–14.

MARCOTTE, A.C and La BARBA, R.C. 1985: Cerebral lateralization for speech in deaf and normal children. *Brain and Language* 26, 244–58.

MARKIDES, A. 1977: *Binaural hearing aids.* London: Academic Press.

MARTIN, F.N. and CLARK, J.G. 1977: Audiologic detection of auditory processing disorders in children. *Journal of the American Audiology Society* 3, 140–6.

MARTIN, J.A.M. 1982: Aetiological factors relating to childhood deafness in the European Community. *Audiology* 21, 149–158.

MARTIN, J.A.M. 1983: Normal patterns of early vocalization and their significance for the deaf child. *Proceedings of the IV British conference on audiology,* London.

MARTIN, M.C. 1973: Hearing aid gain requirements in sensorineural hearing loss. *British Journal of Audiology* 7, 21–4.

MARTIN, M.C. 1974: Critical bands in sensori-neural hearing loss. *Scandinavian Audiology* 3, 133–40.

MASTERS, L. and MARSH, G.E. 1978: Middle ear pathology as a factor in learning disabilities. *Journal of Learning Disabilities* 11, 54–7.

MATKIN, N.D. and HOOK, P.E. 1983: A multidisciplinary approach to central auditory evaluations. In Lasky, E.J. and Katz, J. (eds.) *Central auditory processing disorders.* (Baltimore: University Park Press).

MATZKER, J. 1959: Two new methods for the assessment of central auditory functions in cases of brain disease. *Annals of Otology, Rhinology and Laryngology* 68, 1185–97.

MAULDIN, L. and JERGER, J. 1979: Auditory brainstem evoked responses to bone conducted signals. *Arch. Otolaryngology* 105, 656–61.

McCORMICK, B., CURNOCK, D.A. and SPAVINS, F. 1984a: Auditory screening of special care neonates using the auditory response cradle. *Archives of Disease in Childhood* 59, 1168–72.

McCORMICK, B., WOOD, S.A., COPE, Y. and SPAVINS, F.M. 1984b: Analysis of records from an open access audiology service. *British Journal of Audiology* 18, 127–32.

McGURK, H., TUNMORE, C. and CREIGHTON, S.J. 1977: Auditory visual coordination in neonates. *Child Development* 48, 138–43.

McKIRDY, L.S. and BLANK, M. 1973: Dialogue in deaf and hearing pre-schoolers.

Journal of Speech and Hearing Research 25, 487–99.

McTEAR, M.F. 1981: Investigating children's conversational development. *First Language* 2, 117–30.

MEDICAL RESEARCH COUNCIL: 1957: Acute otitis in general practice: report of a survey by the Medical Research Council Party for research in general practice. *Lancet,* vol. 2, 14th September, 510–14.

MENYUK, P. 1979: Design factors in the assessment of language development in children with otitis media. *Annals of Otology, Rhinology and Laryngology Supplement* 60, 78–87.

MENYUK, P. and MENN, L. 1979: Early strategies for the perception and production of words and sounds. In Fletcher, P. and Garman, M. (eds), *Language acquisition* (Cambridge: Cambridge University Press, 49–70).

MERRILL, E.C. 1979: A deaf presence in education. *Proceedings of the 8th world congress of the world federation of the deaf,* 194–5.

MILLER, G.A. and LICKLIDER, J.C.R. 1950: The intelligibility of interrupted speech. *Journal of the Acoustical Society of America* 22, 167–73.

MILLER, C.L. and MORSE, P.A. 1979: Selective adaptation effects in infant speech perception paradigms. *Journal of the Acoustical Society of America* 65 (3), 789–98.

MILLER, G.A. and NICELY, P.E. 1955: An analysis of perceptual confusions among some English consonants. *Journal of the Acoustical Society of America* 27, 338–52.

MILLS, J. 1977: Noise and children: a review of the literature. *Journal of the Acoustical Society of America* 58, 767–79.

MOFFITT, A.R. 1971: Consonant cue perception by 20–24 week old infants. *Child Development* 42, 717–32.

MOFFITT, A.R. 1972: Intensity discrimination and cardiac reaction in young infants. *Developmental Psychology* 8, 357–9.

MOGFORD, K. 1988: Oral language acquisition in the prelingually deaf. In Bishop, D. and Mogford, K. (eds.), *Language development in exceptional circumstances* (London: Churchill Livingstone).

MOGFORD, K. and BISHOP, D. 1988: Language development in unexceptional circumstances. In Bishop, D. and Mogford, K. (eds.), *Language development in exceptional circumstances* (London: Churchill Livingstone).

MOORE, B.C.J. 1989: *An introduction to the psychology of hearing.* London: Academic Press.

MOORE, B.C.J. and GLASBERG, B.R. 1982: Interpreting the role of suppression in psychophysical tuning curves. *Journal of the Acoustical Society of America* 68, 814–25.

MOORE, B.C.J. and GLASBERG, B.R. 1983: Suggested formulae for calculating auditory-filter bandwidths and excitation patterns. *Journal of the Acoustical Society of America* 74, 750–3.

MOORE, B.C.J., GLASBERG, B.R., HESS, R.F. and BIRCHALL, J.P. 1985: Effects of flanking noise bands on the rate of growth of loudness of tones in normal and recruiting ears. *Journal of the Acoustical Society of North America* 77, 1505–13.

MOORE, J.M. and WILSON, W.R. 1978: Visual reinforcement audiometry (VRA) with infants. In Gerber, S.E. and Mencher, G.T. (eds.) *Early diagnosis of hearing loss*. (New York: Grune and Stratton).

MOORE, J.M., WILSON, W.R. and THOMPSON, G. 1977: Visual reinforcement of head-turn responses in infants under 12 months of age. *Journal of Speech and Hearing Disorders* 42, 328–38.

MORALES-GARCIA, C. and POOLE, J.P. 1972: Masked speech audiometry in central deafness. *Acta Otolaryngologica* 74, 307–16.

MORRIS, T. 1978: Some observations on the part played by oral teaching methods in perpetuating low standards of language achievement in severely and pro-foundly deaf pupils. *Journal of the British Association of Teachers of the Deaf* 2, 130–5.

MORSE, P.A. 1972: The discrimination of speech and non-speech stimuli in early infancy. *Journal of Experimental Child Psychology* 14, 477–92.

MOSCOVITCH, M. 1977: The development of lateralisation of language function and its relation to cognitive and linguistic development: a review and some theoretical speculations. In Segalowitz, S. and Gruber, F. (eds.) *Language, Developmental and Neurological Theory*, (N.Y.: Academic Press, Inc.).

MUIR, D. and FIELD, J. 1979: Newborn infant's orientation to sounds. *Child Development* 50, 431–6.

MUIR, D., ABRAHAM, W., FORBES, B. and HARRIS, L. 1979: The otogenesis of an auditory localization response from birth to 4 months. *Canadian Journal of Psychology* 33(4), 320–33.

MULLINS, C.J. and BANGS, J.L. 1957: Relationships between speech discrimination and other audiometric data. *Acta Otolaryngologica* 47, 149–57.

MUSIEK, F.E. 1983: Assessment of three dichotic speech tests on subjects with intra-cranial lesions, *Ear and Hearing* 4, 318–23.

MUSIEK, F.E. 1986: Neuroanatomy, neurophysiology, and central auditory assessment. Part II: The cerebrum. *Ear and Hearing* 7, 283–94.

MUSIEK, F.E. and BARAN, J.A. 1986: Neuroanatomy, neurophysiology, and central auditory assessment. Part I: Brain stem. *Ear and Hearing* 7, 207–19.

MUSIEK, F.E. and PINHEIRO, M.L. 1985: Dichotic speech tasks in the detection of central auditory dysfunction. In Pinheiro, M.L. and Musiek, F.E. (eds) *Assessment of Central Auditory Dysfunction* (Baltimore, MD: Williams and Wilkins, 143–54).

MUSIEK, F.E., GEURKINK, N. and KEITEL, S. 1982: Test battery assessment of auditory perceptual dysfunction in children. *Laryngoscope* 92, 251–7.

MUSIEK, F.E., GOLLEGLY, K. and BARAN, J.A. 1984: Myelination of the corpus callosum and auditory processing problems in children: Theoretical and clinical correlates. *Seminars in Hearing* 5, 231–41.

MYKLEBUST, H.R. 1954: *Auditory Disorders in Children*. New York: Grune and Stratton.

MYKLEBUST, H.R. 1960: The psychological effects of deafness. *American Annals of the Deaf* 105, 372–85.

MYKLEBUST, H.R. 1964: *The Psychology of Deafness*. New York: Grune and Stratton.

MYKLEBUST, H.R. and BRUTTEN, M. 1952: A study of the visual performance of deaf children. *Acta Otolaryngologica* Supplement 105.

NABALEK, I.V. 1978: Temporal summation of constant and gliding tones at masked auditory threshold. *Journal of the Acoustical Society of America* 64, 751–63.

NDCS, 1983: *Discovering deafness.* London: National Deaf Children's Society.

NEEDLEMAN, H. 1977: Effects of hearing loss from early recurrent otitis media on speech and language development. In Jaffe, B. (ed.) *Hearing loss in children* (Baltimore: University Park Press, 640–9).

NEISSER, U. 1967: *Cognitive Psychology.* New York: Appleton-Century-Crofts.

NELSON, D.A. and BILGER, R.C. 1974: Pure tone octave masking in listeners with sensorineural hearing loss. *Journal of Speech and Hearing Research* 17, 252–69.

NELSON, K. 1973: Structure and strategy in learning to talk. *Monograph of the Society for Research in Child Development*, 38.

NEWTON, V.E. 1983: Sound localization in children with a severe unilateral hearing loss. *Audiology* 22, 189–98.

NEWTON, V.E. 1985: Aetiology of bilateral sensorineural hearing loss in young children. *Journal of Laryngology and Otology*, Supplement 10.

NICE, M.M. 1915: The development of a child's vocabulary in relation to environment. *Pedagogic seminars* 22, 36–64.

NOBACK, C.R. 1985: Neuroanatomical correlates of central auditory function. In Pinheiro, M.L. and Musiek, F.E. (eds.), *Assessment of central auditory dysfunction* (Baltimore, MD: Williams & Wilkins) 7–22.

NOFFSINGER, D., OLSEN, W.D., CARHART, R., HART, C.W. and SAHGAL, V. 1972: Auditory and vestibular aberrations in multiple sclerosis. *Acta Otolaryngologica* Supp. 303.

NORDLUND, B. 1964: Directional audiometry. *Acta Otolaryngologica* 57, 1–18.

NORLIN, P.F. and VAN TASELL, D.J. 1980: Linguistic skills of hearing-impaired children. *Monographs in Contemporary Audiology* Volume 2 No. 4.

NORTHERN, J.L. and DOWNS, M.P. 1978: *Hearing in Children.* Baltimore: Williams and Wilkins.

ODOM, P.B. and BLANTON, R.L. 1967: Phrase-learning in deaf and hearing subjects. *Journal of Speech and Hearing Research* 10, 600–5.

OLLER, D.K., WIEMAN, L.A., DOYLE, W.J., and ROSS, C. 1976: Infant babbling and speech. *Journal of Child Language* 3, 1–11.

OLSEN, G.M. 1973: Developmental changes in memory and the acquisition of language. In Moore, T.E. (ed.) *Cognitive development and the acquisition of language.* (N.Y.: Academic Press, 145–57).

OLSHO, L.W., SCHOON, C, SAKAI, R, TURPIN, R. and SPERDUTO, V. 1982: Preliminary data on frequency discrimination in infancy. *Journal of Acoustical Society of America* 71, 509–11.

OWENS, E. and SCHUBERT, E.D. 1968: The development of constant items for speech discrimination testing. *Journal of Speech and Hearing Research* 11, 656–67.

OWRID, H.L. 1960: Measuring spoken language in young deaf children. *Teacher of the Deaf* 58, 24–34, 124–9.

OWRID, H.L. 1970: Hearing impairment and verbal attainments in primary school children. *Education Research* 12, 209–14.

PARADISE, J.L. 1981: Otitis media during early life. How hazardous to development? A critical review of the evidence. *Pediatrics* 68, 868–73.

PARADISE, J.L., SMITH, C.G. and BLUESTONE, C.D. 1977: Tympanometric detection of middle ear effusion in infants and young children. *Pediatrics* 58, 198–210.

PARADY, S., DORMAN, M.H., WHALEY, P. and RAPHAEL, L.J. 1981: Identification and discrimination of synthesized voicing contrast by normal and sensorineural hearing-impaired children. *Journal of the Acoustical Society of America* 69, 783–90.

PARVING, A. 1983: Epidemiology of hearing loss and aetiological diagnosis of hearing impairment in childhood. *International Journal of Pediatric Otorhinolaryngology* 5, 151–65.

PASCOE, D.P. 1978: An approach to hearing-aid selection. *Hearing Instruments* 12–16, 36.

PATTERSON, R.D. 1973: The effects of relative phase and the number of components on residue pitch. *Journal of the Acoustical Society of America* 53, 1565–72.

PATTERSON, R.D. 1974: Auditory filter shape. *Journal of the Acoustical Society of America* 55, 802–9.

PATTERSON, R.D. 1976: Auditory filter shapes derived with noise stimuli. *Journal of the Acoustical Society of America* 59, 640–54.

PATTERSON, R.D. and MILROY, R. 1981: Ageing and the shape of the auditory filter. Paper to British Society of Audiology, Manchester.

PATTERSON, R.D. and MOORE, B.C.J. 1985: Auditory filters and excitation patterns as representations of frequency resolution. In Moore, B.C.J (ed), *Frequency selectivity in hearing*, (London: Academic Press) 123–77.

PATTISON, H. 1983: Literacy skills in hearing-impaired children. Unpublished Ph.D. thesis, University of Reading.

PEARSON, J.C.G. 1977: Prediction of presbyacusis. *Journal of Social and Occupational Medicine* 27, 125–33.

PEARSON, P.D. and JOHNSON, D.D 1978: *Teaching reading comprehension*. New York: Holt Rinehart and Winston.

PEDERSEN, B.C. and PULSEN, T. 1973: Loudness of brief tones in hearing-impaired ears. *Acta Otolaryngologica* 76, 402–9.

PHIPPARD, D. 1977: Hemifield differences in visual perception in deaf and hearing subjects. *Neuropsychologia* 15, 555–61.

PIAGET, J. 1952: *The language and thought of the child*. London: Routledge und Kegan Paul.

PICK, G.F., EVANS, E.F. and WILSON, J.P. 1977: Frequency resolution in patients with hearing loss of cochlear origin. In Evans, E.F. and Wilson, J.P. (eds.), *Psychophysics and physiology of hearing* (London: Academic Press, 273–83).

PICKETT, J.M., MARTIN, E.S., JOHNSON, D., SMITH, S.B., DANIEL, Z., WILLIS, D. and OTIS, W. 1972: On patterns of speech feature reception of deaf listeners. In Fant, G. (ed.), *Speech communication ability and profound deafness*

(Washington, DC: A.G. Bell, 119–33).

PICKLES, J.O. 1982: *An introduction to the physiology of hearing.* London and New York: Academic Press.

PINHEIRO, M.L. 1977: Tests of central auditory function in children with learning disabilities. In Keith, R.W. (ed.), *Central auditory dysfunction* (New York: Grune and Stratton).

PINHEIRO, M.L. 1978: A central auditory test profile of learning disabled children with dyslexia. *Communicative disorders: An auditory journal for continuing education* (New York: Grune and Stratton).

PINTNER, R. 1928. Psychological survey. In Day, H.E., Fusfeld, I.S. and Pintner, R. (eds.). *A survey of American schools for the deaf* (Washington D.C.: National Research Council, 252–89).

PISONI, D.B. 1973: Auditory and phonetic memory codes in the discrimination of consonants and vowels. *Perception and Psychophysics.* 13, 253–60.

PISONI, D.B. 1977: Identification and discrimination of the relative onset of two-component tones: implications for voicing perception in stops. *Journal of the Acoustical Society of America* 61, 1352–61.

PISONI, D.B. 1980: Adaptation of the relative onset time of two-component tones. *Perception and Psychophysics* 28, 337–46.

PLAKKE, B., ORCHIK, D. and BEASLEY, D. 1981: Children's performance on a binaural fusion task. *Journal of Speech and Hearing Research* 24, 520–5.

PLOMP, R. 1981: Perception of sound signals at low signal-to-noise ratios. In Getty, D.J. and Howard, J.H. (eds.), *Auditory and visual pattern recognition* (Hillsdale, N.J.: Lawrence Erlbaum, 27–35).

POLLACK, I. 1948: Monaural and binaural threshold sensitivity for tones and white noise. *Journal of the Acoustical Society of America* 20, 52–8.

POLLACK, I. and PICKETT, J.M. 1958: Stereophonic listening and speech intelligibility against voice babble. *Journal of the Acoustical Society of America* 30, 131–3.

POLLACK, I. and PICKETT, J.M. 1963: The intelligibility of excerpts from conversation. *Language and Speech* 6, 165–71.

POLLARD, G. and NEUMAIER, R. 1974: Vision characteristics of deaf students. *American Annals of the Deaf* 110, 740–5.

PORTER, R.J. Jr. and BERLIN, C.J. 1975: On interpreting developmental changes in dichotic right ear advantage. *Brain and Language* 2, 186–200.

POWER, D.J. and QUIGLEY, S.P. 1973: Deaf children's acquisition of the passive voice. *Journal of Speech and Hearing Research* 16, 5–11.

POWERS, G.L. and WILCOX, J.C. 1977: Intelligibility of temporally interrupted speech with and without intervening noise. *Journal of the Acoustical Society of America* 61; 195–9.

PRESSNELL, L.M. 1973: Hearing-impaired children's comprehension and production of syntax in oral language. *Journal of Speech and Hearing Research* 16, 12–21.

PROTTI, E. 1983: Brainstem auditory pathways and auditory processing disorders. In Lasky, E.Z. and Katz, J. (eds.) *Central auditory processing disorders,*

(Baltimore: University Park Press).

PROTTI, E. and YOUNG, M. 1980: The evaluation of a child with auditory perceptual deficiencies: an inter-disciplinary approach. *Seminars in Speech, Language and Hearing* 1, 167–80.

PUNCH, J.L. and BECK, E.L. 1980: Low-frequency response of hearing aids and judgements of aided speech quality. *Journal of Speech and Hearing Disorders* 45, 325–35.

PUNCH, J.L., MONTGOMERY, A.A., SCHWARTZ, D.M., WALDEN, B.E., PROSEK, R.A. and HOWARD, M.T. 1980: Multidimensional scaling of quality judgements of speech signals processed by hearing aids. *Journal of the Acoustical Society of America* 68, 458–66.

QUIGLEY, S.P. and KRETSCHMER, R.E. 1982: *The education of deaf children.* Baltimore: University Park Press.

QUIGLEY, S.P. and POWER, D.J. 1972: The development of syntactic structures in the language of deaf children. Report from Institute for Research on Exceptional Children, University of Illinois.

QUIGLEY, S.P., MONTANELLI, D.S. and WILBUR, R.B. 1976b: Some aspects of the verb system in the language of deaf students. *Journal of Speech and Hearing Research* 19, 536–50.

QUIGLEY, S.P., SMITH, N.L. and WILBUR, R.B. 1974a: Comprehension of relativized sentences by deaf children. *Journal of Speech and Hearing Research* 17, 325–41.

QUIGLEY, S.P., WILBUR, R.B. and MONTANELLI, D.S. 1976a: Complement structures in the language of deaf students. *Journal of Speech and Hearing Research* 19, 448–57.

QUIGLEY, S.P., WILBUR, R.B. and MONTANELLI, D.S. 1974b: Question formation in the language of deaf students. *Journal of Speech and Hearing Research* 17, 699–713.

RACH, G.H., ZIELHUIS, G.A. and VAN DEN BROEK, P.D. 1988: The influence of chronic persistent otitis media with effusion on language development of 2- to 4-year olds. *International Journal of Pediatric Otorhinolaryngology* 15, 253–61.

REAMER, J.C. 1921: Mental and educational measurements of the deaf. *Psychological Monographs* 29.

REAY, E.W. 1947: A comparison between deaf and hearing children in regard to the use of verbs and nouns in compositions describing a short motion picture story. *American Annals of the Deaf* 91, 453–91.

REDGATE, G.W. 1972: *The teaching of reading to deaf children.* Manchester: University of Manchester Press.

REED, J.C. 1967: Lateralized finger agnosia and reading achievement at ages six and ten. *Child Development* 38, 247.

REES, N.S. 1981: Saying more than we know: is auditory processing disorder a meaningful concept? In Keith, R.W. (ed.), *Central auditory and language disorders in children* (San Diego: College-Hill Press, 94–120).

REMEZ, R.E., RUBIN, P.E., PISONI, D.B. and CARRELL, T.D. 1981: Speech perception without traditional speech cues. *Science* 212, 947–50.

RENTSCHER, G.I., RUPP, R.R. and PRESLEY, M. 1980: Screening selective auditory deficits in speech and language impaired children. *Journal of Auditory Research* 20, 271–8.

RENVALL, U., LIDEN, G., JUNGERT, S. and NILSSON, E. 1975: Impedance audiometry in the detection of secretory otitis media. *Scandinavian Audiology* 4, 119–24.

REVOILE, S., PICKETT, J.M., HOLDEN, L.D. and TALKIN, D. 1982: Acoustic cues to final stop voicing for impaired- and normal-hearing listeners *Journal of the Acoustical Society of America* 72, 1145–54.

RHODE, W.S. 1971: Observations on the vibration of the basilar membrane in squirrel monkeys using the Mossbauer technique. *Journal of the Acoustical Society of America* 49, 1218–31.

RICHARDS, S.H., KILBY, D. and SHAW, I.D. 1971: Grommets and glue ears; a clinical trial. *Journal of Laryngology and Otolargyngology* 83, 17–22.

RICHARDSON, S.O. 1981: A pediatricians's view of central auditory disorders: bridging the gap between diagnosis and treatment. In Keith, R.W. (ed.), *Central auditory and language disorders in children* (San Diego: College Hill Press, 85–93).

RITTMANIC, P.A. 1962: Pure tone masking by narrow noise bands in normal and impaired ears. *Journal of Auditory Research* 2, 287–304.

ROBERTS, J.E., SANYAL, M.A., BURCHINAL, M.R., COLLIER, A.M., RAMEY, C.Y. and HENDERSON, F.W. 1986: Otitis medis in early childhood and its relationship to later verbal and academic performance. *Pediatrics* 78, 423–30.

ROBERTSON, E, PETERSON, J. and LAMB, C. 1968: Relative impedance measurements in young children. *Archives of Otolaryngology* 88, 162–8.

RODGON, M.M. 1976: *Single-word usage, cognitive development and the beginnings of combinatorial speech.* Cambridge: Cambridge University Press.

ROSE, J.E., BRUGGE, J.F., ANDERSON, D.J. and HIND, J.E. 1967: Phase-locked response to low-frequency tones in single auditory nerve fibres of the squirrel monkey. *Journal of Neurophysiology* 30, 769–93.

ROSE, R.J., SOH, J., DUNCKEL, D.C. and ADAMS, R. 1977: Comparison of tympanometry and otoscopy in establishing pass/fail criteria. *Journal of American Audiological Society* 3, 20–5.

ROSEN, S.M. and FOURCIN, A.J. 1986: Frequency selectivity and the perception of speech. In Moore, B.C.J. (ed.) *Frequency selectivity in hearing* (London: Academic Press).

ROUSH, J. and TAIT, C.A. 1984: Binaural fusion, masking level differences, and auditory brain-stem responses in children with language-learning disabilities. *Ear and Hearing* 5, 37–41.

RUBEN, R.J. 1980: A review of transneuronal changes of the auditory central nervous system as a consequence of auditory defects. *International Journal of Pediatric Otorhinolaryngology* 1, 269–77.

RUSSELL, I.J. and SELLICK, P.M. 1978: Intracellular studies of hair cells in the mammalian cochlea. *Journal of Physiology* 284, 261–90.

RUTHERFORD, W. 1886: A new theory of hearing. *Journal of Anatomy and Physiology* 21, 166–8.

SADE, J. 1979: Inflammatory and non-inflammatory factors related to secretory otitis media. *International Journal of Pediatric Otolaryngology* 1, 41–59.

SAK, R. and RUBEN, R.J. 1981: Recurrent middle-ear effusion in childhood: implication of temporary auditory deprivation for language learning. *Annals of Otology, Rhinology, and Laryngology* 89, 303–11.

SALAMY, A, MENDLESON, T. and TOOLEY, W.H. 1982: Developmental profiles of the brainstem auditory evoked potential. *Early Human Development* 6, 331–9.

SANCHEZ-LONGO, L.P., FORSTER, F.M. and AUTH, T.L. 1957: A clinical test for sound localisation and its application. *Neurology* 7, 655–63.

SANCHO, J., HUGHES, E., DAVIS, A. and HAGGARD, M. 1988: Epidemiological basis for screening hearing. In McCormick, B. (ed.) *Pediatric audiology 0– 5 years* (London: Taylor & Francis).

SANDEL, T.T., TEAS, D.C., FEDDERSON, W.E. and JEFFRESS, L.A. 1955: Localization of sound from single and paired sources. *Journal of the Acoustical Society of America* 27, 842–52.

SARACHAN-DEILY, A.B. and LOVE, R.J. 1974: Underlying grammatical rule structure in the deaf. *Journal of Speech and Hearing Research* 17, 689–98.

SAUNDERS, J.C., BOCK, G.R., JAMES, R. and CHEN, C.S. 1972: Effects of priming for audiogenic seizure on auditory evoked responses in the cochlear nucleus and inferior colliculus of BALB/C mice. *Exp. Neurol.* 37, 388–94.

SAVIN, H.B. and BEVER, T.G. 1970: The nonperceptual reality of the phoneme. *Journal of Verbal Learning and Verbal Bahaviour* 9, 295–302.

SCAIFE, B.K. and BRUNER, J.S. 1975: The capacity for joint visual attention in the infant. *Nature* 253, 265–6.

SCHARF, B. and HELLMAN, R.P. 1966: A model of loudness summation applied to impaired ears. *Journal of the Acoustical Society of America* 40, 71–8.

SCHLESINGER, H.S. and MEADOW, K.P. 1972: *Sound and sign: childhood deafness and mental health.* Berkeley: University of California Press.

SCHLESINGER, I.M. and NAMIR, L. (eds.) 1978: *Sign language of the deaf.* London: Academic Press.

SCHLIEPER, A., KISILEVSKY, H., MATTINGLY, S. and YORKE, L. 1985: Mild conductive hearing loss and language development: A one year follow-up study. *Developmental and Behavioural Pediatrics* 6, 65–8.

SCHNEIDER, B., TREHUB, S.E. and BULL, D. 1979: The development of basic auditory processes in infants. *Canadian Journal of Psychology* 33, 306–19.

SCHOENY, Z. and CARHART, R. 1971: Effects of unilateral Menière's disease on masking-level differences. *Journal of the Acoustical Society of America* 50, 1143–50.

SCHOUTEN, J.F. 1940: The residue and the mechanism of hearing. *Proceedings of the Koninklijke Nederlandse Akademie van Wetenschappen* 43, 991–9.

SEIGENTHALER, B.M. and STRAND, R. 1964: Audiogram-average methods and SRT scores. *Journal of the Acoustical Society of America* 36, 589–93.

SELLICK, P.M., PATUZZI, R. and JOHNSTONE, B.M. 1982: Measurement of basilar membrane motion in the guinea pig using the Mössbauer technique. *Journal of the Acoustical Society of America* 72, 131–41.

SHAFER, D. and LYNCH, J. 1981: Emergent language of six prelingually deaf children. *Journal of the British Association of Teachers of the Deaf* 4, 94–111.

SHANKWEILER, D. and STUDDERT-KENNEDY, M. 1967: Identification of consonants and vowels presented to left and right ears. *Quarterly Journal of Experimental Psychology* 19, 59–63.

SHEPARD, N.T. 1983: Newborn hearing screening using the Linco-Bennett Auditory Response Cradle. *Ear and Hearing* 4, 5–10.

SILVA, P.A., KIRKLAND, C., SIMPSON, A., STEWART, I.A. and WILLIAMS, S.M. 1983: Some developmental and behavioural problems associated with bilateral otitis media with effusion. *Journal of Learning Disabilities* 15, 417–21.

SIMMONS, A.A. 1962: A comparison of the type-token ratio of spoken and written language of deaf and hearing children. *Volta Review* 64, 417–21.

SIMON, C. and FOURCIN, A.J. 1978: Cross language study of speech pattern learning. *Journal of the Acoustical Society of America* 63, 925–35.

SKINNER, B.F. 1957: *Verbal behaviour.* New York: Appleton-Century-Crofts.

SMITH, B.L. 1982: Some observations concerning premeaningful vocalizations of hearing-impaired infants. *Journal of Speech and Hearing Research* 47, 439–41.

SMITH, F. 1971: *Understanding reading.* New York: Holt, Rinehart and Winston.

SMITH, F. 1975: *Comprehension and learning.* New York: Holt, Rinehart and Winston.

SNOW, C. 1977: The development of conversation between mothers and babies. *Journal of Child Language* 4, 1–22.

SOKOLOV, A.N. 1972: *Inner speech and thought.* New York: Plenum Press.

SPEAKES, C., NICCUM, N. and CARNEY, E. 1982: Statistical properties of responses to dichotic listening with nonsense syllables. *Journal of the Acoustical Society of America* 72, 1185–94.

SPRING, D.R. and DALE, P.S. 1977: The discrimination of linguistic stress in early infancy. *Journal of Speech and Hearing Research* 20, 224–32.

STARR, A, AMLIE, R.N., MARTIN, W.H. and SANDERS, S. 1977: Development of auditory function in newborn infants revealed by auditory brainstem potentials. *Pediatrics* 60, 831–9.

STEPHENS, S.D.G. 1973: Some experiments on the detection of short duration stimuli. *British Journal of Audiology* 7, 81–97.

STERN, D. 1977: *The first relationship.* London: Fontana.

STEVENS, J.C., WEBB, H.D., HUTCHINSON, J., CONNELL, J., SMITH, M.F. and BUFFIN, J.T. 1989: Click evoked otoacoustic emissions compared with brainstem electric response. *Archives of Disease in Childhood* 64, 1105–11.

STEVENS, K.N. and KLATT, D.H. 1974: Role of formant transitions in the voiced-voiceless distinction for stops. *Journal of the Acoustical Society of America* 55, 653–9.

STEVENS, S.S. 1957: On the psychophysical law. *Psychological Review* 64, 153–81.

STEVENS, S.S. and NEWMAN, E.B. 1936: The localization of actual sources of sound. *American Journal of Psychology* 48, 297–306.

STOKES, J. 1990: Evaluation of an early language programme for hearing-impaired infants. *British Journal of Audiology* (in press).

STOKES, J. and BAMFORD, J.M. 1990: Transition from pre-linguistic to linguistic communication in hearing-impaired infants. *British Journal of Audiology* (in press).

STREETER, L.A. 1976a: Kikuyu labial and apical stop discrimination. *Journal of Phonetics* 4, 43–9.

STREETER, L.A. 1976b: Language perception of two-month-old infants shows effects of both innate mechanism and experience. *Nature* 259, 39–41.

STUDDERT-KENNEDY, M. 1976: Speech perception. In Lass, N.J. (ed.), *Contemporary issues in experimental phonetics* (New York: Academic Press, 243–93).

STUDDERT-KENNEDY, M. and SHANKWEILER, D. 1970: Hemispheric specialization for speech perception. *Journal of the Acoustical Society of America* 48, 579–94.

STUDDERT-KENNEDY, M, LIBERMAN, A.M., HARRIS, K.S., and COOPER, F.S.: 1970: Motor theory of speech perception: A reply to Lane's critical review. *Psychological Review* 77, 234–49.

SUMMERFIELD, Q. 1982: Differences between spectral dependencies in auditory and phonetic temporal processing. Relevance to the perception of voicing in initial stops. *Journal of the Acoustical Society of America* 72(1), 51–61.

SUMMERFIELD, Q., TYLER, R., FOSTER, J., WOOD, E. and BAILEY, P.J. 1981: Failure of formant-bandwidth-narrowing to improve speech reception in sensorineural impairments. *Paper to British Society of Audiology*.

SUPPLE, M. de M. 1983: Auditory perceptual function in relation to phonological development. *British Journal of Audiology* 17, 59–68.

SUZUKI, T. and OGIBA, Y. 1960: A technique of pure tone audiometry for children under three years of age. Conditioned orienting reflex (COR) audiometry. *Review Laryngology* 81, 33–43.

SWOBODA, P.J., MORSE, P.F. and LEAVITT, L. 1976: Continuous vowel discrimination in normal and at risk infants. *Child Development* 47, 459–65.

SWOBODA, P.J., KASS, J., MORSE, P.F. and LEAVITT, L.C. 1978: Memory factors in vowel discrimination of normal and at-risk infants. *Child Development* 49, 332–9.

TALLAL, P. 1976: Rapid auditory processing in normal and disordered language development. *Journal of Speech and Hearing Research* 19, 561–71.

TALLAL, P. 1980: Auditory processing disorders in children. In Levinson, P. and Sloan, C. (eds.) *Processing and language: clinical and research perspectivies* (London and N.Y.: Grune and Stratton, 81–100).

TALLAL, P. and NEWCOMBE, F. 1978: Impairment of auditory perception and language comprehension in dysphasia. *Brain and Language* 5, 13–24.

TALLAL, P. and PIERCY, M. 1975: Developmental aphasia: the perception of brief vowels and extended stop consonants. *Neuropsychologia* 13, 69–74.

TALLAL, P. and STARK, R.E. 1981: Speech acoustic-cue discrimination abilities of normally developing and language-impaired children. *Journal of the Acoustical Society of America* 69, 568–74.

TARKKANEN, J. and AHO, J. 1966: Unilateral deafness in children. *Acta otolaryngologia* 61, 270–8.

TASK FORCE ON IMPEDANCE SCREENING 1978: Report in Proceedings of the Symposium on Impedance Screening for Children. New York: Grune and Stratton.

TAYLOR, I.G. 1980: The prevention of congenital sensorineural deafness. In Taylor, I.G. and Markides, A. (eds.), *Disorders of auditory function III* (London: Academic Press, 25–31).

TEELE, D.W., KLEIN, J.O. and ROSNER, B.A. 1984: Otitis media with effusion during the first three years of life and development of speech and language. *Pediatrics* 74, 282–7.

TEES, R.C. 1967: The effects of early auditory restrictions in the rat on adult auditory discrimination. *Journal of Auditory Research* 7, 195–207.

TEMPLIN, M.C. 1966: Vocabulary problems of the deaf child. *International Audiology* 4, 349–54.

TENG, E.L. 1981: Dichotic ear difference is a poor index for the functional asymmetry between the cerebral hemispheres. *Neuropsychologia* 19, 235–40.

TERHAPDT, E. 1974: Pitch, consonance and harmony. *Journal of the Acoustical Society of America* 1061–69.

THATCHER, J. 1976: An analysis of the structure, function and content of the vocabularies of babies: the first hundred words. Unpublished MA thesis, University of Nottingham (quoted by Gregory and Mogford, 1981).

THYER, N. 1984: An investigation into the discrimination of unidirectional linear frequency transitions in normal and hearing-impaired listeners: acoustic and linguistic considerations. M.Sc. thesis, University of Southampton.

TILLMAN, T.W., KASTEN, R.N. and HORNER, J.S. 1963: Effect of head shadow on reception of speech. *Journal of the American Speech and Hearing Association* 5, 778–9.

TOBIAS, J.V. 1972: Curious binaural phenomena. In Tobias, J.V. (ed.), *Foundations of Modern Auditory Theory* (New York: Academic Press, 463–86).

TOBIN, H. 1985: Binaural interaction tasks. In Pinheiro, M.L. and Musiek, F.E. (eds.), *Assessment of central auditory dysfunction* (Baltimore, MD: Williams & Wilkins) 155–72.

TONNING, F. 1971: Directional audiometry, III. The influence of azimuth on the perception of speech in patients with monaural hearing loss. *Acta Otolaryngologica* 72, 404–12.

TONNING, F. 1972a: Directional audiometry, IV. The influence of azimuth on the perception of speech in aided and unaided patients with monaural hearing loss. *Acta Otolaryngologica* 73, 44–52.

TONNING, F. 1972b: Directional audiometry, VI. Directional speech audiometry in patients with practical deafness in one ear and impaired hearing in the other ear treated with hearing aids. *Acta Otolaryngologica* 74, 206–11.

TOS, M. and POULSEN, G. 1976: Secretory otitis media. *Archives of Otolaryngology* 102, 672-5.

TREHUB, S.E. 1973: Infants' sensitivity to vowel and tonal contrasts. *Developmental Psychology* 9, 91-6.

TREHUB, S.E. 1979: Reflections on the development of speech perception. *Canadian Journal of Psychology* 33(4), 368-81.

TREHUB, S.E., SCHNEIDER B.A. and ENDMAN, M. 1980: Developmental changes in infants, sensitivity to octave-band noises. *Journal of Experimental Child Psychology* 29, 282-93.

TREHUB, S.E., SCHNEIDER, B.A. and BULL, D. 1981: Effect of reinforcement on infants performance in an auditory detection task. *Development Psychology* 17, 872-7.

TREISMAN, A.M. 1960: Contextual cues in selective listening. *Quarterly Journal of Experimental Psychology* 12, 242-8.

TREVARTHEN, C. 1974: Conversations with a two month-old. *New Scientist* 62, 230-3.

TREVOORT, B. 1970: The understanding of passive sentences by deaf children. In D'Arcais, G.B.F. and Levett, W.J.M. (eds.), *Advances in psycholinguistics* (New York: American Elsevier, 166-73).

TUMIM, W. 1982: Intonation as a clue to first language learning in hearing-impaired children. *Paper to British Society of Audiology and College of Speech Therapists*, London.

TUREK, S.V. de G., DORMAN, K.F., FRANKS, J.R. and SUMMERFIELD, Q. 1980: Identification of synthetic /bdg/ by hearing-impaired listeners under monotic and dichotic formant presentation. *Journal of the Acoustical Society of America* 67, 1031-40.

TURKEWITZ, G, BIRCH, H.G., MOREAU, T, LEVY, L. and CORNWELL, A.C. 1966: Effect of intensity of auditory stimulation on directional eye movements in the human neonate. *Animal Behaviour* 14, 93-101.

TURNER, C.W. and NELSON, D.A. 1982: Frequency discrimination in regions of normal and impaired sensitivity. *Journal of Speech and Hearing Research* 25, 34-41.

TURNER, E.A. and ROMMETVEIT, R. 1967: The acquisition of sentence voice and reversibility. *Child Development* 38, 649-60.

TYLER, R.S. 1976: Temporal integration and cochlear hearing loss. *Human Communication* 4, 9-24.

TYLER, R.S. 1986: Frequency resolution in hearing-impaired listeners. In Moore, B.C.J. and Glasberg, B.R. (eds.), *Frequency selectivity in hearing* (London: Academic Press).

TYLER, R.S. and SUMMERFIELD, Q. 1980: Psychoacoustical and phonetic measures of temporal processing in normal and hearing-impaired listeners. In van den Brink, G. and Bilsen, F.A. (eds.), *Psychophysical, physiological and behavioural studies in hearing* (Delft: Delft University Press, 458-65).

TYLER, R.S., WOOD, E.J. and FERNANDES, M. 1982: Frequency resolution and hearing loss. *British Journal of Audiology* 16, 45-63.

TYLER, R.S., SUMMERFIELD, Q., WOOD, E.J. and FERNANDES, M.A. 1982: Psychoacoustic and phonetic temporal processing in normal and hearing-impaired listeners. *Journal of the Acoustical Society of America* 72, 740–52.

TYLER, R.S., WOOD, E.J. and FERNANDES, M. 1983: Frequency resolution and discrimination of constant and dynamic tones in normal and hearing-impaired listeners. *Journal of the Acoustical Society of America* 74, 1190–9.

TZENG, O.J.L., HUNG, D.L. and WANG, W.S.Y. 1977: Speech recording in reading Chinese characters. *Journal of Experimental Psychology: Human Learning and Memory* 3, 621–30.

UPFOLD, L.J. and ISEPY, J. 1982: Childhood deafness in Australia: incidence and maternal rubella, 1949–1980. *Medical Journal of Australia* 2, 323–6.

VAN BERGEIJK, W.A. 1964: Sonic pulse compression in bats and people: a comment. *Journal of the Acoustical Society of America* 36, 594–7.

VAN ZYL, F.J. and IVES, L.A. 1971: Visual perception and eye-motor co-ordination in a group of young deaf children. *Developmental Medicine and Child Neurology* 13, 373–9.

VELMANS, M. 1979: A new frequency transposing aid. *Hearing Aid Journal* 32, 9, 51–3.

VENTRY, I.M. 1980: Effects of conductive hearing loss: fact or fiction. *Journal of Speech and Hearing Disorders* 45, 143–56.

VIEHWEG, R. and CAMPBELL, R.A. 1960: Localization difficulty in monaurally impaired listeners. *Transactions of the American Otolaryngological Society* 48, 339–50.

VYGOTSKY, L.S. 1978: Play and its role in the mental development of the child. In Cole, M., John-Steiner, V., Scribner, S. and Souberman, E. (eds.), *Mind in society* (Cambridge, Mass: Harvard University Press).

WALES, R. 1979: Deixis. In Fletcher, P. and Garman, M. (eds.), *Language acquisition* (Cambridge: Cambridge University Press), 241–60.

WALLACH, H., NEWMAN, E.B. and ROSENSWEIG, M.R. 1949: The precedence effect in sound localization. *American Journal of Psychology* 62, 315–36.

WANG, M.D., REED, C. and BILGER, R.C. 1978: A comparison of the effects of filtering and sensorineural hearing loss on patterns of consonant confusions. *Journal of Speech and Hearing Research* 21, 5–36.

WARREN, R.M. 1970: Perceptual restoration of missing speech sounds. *Science* 167, 392–3.

WARREN, R.M. 1976: Auditory illusions and perceptual processes. In Lass, N.J. (ed.) *Contemporary issues in experimental phonetics* (London, Academic Press, 389–417).

WARREN, R.M., OBUSEK, C.J., FARMER, R.M.1 and WARREN, R.P. 1969: Auditory sequence: confusion of patterns other than speech or music. *Science* 164, 586–7.

WEBSTER, A. 1983: Reading and writing in severely hearing-impaired children. Unpublished Ph.D. thesis, University of Nottingham.

WEBSTER, A., WOOD, D.J. and GRIFFITHS, A.J. 1981: Reading retardation or linguistic deficit? I: interpreting reading test performances of hearing-impaired adolescents. *Journal of Research in Reading* 4, 136–47.

WEBSTER, D.B. 1982: Effects of neonatal sound deprivation in animal research. *Seminars in Speech, Language and Hearing* 3, 336–43.

WEBSTER, D.B. and WEBSTER, A.B. 1979: Effects of neonatal conductive hearing loss on brain stem auditory nuclei. *Annals of Otology* 88, 684–8.

WEBSTER, F.A. 1951: Influence of interaural phase on masked thresholds. *Journal of the Acoustical Society of America* 23, 452–62.

WELLS, G. 1979: Variation in child language. In Fletcher, P. and Garman, M. (eds.) *Language acquisition* (Cambridge: Cambridge University Press, 377–96).

WELSH, L., WELSH, J. and HEALEY, M. 1980: Auditory testing and dyslexia. *Laryngoscope* 90, 972–84.

WERTHEIMER, M. 1961: Psychomotor co-ordination of auditory and visual space at birth. *Science* 134, 1692.

WEVER, E.G. 1949: Theory of hearing. New York: Wiley.

WHITFIELD, I. 1967: *The auditory pathway.* Baltimore: Williams and Wilkins Co.

WHORF, B.L. 1956: *Language, thought and reality.* Cambridge, Mass: MIT Press.

WIEDERHOLD, M.L., ZAJTCHUK, J.T. and VAP, J.G. 1980: Hearing loss relating to physical properties of middle ear conditions. *Annals of Otorhinolaryngology* 89 (Suppl 60), 185–9.

WIENER, F.N. 1947: On the diffraction of a progressive sine wave by the human head. *Journal of the Acoustical Society of America* 19, 143–6.

WIENER, F.N. and ROSS, D.A. 1946: The pressure distribution in the auditory canal in a progressive sound field. *Journal of the Acoustical Society of America* 18, 401–8.

WIGHTMAN, F.L. 1973: The pattern-transformation model of pitch. *Journal of the Acoustical Society of America* 54, 407–12.

WIGHTMAN, F.L. 1981: Pitch perception: an example of auditory pattern recognition. In Getty, D.J. and Howard, J.H. (eds.) *Auditory and visual pattern recognition* (New Jersey: Lawrence Erlbaum, 3–25).

WILBUR, R. 1977: An explanation of deaf children's difficulty with certain syntactic structures in English. *Volta Review* 79, 85–92.

WILBUR, R.B., MONTANELLI, D.S. and QUIGLEY, S.P. 1976: Pronominalization in the language of deaf students. *Journal of Speech and Hearing Research* 19, 120–40.

WILBUR, R.B., QUIGLEY, S.P. and MONTENELLI, D.S. 1975: Conjoined structures in the language of deaf students. *Journal of Speech and Hearing Research* 18, 319–35.

WILCOX, J. and TOBIN, H. 1974: Linguistic performance of hard-of-hearing and normal-hearing children. *Journal of Speech and Hearing Research* 17, 286–93.

WILKENFELD, D. 1981: Reading, prosody and orthography. *Haskins Laboratories: Status Report on Speech Research* SR 67/68, 145–53.

WILLEFORD, J.A. 1976: Central auditory function in children with learning disabilities. *Audiology Hearing Education* 2, 12–20.

WILLEFORD, J.A. 1977: Assessing central auditory behaviour in children: a test battery approach. In Keith, R.W. (ed.) *Central auditory dysfunction.* New York: Grune and Stratton.

WILLEFORD, J.A. 1985: Assessment of central auditory disorders in children. In Pinheiro, M.L. and Musiek, F.E. (eds.), *Assessment of central auditory dysfunction* (Baltimore, MD: Williams & Wilkins) 239–56.

WILLS, R. 1987: Classroom reverberation times and implications for hearing aid use. Paper to British Society of Audiology, Birmingham, UK.

WILSON, J.P. 1974: Psychoacoustical and neurophysiological aspects of auditory pattern recognition. In Schmitt, F.P. and Worden, F.G. (eds.), *The*

WINDHAM, R., PARKS, M. and MITCHENER-COLSTON, W. 1986: Central auditory processing in urban black children: a normative study. *Developmental and Behavioral Pediatrics* 7, 8–13.

neurosciences: third study program (Cambridge, Mass.: MIT Press).

WOLL, B., KYLE, J. and DEUCHER, M. (eds). 1981: *Perspectives on British sign language and deafness.* London: Croom Helm.

WOOD, D.J. 1981: Some developmental aspects of prelingual deafness: In Woll, B., Kyle, J. and Deuchar, M. (eds.), *Perspectives on British sign language and deafness* (London: Croom Helm, 27–42).

WOOD, D.J. 1982: Fostering language development in hearing-impaired children. Paper to 5th Priorsfield Symposium, University of Birmingham.

WOOD, H.A. and WOOD, D.J. 1984: An experimental evaluation of the effects of five styles of teacher conversation on the langauge of hearing-impaired children. *Journal of Child Psychology and Psychiatry* 25, 45–62.

WOOD, D.J., GRIFFITHS, A.J. and WEBSTER, A. 1981: Reading retardation or linguistic deficit? II: test-answering strategies in hearing and hearing-impaired school children. *Journal of Research in Reading* 4, 148–56.

WOOD, D.J., WOOD, H.A., GRIFFITHS, A.J., HOWARTH, SP. and HOWARTH, C.I. 1982: The structure of conversations with 6- to 10-year old deaf children. *Journal of Child Psychology and Psychiatry* 23, 295–308.

WRIGHT, J. 1984: Personal Communication.

WRIGHTSTONE, J.W., ARONOW, M.S. and MOSKOWITZ, S. 1963: Developing reading test norms for deaf children. *American Annals of the Deaf* 108, 311–16.

YATES, G.K. 1986: Frequency selectivity in the auditory periphery. In Moore, B.C.J. (ed.), *Frequency selectivity in hearing* (London: Academic Press) 1–50.

YOUNG, M.A. and GIBBONS, E.W. 1962: Speech discrimination scores and threshold measurements in a non-normal hearing population. *Journal of Auditory Research* 2, 21–33.

YOUNG, M.L. 1983: Neuroscience, pragmatic competence and auditory processing. In Lasky, E. and Katz, J. (eds.) *Central auditory processing disorders,* (Baltimore: University Park Press, 141–61).

ZINKUS, P.W. and GOTTLIEB, M.I. 1980: Patterns of perceptual and academic deficits related to early chronic otitis media. *Pediatrics* 66, 246–53.

ZINKUS, P.W., GOTTLIEB, M.I. and SCHAPIRO, M. 1978: Developmental and psycho-educational sequelae of chronic otitis media. *American Journal Dis. Child*

132, 1100-4.

ZLATIN, M.A. and KOENIGSKNECHT, R.A. 1976: Development of the voicing contrast: a comparison of voice onset time in stop perception and production. *Journal of Speech and Hearing Research* 19, 93–111.

ZWICKER, E. and SCHORN, K. 1978: Psychoacoustical tuning curves in audiology. *Audiology* 17, 120–40.

ZWICKER, E. and SCHORN, K. 1982: Temporal resolution in hard-of-hearing patients. *Audiology* 21, 474–92.

ZWISLOCKI, J. 1969: Temporal summation of loudness; an analysis. *Journal of the Acoustical Society of America* 46, 431–41.

Index